Essentials of Veterinary Science

Essentials of Veterinary Science

Edited by **Mel Roth**

SYRAWOOD
PUBLISHING HOUSE

New York

Published by Syrawood Publishing House,
750 Third Avenue, 9th Floor,
New York, NY 10017, USA
www.syrawoodpublishinghouse.com

Essentials of Veterinary Science
Edited by Mel Roth

International Standard Book Number: 978-1-68286-121-9 (Hardback)

The publisher's policy is to use permanent paper from mills that operate a sustainable forestry policy. Furthermore, the publisher ensures that the text paper and cover boards used have met acceptable environmental accreditation standards.

Trademark Notice: Registered trademark of products or corporate names are used only for explanation and identification without intent to infringe.

Printed in the United States of America.

Contents

Preface

Veterinary Science is a rapidly expanding branch of science. Encompassing all species of animals, both wild and domesticated, veterinary science has a wide scope of research. Veterinary medicine has evolved as a self-sustaining science in the modern times. Students all around the world are interested in this discipline and are studying as well as practicing it. This book caters to such pool of students as well as practitioners or researchers who are interested in this field and want to explore this advancing science. In the recent years, there have been some revolutionizing researches in this field which have paved the way for new concepts and methods of treatments in animals. Such researches have been discussed in detail in this book. It presents diverse researches from different parts of the world which will help students understand the existing medicines better and also find new methods and techniques to treat animals better.

This book is a comprehensive compilation of works of different researchers from varied parts of the world. It includes valuable experiences of the researchers with the sole objective of providing the readers (learners) with a proper knowledge of the concerned field. This book will be beneficial in evoking inspiration and enhancing the knowledge of the interested readers.

In the end, I would like to extend my heartiest thanks to the authors who worked with great determination on their chapters. I also appreciate the publisher's support in the course of the book. I would also like to deeply acknowledge my family who stood by me as a source of inspiration during the project.

Editor

Effects of corticosterone on the metabolic activity of cultured chicken chondrocytes

Hua Zhang, Zhenlei Zhou[*], Jingwen Luo and Jiafa Hou

Abstract

Background: Corticosterone is one of the most crucial glucocorticoids (GCs) in poultry. Our previous study shows that corticosterone can retard the longitudinal growth of bones by depressing the proliferation and differentiation of chondrocytes in broilers. The present study was designed to investigate whether corticosterone affect the development of chondrocytes and the synthesis of collagen *in vitro*. The chondrocytes were isolated from proximal tibial growth plates of 6-week-old broiler chickens and cultured with different doses of corticosterone for 48 h. Then the cell viability, alkaline phosphatase (ALP) activity and the expression of parathyroid hormone-related peptide (PTHrP) and type X collagen (Col X) were detected.

Results: At 10^{-9}-10^{-6} M concentration, corticosterone significantly inhibited the viability and differentiation of chondrocytes, as indicated by decreases in ALP and type X collagen expression. Conversely, there was completely opposite effect at 10^{-10} M. In addition, the expression of PTHrP was significantly downregulated at 10^{-6} M and 10^{-8} M, and was upregulated at 10^{-10} M.

Conclusions: The results suggested that corticosterone regulated chicken chondrocytes performance depending on its concentration with high concentrations inhibiting the viability and differentiation of chondrocytes and light concentrations promoting them, and these roles of corticosterone may be in part mediated through PTHrP.

Keywords: Corticosterone, Chondrocytes, ALP, Col X, PTHrP

Background

Longitudinal bone growth depends on the proliferation, differentiation of growth plate chondrocytes by complex endocrine regulation [1]. It is well known that glucocorticoids (GCs) have complex effects on bone metablism. Prolonged or high dose glucocorticoid administration as well as an excess of endogenous production of GCs increases the risk of bone disorders [2]. Corticosterone (CORT) is the main glucocorticoid hormone in birds [3] and in charge of bone metabolism [2]. Numerous studies had been conducted concerning the effects of GCs on growth retardation in mammals [4-15] and were to some extent controversial [16,17], whereas relatively few data were available with regard to its roles in bone development in avian.

It was reported that parathyroid hormone-related peptide (PTHrP) was one of the important cytokines. Both the periarticular perichondrium and growth plate chondrocytes are the source of PTHrP [18,19]. Ablation of the PTHrP gene exhibits a delay in chondrocyte differentiation and leads to distinct abnormalities in bone development [20]. PTHrP directly stimulates chondrocyte proliferation and prevents the differentiation of proliferating chondrocytes to prehypertrophic cells [21,22]. Type X collagen (Col X) expressing exclusively in the matrix of the hypertrophic zone [23,24] is one of the well-known markers of chondrocyte hypertrophy [25,26].

Previous studies from our laboratory showed that exposure to CORT depressed the longitudinal growth of the long bones by inhibiting the proliferation and differentiation of chondrocytes in growth plate in broilers [27], but the effects of CORT on the cellular events that occurred during this process in birds were uncertain, the present study was designed to investigate whether CORT affect the performance of chondrocytes obtained from the epiphyseal growth plates of broiler chickens by determining the ALP activity and expression of PTHrP and ColX.

* Correspondence: zhouzl@njau.edu.cn
College of Veterinary Medicine, Nanjing Agricultural University, Nanjing, Jiangsu 210095, China

Results

Effect of CORT on cell viability and ALP activity in cultured chicken chondrocytes

The results showed that CORT inhibited chondrocytes viability and ALP activity significantly at concentrations of 10^{-9} M to 10^{-6} M in a dose-dependent manner (Figures 1 and 2). The lowest chondrocytes viability was observed at 10^{-6} M CORT reducing the cell viability as great as to 64.2% of the control. And the lowest ALP activity (150.57 ± 10.591 nmol/min/mg) was also measured at 10^{-6} M CORT. However, 10^{-10} CORT administration did not affect chondrocytes viability and ALP activity. Additional tables file show this in more detail [see Additional files 1 and 2]. Based on these results, 10^{-10} M, 10^{-8} M and 10^{-6} M CORT (as low, middle and high concentration, respectively) were determined to evaluate its roles in the regulation of gene expression in cultured growth plate chondrocytes.

Effect of CORT on expression of PTHrP and ColX in cultured chicken chondrocytes

Expression of related genes was investigated after 48 h exposure of different doses of CORT (10^{-10} M, 10^{-8} M and 10^{-6} M). Real-time RT-PCR showed that 10^{-10} M CORT resulted in obviously increasing the expression of PTHrP and Col X (Figure 3A and B). Furthermore, 10^{-8} M and 10^{-6} M CORT significantly declined PTHrP and Col X mRNA levels, and the inhibition exerted at the concentration of 10^{-6} M CORT was more effective. The Col X protein levels (expressed as the Col X: Gapdh ratio) displayed the same changes as its mRNA expression after CORT treatment (Figure 4).

Discussion

In the present study, we investigated the effects of CORT on cultured chicken growth plate chondrocytes in terms of cell viability, ALP activity and the expression of Col X and PTHrP. Growth plate chondrocytes were exquisitely sensitive to GCs [6,27,28]. The results showed that PTHrP signaling could play a crucial role in regulating the viability and differentiation of growth plate chondrocytes of chickens.

Based on the present study, MTT assay was performed to evaluate the effect of CORT on the viability of chondrocytes for 48 h. Interestingly, CORT at the concentration of 10^{-10}-10^{-6} M didn't have a clear dose-dependent effect on cell viability. CORT could inhibit chondrocytes viability at the concentration of 10^{-9}-10^{-6} M and have no effect with 10^{-10}. M. R. Quarto et al. [17] suggested that GCs can support chondrocytes viability. However, it was difficult to compare our observations with other studies because the origin of the investigated chondrocytes, the culture conditions, the types and doses of GCs and the exposure times were distinct.

The process of endochondral ossification which consists of cartilage formation and replacement of cartilage by bone plays a major role in bone development [29]. The chondrocytes actively proliferate and synthesize a large amount of extracellular matrix components undergo a series of maturation events. They advance to

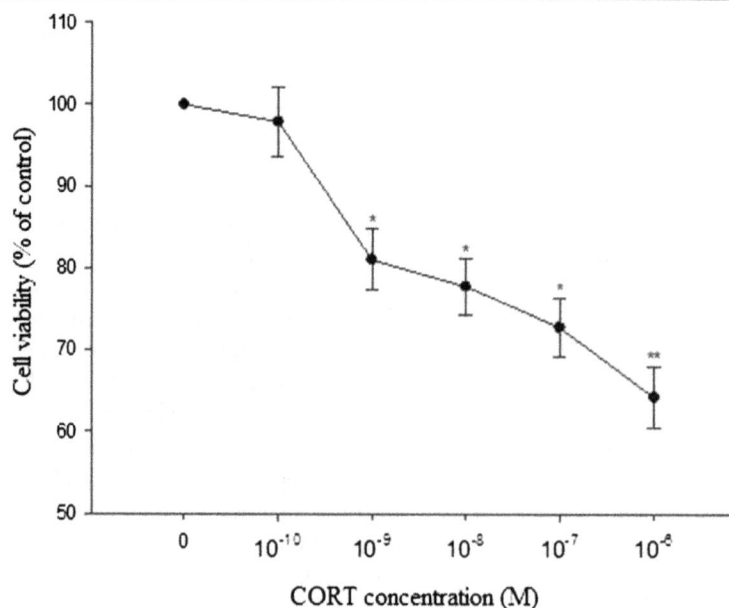

Figure 1 Effects of various doses CORT on cell viability measured by MTT assay. The cells were incubated with increasing concentrations of CORT for 48 h. Treated cell viabilities were expressed as a percentage of control (100%). Data were mean ± SEM from at least three separate experiments, each performed in triplicates. *P < 0.05 and **P < 0.01 versus control (0 M CORT).

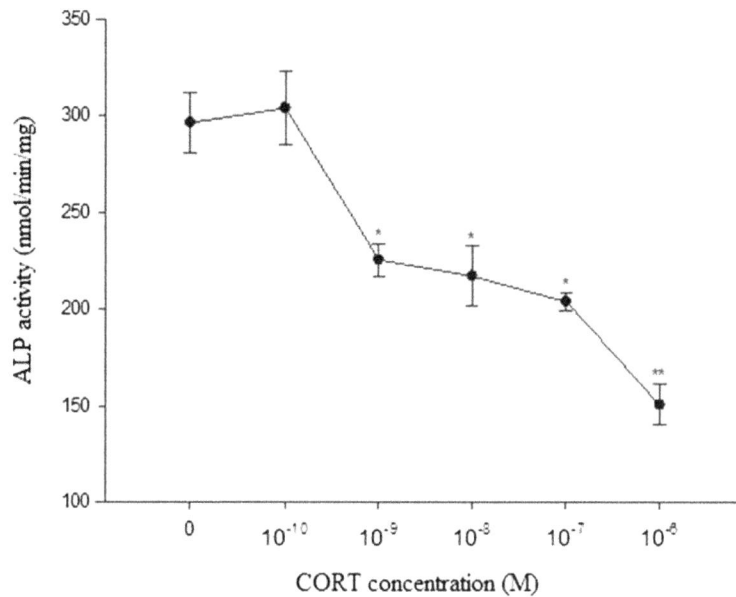

Figure 2 Effects of various doses CORT on intracellular ALP activity. The cells were incubated with increasing concentrations of CORT for 48 h. Values were mean ± SEM from at least three separate experiments, each performed in triplicates. *P < 0.05 and **P < 0.01 versus control (0 M CORT).

the hypertrophic stage, which is characterized by the expression of type X collagen and ALP [30]. In the process of chondrocytes maturation, ALP secreted from chondrocytes could convert organic phosphorus esters to inorganic phosphates by hydrolysis, forming a hydroxyapatite precursor which then undergoes calcification [31]. Therefore, ALP is recommended as a marker of chondrocyte maturation [32]. In this study, we observed that the decrease in ALP activity was accompanied by a decline in

the viability of choncrocytes after CORT treatment at 10^{-9} -10^{-6} M. It indicated that the supression of chondrocytes differentiation and the reduction of ALP activity may be due to inhibitory effect of CORT on the viability of chondrocytes.

Col X, which is a recognized marker of chondrocyte hypertrophy, is mainly synthesized by hypertrophic chondrocytes and plays a key role in endochondral ossification. The current study showed that the expression

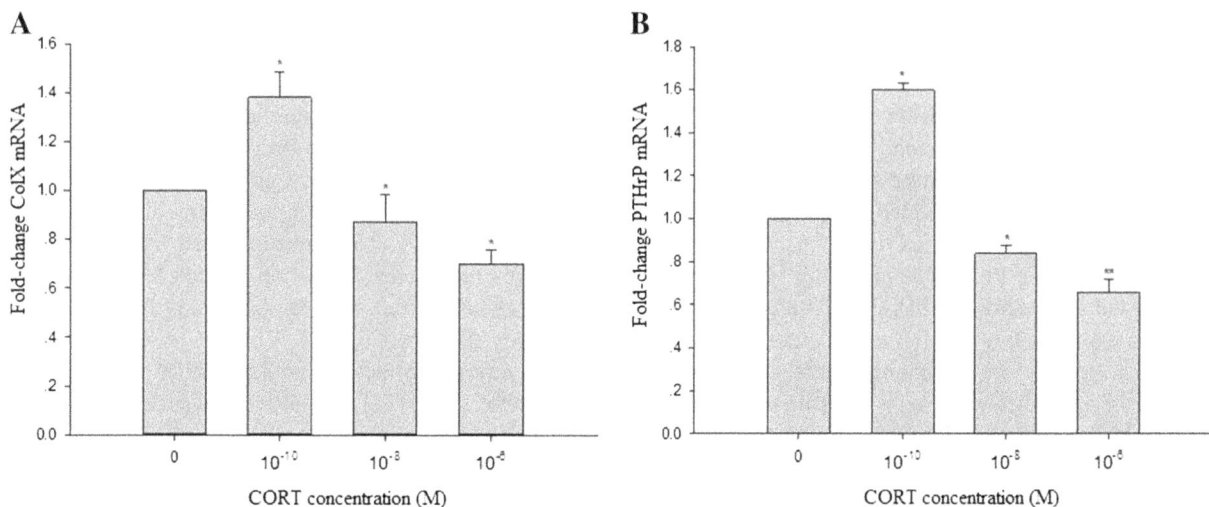

Figure 3 Effects of CORT on PTHrP and Col X mRNAs expression in cultured Chondrocytes (A-B). The cells were incubated with various doses of CORT for 48 h. The relative expression of PTHrP and Col X genes was analysed by real-time PCR. Gene expression was normalized using GAPDH as an internal control. Values were mean ± SEM from at least three separate experiments, each performed in triplicates. *P < 0.05 and **P < 0.01 versus control (0 M CORT).

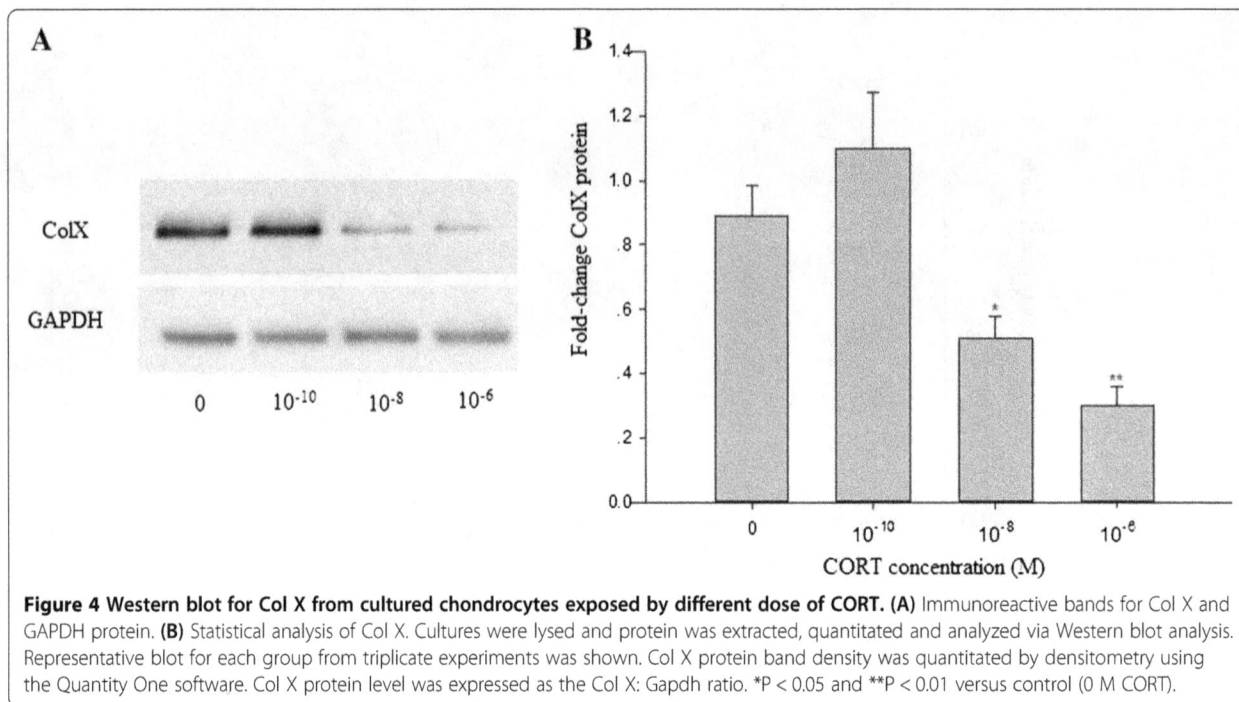

Figure 4 Western blot for Col X from cultured chondrocytes exposed by different dose of CORT. (A) Immunoreactive bands for Col X and GAPDH protein. **(B)** Statistical analysis of Col X. Cultures were lysed and protein was extracted, quantitated and analyzed via Western blot analysis. Representative blot for each group from triplicate experiments was shown. Col X protein band density was quantitated by densitometry using the Quantity One software. Col X protein level was expressed as the Col X: Gapdh ratio. *P < 0.05 and **P < 0.01 versus control (0 M CORT).

of Col X was inhibited by CORT with middle and high concentration, while the expression of Col X was significantly increased with low concentration CORT treatment. These results provided an evidence for our previous study in vivo that excess CORT inhibited the growth of proliferative and prehypertrophic chondrocytes and the synthesis of Col X [27]. This finding, together with the variation of ALP activity and cell viability, clearly indicated that CORT not only affected cell viability, but also inhibited the differentiation process of growth plate chondrocytes.

A number of growth factors are known to be regulators of chondrocytes development. PTHrP plays important roles in longitudinal bone growth, as it is a negative regulator of growth plate chondrocytes terminal differentiation [18]. As a key cytokine, PTHrP maintains chondrocytes in a proliferative state and regulate chondrocytes proliferation [33,34]. PTHrP blocks matrix calcification and decrease ALP activity markedly in chondrocytes through PKC/p38 signaling pathways [30]. The present study showed that CORT had distinct impact on the expression of PTHrP mRNA with various concentrations. In addition, the changes of levers of Col X and ALP in chondrocytes were coordinated with trends of PTHrP expression following treatment with CORT. Our finding indicated that the regulation of the viability and differentiation of chondrocytes by CORT might be in part mediated through by PTHrP. More studies were still needed to further to determine whether there were interactions between CORT and PTHrP.

Conclusions
Based on the outcome, our data confirmed that CORT had profound impacts upon bone growth through orderly process of differentiation of growth plate chondrocytes reported by our previous study but now amongst in vivo circumstances [27]. PTHrP may play a certain role in regulating chondrocytes growth induced by CORT. The effect of CORT may be in part mediated by the expression of PTHrP.

Methods
Chemicals and reagents
Dulbecco's modified eagle's medium (DMEM), penicillin-streptomycin solution, fetal bovine serum (FBS), amphotericin B solution, collagenase type IV and Trizol reagent were procured from Invitrogen, Carlsbad, CA, USA. Bovine testicular hyaluronidase, a nonessential amino acids mixture (100×) and CORT were purchased from Sigma-Aldrich, Shanghai, China. Two-step reverse-transcriptase polymerase chain reaction kit was purchased from TaKaRa Biotechnology (Dalian) Co., Ltd., China. Col X antibody, anti Gapdh mouse monoclonal antibody, HRP conjugated goat anti-rabbit IgG (H+L) and HRP conjugated goat anti-mouse IgG (H+L) were purchased from Otwo Biotech Co., Ltd., China. Cell lysis buffer for Western was procured from Beyotime Institute of Biotechnology, China. Other chemicals and reagents used in the present study were of analytical grade and were obtained from the Jiancheng Bioengineering Institute (Nanjing, China) unless otherwise indicated.

All animal work was performed according to the international animal welfare guidelines, and protocols were approved by Nanjing Agricultural University Animal Care Committee. Animal studies were conducted in accordance with the recommendations in the Guidelines for the Care and Use of Laboratory Animals of the Ministry of Science and Technology of the People's Republic of China ([2006] 398).

Cell culture and treatment

Growth plate cartilage was harvested from the proximal end of the tibia of 6-week-old hybrid broiler chickens and chondrocytes were isolated as previously described [35]. Briefly, tibial growth plate slices were treated in a digest solution (0.1% type IV collagenase, 0.1% hyaluronidase, 5% FBS) and incubated at 37°C overnight. The resulting crude cell preparations were further purified on lymphocyte separation medium (MP Biomedicals, LLC, California, USA), resuspended and counting, then inoculated to multi-well plates containing complete medium with the density for 10^6 cell/cm^2. Culture medium (10% FBS, 1% nonessential amino acids mixture) was changed every other day with a fresh supplement of ascorbic acid (50 μg/ml) from day 3 onward, for the duration of the experiments. To facilitate cell attachment, 4U/mL testicular hyaluronidase was added to the medium. After the attachment of cells, the growth medium was then removed and cells were exposed to different doses of CORT (10^{-10} - 10^{-6} M) using serum-free fresh medium at 37°C and 5% CO_2 for 48 h. All culture media contained 100 IU/ml of penicillin, 100 μg/ml of streptomycin and 0.25 μg/ml of amphotericin B.

MTT assay

Cell viability was assessed by the ability of mitochondrial dehydrogenases to oxidize the 3-(4, 5-dimethylthiazol-2-yl)-2, 5-diphenyltetrazolium bromide (MTT) to a purple formazan product [27]. After 48 h exposure, 20 μl MTT (5 mg/ml) was added into each well and incubated for 4 h at 37°C. Purple formazan crystals were solubilized in dimethyl sulfoxide for 10 min at 37°C. The absorbance at 570 nm was measured in a Bio-Rad microplate reader (Bio-Rad Laboratories, Hercules, CA) and results were expressed as a percentage of control.

Alkaline phosphatase (ALP) activity

Cell layers were washed twice with cold phosphate buffered saline (PBS pH = 7.4). The cell suspension was homogenized and 50 μl of each sample was aliquoted into a 96-well plate in duplicate to assay ALP activity and protein content [36]. 150 μl of a buffer solution consisting of 10 mM p-nitrophenyl phosphate (pNPP), 0.2 mM $MgCl_2$ and 1 mM diethanolamine was added to each sample [35]. After incubated at 37°C for 30 min and then 100 μl of 0.1 M NaOH was added to stop the reaction. The plates were read in a Bio-Rad microplate reader at 405 nm. The ALP activity was determined by comparing the experimental samples with standard solutions of p-nitrophenol and an appropriate blank. Protein concentrations of the samples were determined using the BCA assay kit (Wuhan Boster Company, Wuhan, China). Each sample was normalized by the total protein content per well to determine specific activity. Total ALP activity was expressed as nmoles pNPP hydrolysed/min/mg protein.

Real-time RT-PCR

Total RNA was isolated from chondrocytes using Trizol reagent after 48 h exposure of different doses of CORT (10^{-10} M, 10^{-8} M and 10^{-6} M). Real-time RT-PCR was carried out using two-step RT-PCR kit per the instructions of the manufacturer. Gapdh, the house-keeping gene, was used as an internal control of the quantity and quality of the cDNAs. The primer sequences used for PCR amplification for Col X, PTHrP and Gapdh were listed in Table 1. Real-time PCR amplification was performed on LightCycler (Applied Biosystems, Inc., Foster City, CA). A Light Cycler melting curve was constructed to test for a single product at the end of each PCR reaction. Analysis of the relative gene expression level was achieved by using the $2_T^{-\Delta\Delta C}$ method for fold induction, and C_T (the threshold cycle) indicated the fractional cycle number at which the amount of amplified target reached a fixed threshold [37].

Western blot analysis

After 48 h exposure of CORT (10^{-10} M, 10^{-8} M and 10^{-6} M), chondrocyte lysates were prepared with RIPA

Table 1 Sequence of primers used to amplify specific mRNA by real-time RT-PCR

Name	Primer sequence (5'-3')	Product size (bp)	NCBI Genbank
Col X[#]	Sense: AGTGCTGTCATTGATCTCATGGA	83	L11BB9.1
	Anti-sense: TCAGAGGAATAGAGACCATTGGATT		
PTHrP	Sense: CGGAGGATATGATGTTCAC	79	AB175678.1
	Anti-sense: TAGGAGGGCACAGAATAAC		
GAPDH	Sense: GAACATCATCCCAGCGTCCA	132	NM_204305.1
	Anti-sense: CGGCAGGTCAGGTCAACAAC		

[#]The primers of Col X was quoted from Reference [38].

Lysis buffer (Beyotime, Nanjing, China), and centrifuged at 12,000 g. Protein concentration was determined by using the BCA assay kit. Fifty micrograms of total protein (per lane) were resolved by sodium dodecyl sulphate-polyacrylamide gel electrophoresis (SDS-PAGE; 10% acrylamide) and transferred onto a nitrocellulose membrane. The membranes were blocked with 5% skimmed milk in Tris-buffered saline-Tween (TBS-T) for 2 hours and then probed with antibodies. The primary antibodies to Col X (diluted 1:200), and anti-Gapdh (diluted 1:5000) were used. HRP conjugated goat anti-rabbit or mouse IgG (H+L) (diluted 1:5000) was used as a secondary antibody. Visualization of immunoreactive proteins was achieved using the ECL Western blotting detection reagents (Millipore Corporation, Billerica, USA). Molecular weights of the immunoreactive proteins were determined against a protein marker ladder. Band density was quantitated using the Quantity One software (Bio-Rad Laboratories, Hercules, CA).

Statistical analysis

Tests were carried out in triplicate and all experiments were performed a minimum of three times, and the mean and standard error of the mean (SEM) were determined. Statistical analyses were conducted using SPSS 11.0 for Windows (SPSS Inc., Chicago, IL, USA). Data were analyzed by one-way Analysis of variance (ANOVA) followed by Duncan's multiple range tests to assess the significance between the control and experimental groups. Statistical significance was considered at the level of $P < 0.05$.

Additional files

Additional file 1: Additional numerical data for effects of various doses CORT on cell viability measured by MTT assay.

Additional file 2: Additional numerical data for effects of various doses CORT on intracellular ALP activity.

Abbreviations

ALP: Alkaline phosphatase; ANOVA: Analysis of variance; Col X: Type X collagen; CORT: Corticosterone; DMEM: Dulbecco's modified eagle's medium; FBS: Fetal bovine serum; GCs: Glucocorticoids; MTT: 3-(4, 5-dimethylthiazol-2-yl)-2, 5-diphenyltetrazolium bromide; PBS: phosphate buffered saline; PNPP: P-nitrophenyl phosphate; PTHrP: Parathyroid hormone-related protein; SDS-PAGE: Sodium dodecyl sulphate-polyacrylamide gel electrophoresis; SEM: Standard error of the mean; TBST: Tris-buffered saline-Tween.

Competing interests

The authors declare that they have no competing interests.

Authors' contributions

HZ carried out most of the studies, arranged the data for statistical analysis and drafted the manuscript. JWL participated in writing, JFH revised the manuscript. ZLZ designed the study and revised the manuscript. All authors read and approved the final manuscript.

Acknowledgments

This work was supported by the Natural Science Foundation of Jiangsu Province (no. BK2011648), a project funded by the Priority Academic Program Development of Jiangsu Higher Education Institutions (PAPD) and the Fundamental Research Funds for the Central Universities.

References

1. Nilsson O, Marino R, De Luca F, Phillip M, Baron J. Endocrine regulation of the growth plate. Horm Res. 2005;64:157–65.
2. Castro M, Elias LL, Conde P, Elias L, Moreira AC. Physiology and pathophysi-ology of the HPA. In: Cushing's Syndrome. New Jersey: Humana Press; 2011. p. 1–20.
3. Costantini D, Fanfani A, Dell'omo G. Effects of corticosteroids on oxidative damage and circulating carotenoids in captive adult kestrels (Falco tinnunculus). J Comp Physiol B. 2008;178:829–35.
4. Gafni RI, Weise M, Robrecht DT, Meyers JL, Barnes KM, De-Levi S, et al. Catch-up growth is associated with delayed senescence of the growth plate in rabbits. Pediatr Res. 2001;50:618–23.
5. Miyazaki Y, Tsukazaki T, Hirota Y, Yonekura A, Osaki M, Shindo H, et al. Dexamethasone inhibition of TGF beta-induced cell growth and type II collagen mRNA expression through ERK-integrated AP-1 activity in cultured rat articular chondrocytes. Osteoarthr Cartil. 2000;8:378–85.
6. Siebler T, Robson H, Shalet SM, Williams GR. Dexamethasone inhibits and thyroid hormone promotes differentiation of mouse chondrogenic ATDC5 cells. Bone. 2002;31:457–64.
7. Smink JJ, Buchholz IM, Hamers N, van Tilburg CM, Christis C, Sakkers RJB, et al. Short-term glucocorticoid treatment of piglets causes changes in growth plate morphology and angiogenesis. Osteoarthr Cartil. 2003;11:864–71.
8. Rauch A, Seitz S, Baschant U, Schilling AF, Illing A, Stride B, et al. Glucocorticoids suppress bone formation by attenuating osteoblast differentiation via the monomeric glucocorticoid receptor. Cell Metab. 2010;11:517–31.
9. Sanchez CP, He YZ. Alterations in the growth plate cartilage of rats with renal failure receiving corticosteroid therapy. Bone. 2002;30:692–8.
10. Hofbauer LC, Zeitz U, Schoppet M, Skalicky M, Schuler C, Stolina M, et al. Prevention of glucocorticoid-induced bone loss in mice by inhibition of RANKL. Arthritis Rheum. 2009;60:1427–37.
11. McLaughlin F, Mackintosh J, Hayes BP, Mclaren A, Uings IJ, Salmon P, et al. Glucocorticoid-induced osteopenia in the mouse as assessed by histomorphometry, microcomputed tomography, and biochemical markers. Bone. 2002;30:924–30.
12. Blondelon D, Adolphe M, Zizine L, Lechat P. Evidence for glucocorticoid receptors in cultured rabbit articular chondrocytes. FEBS Lett. 1980;117:195–9.
13. Ranz FB, Aceitero J, Gaytan F. Morphometric study of cartilage dynamics in the chick embryo tibia. II. Dexamethasone-treated embryos. J Anat. 1987;154:73–9.
14. Guerne PA, Desgeorges A, Jaspar JM, Relic B, Peter R, Hoffmeyer P, et al. Effects of IL-6 and its soluble receptor on proteoglycan synthesis and NO release by human articular chondrocytes: comparison with IL-1. Modulation by dexamethasone. Matrix Biol. 1999;18:253–60.
15. Abbadia Z, Amiral J, Trzeciak MC, Delmas PD, Clezardin P. The growth-supportive effect of thrombospondin (TSP1) and the expression of TSP1 by human MG-63 osteoblastic cells are both inhibited by dexamethasone. FEBS Lett. 1993;335:161–6.
16. Kato Y, Gospodarowicz D. Stimulation by glucocorticoid of the synthesis of cartilage-matrix proteoglycans produced by rabbit costal chondrocytes in vitro. J Biol Chem. 1985;260:2364–73.
17. Quarto R, Campanile G, Cancedda R, Dozin B. Thyroid hormone, insulin, and glucocorticoids are sufficient to support chondrocyte differentiation to hypertrophy: a serum-free analysis. J Cell Biol. 1992;119:989–95.
18. Farquharson C, Seawright E, Jefferies D. Parathyroid hormone-related peptide expression in tibial dyschondroplasia. Avian Pathol. 2001;30:327–35.
19. Medill NJ, Praul CA, Ford BC, Leach RM. Parathyroid hormone-related peptide expression in the epiphyseal growth plate of the juvenile chicken: evidence for the origin of the parathyroid hormone-related peptide found in the epiphyseal growth plate. J Cell Biochem. 2001;80:504–11.
20. Lanske B, Amling M, Neff L, Guiducci J, Baron R, Kronenberg HM. Ablation of the PTHrP gene or the PTH/PTHrP receptor gene leads to distinct abnormalities in bone development. J Clin Invest. 1999;104:399–407.

21. Kronenberg HM, Lanske B, Kovacs CS, Chung UI, Lee K, Segre GV, et al. Functional analysis of the PTH/PTHrP network of ligands and receptors. Recent Prog Horm Res. 1998;53:283–301. discussion 301–283.

22. Lanske B, Karaplis AC, Lee K, Luz A, Vortkamp A, Pirro A, et al. PTH/PTHrP receptor in early development and Indian hedgehog-regulated bone growth. Science. 1996;273:663–6.

23. Shen G. The role of type X collagen in facilitating and regulating endochondral ossification of articular cartilage. Orthod Craniofac Res. 2005;8:11–7.

24. Kwan AP, Cummings CE, Chapman JA, Grant ME. Macromolecular organization of chicken type X collagen in vitro. J Cell Biol. 1991;114:597–604.

25. Cancedda R, Cancedda FD, Castagnola P. Chondrocyte differentiation. Int Rev Cytol Survey Cell Biol. 1995;159:265–358.

26. Linsenmayer TF, Long F, Nurminskaya M, Chen Q, Schmid TM. Type X collagen and other up-regulated components of the avian hypertrophic cartilage program. Prog Nucleic Acid Res Mol Biol. 1998;60:79–109.

27. Luo JW, Zhou ZL, Zhang H, Ma RS, Hou JF. Bone response of broiler chickens (Gallus gallus domesticus) induced by corticosterone. Comp Biochem Physiol A Mol Integr Physiol. 2013;164:410–6.

28. Silvestrini G, Ballanti P, Patacchioli FR, Mocetti P, Di Grezia R, Wedard BM, et al. Evaluation of apoptosis and the glucocorticoid receptor in the cartilage growth plate and metaphyseal bone cells of rats after high-dose treatment with corticosterone. Bone. 2000;26:33–42.

29. Ma RS, Zhou ZL, Luo JW, Zhang H, Hou JF. The Ihh signal is essential for regulating proliferation and hypertrophy of cultured chicken chondrocytes. Comp Physiol B-Biochem Mol Biol. 2013;166:117–22.

30. Iwamoto M, Kitagaki J, Tamamura Y, Gentili C, Koyama E, Enomoto H, et al. Runx2 expression and action in chondrocytes are regulated by retinoid signaling and parathyroid hormone-related peptide (PTHrP). Osteoarthritis Cartilage. 2003;11:6–15.

31. Sanchez C, Deberg MA, Piccardi N, Msika P, Reginster JY, Henrotin YE. Subchondral bone osteoblasts induce phenotypic changes in human osteoarthritic chondrocytes. Osteoarthritis Cartilage. 2005;13:988–97.

32. Henson FM, Davies ME, Skepper JN, Jeffcott LB. Localisation of alkaline phosphatase in equine growth cartilage. J Anat. 1995;187(Pt 1):151–9.

33. Harrington EK, Lunsford LE, Svoboda KKH. Chondrocyte terminal differentiation, apoptosis, and type X collagen expression are downregulated by parathyroid hormone. Anat Rec Part Discov Mol Cell Evol Biol. 2004;281A:1286–95.

34. Kobayashi T, Chung UI, Schipani E, Starbuck M, Karsenty G, Katagiri T, et al. PTHrP and Indian hedgehog control differentiation of growth plate chondrocytes at multiple steps. Development. 2002;129:2977–86.

35. He SJ, Hou JF, Dai YY, Zhou ZL, Deng YF. N-acetyl-cysteine protects chicken growth plate chondrocytes from T-2 toxin-induced oxidative stress. J Appl Toxicol. 2012;32:980–5.

36. Kinney RC, Schwartz Z, Week K, Lotz MK, Boyan BD. Human articular chondrocytes exhibit sexual dimorphism in their responses to 17 beta-estradiol. Osteoarthr Cartil. 2005;13:330–7.

37. Livak KJ, Schmittgen TD. Analysis of relative gene expression data using real-time quantitative PCR and the 2 (−Delta Delta C (T)) Method. Methods. 2001;25:402–8.

38. Wang W, Xu JP, Kirsch T. Annexin-mediated Ca2+ influx regulates growth plate chondrocyte maturation and apoptosis. J Biol Chem. 2003;278:3762–9.

2

Systemic and mammary gland disposition of enrofloxacin in healthy sheep following intramammary administration

Cristina López[1], Juan José García[1], Matilde Sierra[1], María José Diez[1], Claudia Pérez[2], Ana Maria Sahagún[1]* and Nélida Fernández[1]

Abstract

Background: Mastitis is one of the most important diseases affecting dairy sheep. Antimicrobial drugs are often administered directly through teat to treat or prevent this disease, but data on drug distribution within glandular tissue are scarce and it cannot be estimated from concentrations in milk. Thus, the aim of this study was to investigate systemic and mammary gland distribution of enrofloxacin after intramammary administration. The drug was administered to 6 healthy lactating Assaf sheep with an injector containing an enrofloxacin preparation (1 g drug/5 g ointment). Blood samples were collected at 0, 30, 60, 90, 120, 150 and 180 min. Animals were then sedated and sacrificed, and glandular tissue samples were obtained from treated udders at 2, 4, 6 and 8 cm height. Enrofloxacin concentrations were measured in plasma and tissue samples by UV high-performed liquid chromatography.

Results: Mean enrofloxacin plasma concentrations were below 0.5 µg/mL. Mean tissue concentrations decreased in mammary gland with vertical distance from the teat, ranging from 356.6 µg/g at 2 cm to 95.60 µg/g at the base of the udder. Glandular tissue concentrations best fitted to a decreasing monoexponential model, and showed a good correlation with an ex vivo model previously developed.

Conclusions: Enrofloxacin concentrations were effective in the entire glandular tissue against the main pathogens causing mastitis in sheep. These results suggest that this drug may be suitable to treat mastitis in sheep by intramammary administration.

Keywords: Enrofloxacin, Sheep, Intramammary, Systemic, Glandular tissue, Disposition

Background

Mastitis is one of the most important and costly diseases affecting dairy sheep, resulting in substantial health and economic problems worldwide. The two major forms of this disease are clinical mastitis, which results in signs of inflammation in infected mammary glands, changes in milk composition and altered systemic condition of the animal, and subclinical mastitis, without readily apparent signs in animals but with altered somatic cell count of the milk. From both types of mastitis, the subclinical one is not only very frequent but also economically important as it reduces the quantity and quality of milk produced. Prevalence values of this form average 5-30% in small ruminants, whereas for clinical mastitis they are generally lower than 5% [1-3].

Although a variety of microorganisms can cause mastitis in sheep, *Staphylococcus* spp. are the most frequently isolated agents involved in both acute clinical and subclinical forms. Other pathogens such as *Enterobacteriaceae*, *Streptococcus* spp., *Mycoplasma* spp., *Mannheimia haemolytica* or *Pseudomonas* spp. are also found.

Fluoroquinolones are considered among the most effective drugs for the treatment of bacterial infections, and they should be reserved to those situations with poor response to other antimicrobial agents, in order to prevent increasing the risk of quinolone-resistant bacteria. Although this pharmacological group should not

* Correspondence: amsahp@unileon.es
[1]Pharmacology, Department of Biomedical Sciences, Institute of Biomedicine (IBIOMED), University of León, Campus de Vegazana s/n, 24071 León, Spain
Full list of author information is available at the end of the article

be used as first-line agents against mastitis, it is important to establish its pharmacokinetics and efficacy in animals in which it could be employed. Enrofloxacin, 1-cyclopropyl-7-(4-ethyl-1-piperazinyl)-6-fluoro-1,4-dihidro-4-oxo-3-quinoline carboxylic acid, is a fluoroquinolone exclusively developed to be used in veterinary medicine [4,5]. It is characterized by a low host toxicity, a high bioavailability, an excellent tissue penetration, a long serum half-life and a broad antibacterial spectrum together with a high bactericidal activity against major pathogenic bacteria (both Gram-positive and Gram-negative) and intracellular microorganisms found in sick animals [6,7].

The pharmacokinetics of enrofloxacin have been widely described in several species including cattle [8-11], buffaloes [12,13], sheep [14-16] and goats [5,17,18]. In most of these species enrofloxacin shows good absorption after parenteral administration, although oral absorption drops to approximately 10% in adult ruminants [19]. This drug exhibits a large volume of distribution, suggesting wide tissue penetration, and a terminal half-life of 2–6 h. Furthermore, enrofloxacin is partially metabolized in the liver to ciprofloxacin, a primary metabolite which is a potent antimicrobial agent itself [8].

It is well known that the strategies to control mastitis include teat dip disinfection, milking procedures and selective dry-off therapy, but studies on the effectiveness of intramammary antimicrobial drugs are especially important, as many antimicrobial drugs are often administered directly through the streak canal to treat or prevent clinical or subclinical mastitis in dairy sheep. Regarding intramammary administration, to establish rational therapeutic dosage regimens, it is necessary to determine drug concentrations achieved within the udder and if these concentrations are sufficient to kill or inhibit microorganism growth, taking into account that drug distribution in tissue udder can vary according to its liposolubility, its affinity for the tissue and the formulation or the vehicle used. Milk and blood sampling are often employed in vivo to assess local concentrations for practical, ethical and economic reasons, although drug concentrations at different areas of the udder cannot be estimated in this way. In a previous study [20] we have developed an ex vivo model of isolated and perfused udder in sheep to investigate the pharmacokinetic behavior of enrofloxacin. In order to complete this former one, the objective of the present study was to determine plasma and tissue mammary gland concentrations of enrofloxacin in healthy sheep after single intramammary administration of 1 g enrofloxacin (1 g drug/5 g ointment) to evaluate, on one hand, the degree of distribution of enrofloxacin in the mammary gland and, on the other one, the transfer of this drug to systemic circulation. Moreover, the study will allow us to confirm the validity of the isolated and perfused model previously carried out in sheep.

Methods

Animals

The study was carried out in six healthy female lactating Spanish Assaf sheep weighing 45–57 kg and aged 4–5 years. Sheep were acclimatized and fed with an antibacterial-free diet of alfalfa hay and pelleted feed concentrate, and unlimited access to water and saltlick. The Institutional Animal Care and Use Committee of the University of León approved in advance all animal procedures described here.

Clinical signs of mastitis, changes in milk or skin lesions were not observed in any gland. Sheep were completely milked previously to drug administration. Intramammary administration was made through teat with a single injector containing an enrofloxacin suspension (1 g of enrofloxacin/5 g of ointment) via the teat canal, massaging afterwards into the gland cistern. Ointment was administered only in one gland. Enrofloxacin preparation was developed by Syva S.A. Laboratories (Leon, Spain), and it is still at the research stage. Up to date, and to our knowledge, there is no enrofloxacin medicine for intramammary use.

Blood samples (10 mL) were collected into heparinized vacuum tubes from a catheter laid in the jugular vein just prior to drug administration, and at 30, 60, 90, 120, 150 and 180 min. Plasma was immediately separated by centrifugation (1500 rpm for 20 min).

After 180 min sampling time, sheep were slaughtered with the following protocol: sedation was carried out with propofol (Propovet (10 mg/mL), Esteve, Barcelona, Spain) (3 mg/kg, intravenous (IV) route) prior to administration of the euthanasia medicine containing embutramide, mebezonium iodide and tetracaine hydrocloride (T-61©, Merck Sharp & Dohme Animal Health, Salamanca, Spain) (100 mg/kg, IV route). Samples of glandular tissue were obtained at four different distances (2, 4, 6 and 8 cm) from the base of the teat. All plasma and tissue samples were frozen at –20°C and stored at –80°C until analysis.

Analysis of enrofloxacin concentrations

Enrofloxacin concentrations in plasma and glandular tissue samples were measured by reversed phase high performance liquid chromatography (HPLC) with UV detection (LC Module I Plus, Waters Corporation, Mildford, MA, USA). 1 mL plasma sample was deproteinized with 0.5 mL 10% acetic acid, centrifuging at 3000 rpm for 10 min. Samples were then extracted and purified according to a method previously reported [21] with minor modifications. Mammary tissue samples were also extracted and purified using a method previously described [22] with minor modifications. 4 mL dichlorometane were added to 1 g tissue and homogenized at 13500 rpm for 30 seconds (Ultra-Turrax T-25, IKA Works Inc, Wilmington, OH). 4 mL dichlorometane and 0.5 mL sodium phosphate buffer 0.5 M (pH = 7.5) were then added to homogenate, which was shaken and centrifuged at 2500 rpm for 10 min. The organic phase was collected and mixed with 1 mL NaOH 0.5 M, centrifuging again at 2500 rpm for 10 min. This latter step was repeated twice, collecting the aqueous phase, which was injected into the chromatograph.

Chromatographic analysis was carried out with a separation Nova Pak C_{18} column (4 μm, 250 × 4 mm) (Waters Corporation, Mildford, MA, USA) at room temperature. The mobile phase consisted of a mixture of a solution of sodium acetate (pH 4.7; 0.1 M) and acetonitrile 60:40 (v/v), with pH adjusted to 5 by addition of acetic glacial acid. The flow rate of the mobile phase was 1 mL/min, and the wavelength was set at 278 nm. Under these conditions, the retention time of enrofloxacin was 2.68 min. Recovery was 73.5 ± 9.1% and 83.8 ± 7.9% in tissue and plasma samples, respectively. Interday and intraday accuracy and precision were within 10%. The limit of quantification was 0.08 μg/mL in both plasma and tissue and the limit of detection was 0.04 μg/mL in plasma and 0.08 μg/mL in tissue.

Statistical evaluation
Data were reported as mean ± standard deviation (mean ± SD) or median and quartiles. Normality of the data and uniformity of the variance were determined by asymmetry and Levene's test, respectively. When data

were normally distributed two-way ANOVA and Duncan test were used to evaluate the significance of differences in drug concentrations of treated udders. If data were not normally distributed, Friedman and Wilcoxon tests were then employed. A value of $P \leq 0.05$ was considered as level of significance for all analyses.

Results
Mean enrofloxacin plasma concentrations after intramammary administration are shown in Figure 1. Concentrations measured were low in these first 3 h after administration, remaining nearly constant from 60 min onwards. At 180 min concentrations ranged from 0.077 to 0.569 μg/mL. In one of the animals the drug was not detected at any sampling time, and at 30 min enrofloxacin was detected only in two sheep.

Regarding tissue concentrations, Figure 2 summarizes enrofloxacin concentrations in glandular tissue taken at 180 min at the different sampling heights. Animals were evaluated hourly during the assay, and neither general signs nor local irritation reactions (swelling or tissue hardening) were observed. Drug concentrations always decreased with increasing distance from the teat. Enrofloxacin concentrations were 356.6 ± 109.3 μg/g tissue near the teat (2 cm distance), declining to 172.34 ± 97.3; 113.06 ± 81.8 and 95.60 ± 74.0 μg/g at 4; 6 and 8 cm distances, respectively. At this latter point, at the base of the udder, values ranged from 8.42 to 188.84 μg/g. Significant differences were found among enrofloxacin concentrations determined at 2 cm and those measured at the other heights (Duncan test, $P \leq 0.05$).

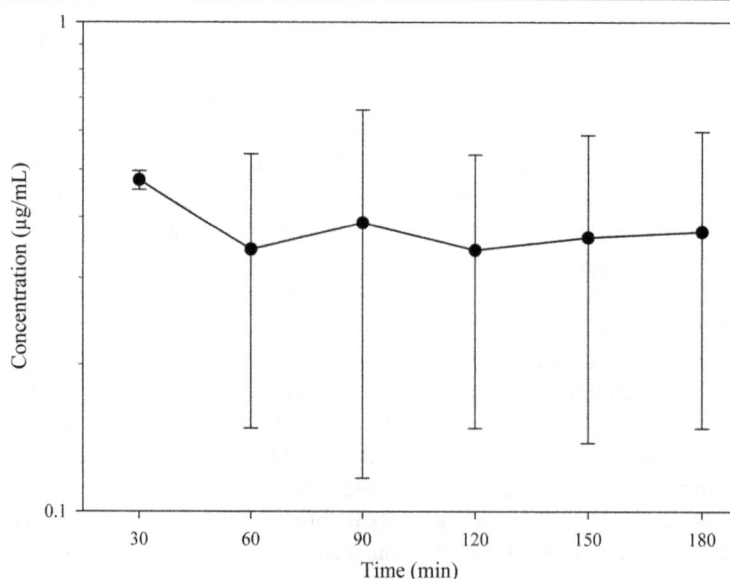

Figure 1 Plasma enrofloxacin concentrations after intramammary administration to 6 sheep. Administration was made with an injector containing 1 g enrofloxacin/5 g ointment. Data are given as mean ± SD (semilogarithmic scale).

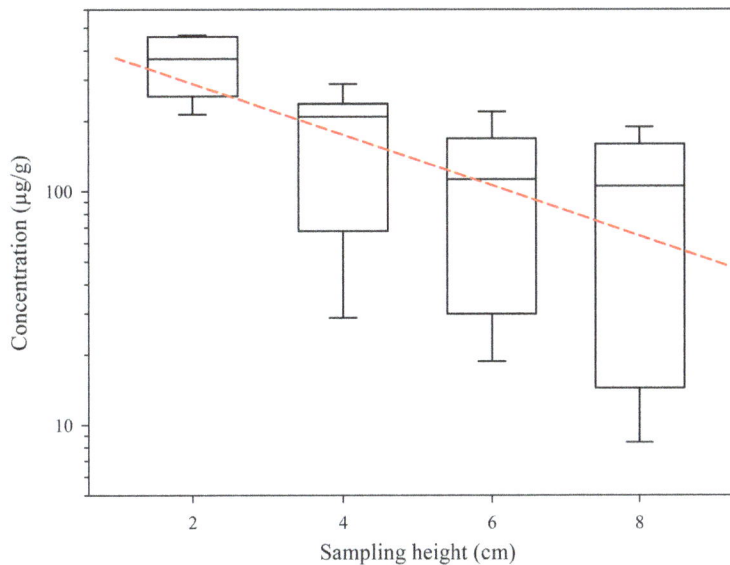

Figure 2 Enrofloxacin concentrations in glandular tissue after intramammary administration to 6 sheep. Administration was made with an injector containing 1 g enrofloxacin/5 g ointment. Samples were taken at constant vertical distances from the base of the teat. Significant differences were found between concentrations determined at 2 cm and at the rest of the heights. Theoretical values predicted with the equation Concentration $= 478.804 \cdot e^{-0.251 \cdot \text{height}}$ are also included (short dash line). Data are given as box plots with median and quartiles (semilogarithmic scale).

Tissue concentrations obtained in healthy animals were also compared with those determined in the ex vivo isolated and perfused udders after intramammary administration [20], and modelled. In both, healthy sheep and isolated udders, the best fit was obtained with a decreasing monoexponential model, described by the following equations:

$$\text{Ex vivo model}: \text{Concentration} = 177.776 \cdot e^{-0.251 \cdot \text{height}} \left(r^2 = 0.924; \ p = 0.039\right)$$

$$\text{Healthy sheep}: \text{Concentration} = 478.804 \cdot e^{-0.219 \cdot \text{height}} \left(r^2 = 0.950; \ p = 0.025\right)$$

In both equations the slopes are very similar (0.251 for the ex vivo model and 0.219 for healthy sheep), which would reveal a similar diffusion kinetics. Thus, taking into account the coefficients obtained in both equations, it would be possible to predict concentrations in alive animals at different heights of mammary gland by multiplying ex vivo tissue concentrations by 2.693 or by using a new equation obtained from that used to describe the ex vivo model concentrations, multiplying the intercept (177.776) by 2.7:

$$\text{Concentration} = 478.804 \cdot e^{-0.251 \cdot \text{height}}$$

Figure 2 shows the close correspondence among the theoretical enrofloxacin concentrations in mammary gland predicted with this latter equation and the experimental values determined in the same tissue but in healthy animals.

Discussion

As expected, enrofloxacin plasma concentrations were low after intramammary administration, showing that most drug remains in the udder carrying out its bactericidal action. These low concentrations would minimize the risk for consumers due to residues in meat or in other tissues. The drug was detected after 30 min administration only in two animals, which would indicate that in the other sheep the rate of absorption was slower that in these two animals. In one sheep absorption was too small to determine detectable levels in plasma at any sampling time. On the other hand, plasma drug concentrations determined in healthy animals were always lower than those obtained in Tyrode solution with the ex vivo model of isolated and perfused sheep udder [20]. This may be due to the fact that the ex vivo model exhibits a lower volume of distribution and it does not reflect the actual physiological conditions of drug elimination, as it lacks the organs involved in elimination process such as liver or kidneys. On the other hand, in healthy animals, although a greater transfer of drug from mammary gland into the bloodstream is expected in comparison with the ex vivo model, the proportional increase in the elimination process should explain the lower enrofloxacin plasma levels.

Regarding enrofloxacin concentrations in glandular tissue, they decreased progressive and exponentially with increased vertical distance from the base of the teat. The high variability obtained in tissue concentrations is consistent with those results indicated in other similar studies [23-27], and it can be due to interindividual variations related to gland size or milk secretion volume (related to the degree of drug dilution), even though animals were selected according to similar conformation and udder size, level of milk production or days in milk. Enrofloxacin concentrations determined reflect a good distribution of this drug in the entire mammary gland. We have chosen four locations per quarter as they represent the minimum number of samples to assess drug distribution because antimicrobials distribute unevenly in glandular tissue [23,28].

Comparing with drug concentrations determined in the ex vivo model developed in sheep [20], mammary concentrations in healthy animals are higher than those quantified in the ex vivo model. Again, these differences could be due to disparities between the model and the physiological conditions of healthy animals: composition of Tyrode solution is not exactly similar to blood composition, and there could also be differences between perfusion flow in the ex vivo model and blood flow in alive animals. Moreover, the ex vivo model is static whereas alive sheep were allowed to move during the entire duration of the sampling time. Finally, the formulation used can also have an influence on the distribution of antimicrobials administered locally into the bovine udder. All these factors could contribute to a greater diffusion of drug within the mammary gland in alive sheep.

Data on drug distribution in mammary gland are scarce, and drug concentration in milk after intramammary administration cannot be used to estimate drug concentration in udder tissue [25]. At present two different approaches have been followed. On one hand, ex vivo perfused models have been designed to establish drug concentrations in bovine and ovine udders [20,24,25,29] but it remained unclear if they accurately reflect the situation in vivo [26,30]. On the other one, anesthetized alive animals have been used to determine tissue distribution, but its major inconvenient is that quarters can be sampled only once [31], which actually limits its usage. We have chosen an intermediate approach to evaluate if drug concentrations determined in healthy animals are comparable to those obtained in the ex vivo perfused model [20]. In this case, we have fixed 180 min as sampling time to collect tissue samples as it is the time for which the isolated and perfused udders remained viable in sheep.

Finally, to establish if sufficient antibacterial concentrations are reached in the target tissue after enrofloxacin

intramammary administration, a pharmacokinetic/ pharmacodynamic (PK/PD) evaluation was also developed to assess treatment effectivity. Regarding its antibacterial activity, enrofloxacin, as any fluoroquinolone, has a concentration-dependent activity. Minimal inhibitory concentrations that inhibits 90% of bacterial isolates (MIC_{90}) have been categorized as sensitive (<0.25 µg/mL), intermediate (0.5-1 µg/mL) or resistant (>2 µg/mL) [32]. In sheep bacterial isolates a MIC of 0.5 µg/mL has been established for *Mycoplasma agalactiae* [33]. MIC values determined in cattle isolates are 0.12 µg/mL for *Escherichia coli* [34], 0.125 µg/mL for *Mannheimia haemolytica* [35], and 0.25 µg/mL for *Staphylococcus aureus* [36-38] and *Streptococcus* spp. [39]. In all the animals MIC were exceeded in the entire glandular tissue following intramammary administration, whereas in plasma samples mean enrofloxacin concentrations did not achieve the MIC fixed for *Mycoplasma agalactiae*.

Moreover, we have chosen the PK/PD index Concentration/MIC (C/MIC) > 8–10 [40,41] to assess if sufficient antibacterial concentrations are reached after intramammary administration within the glandular tissue. After 3 h drug diffusion, enrofloxacin concentrations in the entire glandular tissue were always more than 8–10 times above the MIC established for the main pathogens causing mastitis in sheep. In the base of the udder, C/MIC was 191.20 for *M. agalactiae*; 382.40 for *S. aureus* and *Streptococcus* spp.; 764.80 for *M. haemolytica* and 796.67 for *E. coli*. Regarding plasma concentrations, intramammary treatment would not be actually effective against any microorganism, as C/MIC was always lower than 8.

Finally, and with respect to the potential presence of enrofloxacin residues in both tissues or milk after intramammary administration, the study has shown that the transference of the drug from the mammary gland to plasma is low, which would diminish the risk of drug residues in meat. In mammary gland tissue, high enrofloxacin concentrations have been determined. Thus, further studies are necessary to ensure that the drug has been completely excreted from the animal, prior to dairy/meat products being available for consumers, in order to avoid the emergence and dissemination of harmful bacteria resistant to fluoroquinolones and/or undesirable effects on consumers.

Conclusions

Fluoroquinolones should be only used to treat serious infections with bacteria resistant to other antibacterial agents. To our knowledge, this is the first time that tissue distribution of enrofloxacin in the mammary gland and its degree of systemic absorption following intramammary administration have been established. The study provides complementary data on enrofloxacin tissue distribution that could be useful to design formulations employed to treat mastitis in this species. The drug shows a low transfer to systemic circulation and a wide distribution throughout the udder, achieving in the entire gland adequate concentrations against the major mastitis pathogens in sheep. Thus, enrofloxacin may be a suitable option for treating this disease in dairy sheep following intramammary administration although further studies are needed to ensure its efficacy and safety.

Abbreviations
IV: Intravenous; HPLC: High performance liquid chromatography; MIC_{90}: Minimal inhibitory concentration that inhibits 90% of bacterial isolates; PK/PD: Pharmacokinetic/pharmacodynamic; C/MIC: Concentration/MIC.

Competing interests
The authors declare that they have no competing interests.

Authors' contributions
CLC, AMSP and NFM contributed to writing the manuscript; JJGV, NFM and MSV designed, coordinated and supervised the study; CLC, AMSP, NFM, CPM, MJDL took part in sampling collection and laboratory work; MJDL developed the statistical analysis. All the authors read and approved the final manuscript

Acknowledgements
We would like to thank Syva S.A. Laboratories for the generous gift of the enrofloxacin preparation.

Author details
[1]Pharmacology, Department of Biomedical Sciences, Institute of Biomedicine (IBIOMED), University of León, Campus de Vegazana s/n, 24071 León, Spain. [2]Department of Animal Health, University of León, Campus de Vegazana s/n, 24071 León, Spain.

References
1. Bergonier D, Berthelot X. New advances in epizootiology and control of ewe mastitis. Livest Prod Sci. 2003;79:1–16.
2. Bergonier D, de Cremoux R, Rupp R, Lagriffoul G, Berthelot X. Mastitis of dairy small ruminants. Vet Res. 2003;34:689–716.
3. Contreras A, Sierra D, Sánchez A, Corrales JC, Marco JC, Paape MJ, et al. Mastitis in small ruminants. Small Rumin Res. 2007;68:145–53.
4. Altreuther P. Data on chemistry and toxicology of Baytril®. Vet Med Rev. 1987;2:87–9.
5. Elsheikh HA, Taha AAW, Khalafallah AI, Osma IAM. Disposition kinetics of enrofloxacin (Baytril® 5%) in sheep and goats following intravenous and intramuscular injection using a microbiological assay. Res Vet Sci. 2002;73:125–9.
6. Scheer M. Studies on the antibacterial activity of Baytril®. Vet Med Rev. 1987;2:90–9.
7. Scheer M. Concentrations of active ingredient in the serum and in tissue after oral and parenteral administration of Baytril®. Vet Med Rev. 1987;2:104–18.
8. Kaartinen L, Salonen M, Älli L, Pyörälä S. Pharmacokinetics of enrofloxacin after single intravenous, intramuscular and subcutaneus injections in lactating cows. J Vet Pharmacol Ther. 1995;18:357–62.
9. Kaartinen L, Pyörälä S, Moilanen M, Raisanen S. Pharmacokinetics of enrofloxacin in newborn and one-week-old calves. J Vet Pharmacol Ther. 1997;20:479–82.
10. Bregante MA, Saez P, Aramayona JJ, Fraile L, Garcia MA, Solans C. Comparative pharmacokinetics of enrofloxacin in mice, rats, rabbits, sheep and cows. Am J Vet Res. 1999;60:1111–6.
11. Varma R, Ahmad AH, Sharma LD, Aggarwal P, Ahuja V. Pharmacokinetics of enrofloxacin and its active metabolite ciprofloxacin in cows following single dose intravenous administration. J Vet Pharmacol Ther. 2003;26:303–5.
12. Kumar N, Singh SD, Jayachandran C. Pharmacokinetic study of diclofenac and its interaction with enrofloxacin in buffalo calves. J Vet Sci. 2003;2:155–9.
13. Sharma PK, Ahmad AH, Sharma LD, Varma R. Pharmacokinetics of enrofloxacin and the rate of formation of its metabolite ciprofloxacin following intravenous and intramuscular single dose administration to male buffalo calves. Vet J. 2003;166:101–4.
14. Mengozzi G, Intorre L, Bertini S, Soldani G. Pharmacokinetics of enrofloxacin and its metabolite ciprofloxacin after intravenous and intramuscular administration in sheep. Am J Vet Res. 1996;57:1040–3.
15. Bermingham EC, Papich MG. Pharmacokinetics after intravenous and oral administration of enrofloxacin in sheep. Am J Vet Res. 2002;63:1012–7.
16. Otero JL, Mestorino N, Errecalde JO. Pharmacokinetics of enrofloxacin after single intravenous administration in sheep. Rev Sci Techn. 2009;28:1129–42.
17. Elmas M, Tras B, Kaya S, Bas AL, Yazar E, Yarsan E. Pharmacokinetics of enrofloxacin after intravenous and intramuscular administration in Angora goats. Can J Vet Res. 2001;65:64–7.
18. Ambros L, Montoya L, Kreil V, Waxman S, Albarellos G, Rebuelto M, et al. Farmacocinética de la enrofloxacina y su metabolito ciprofloxacina en cabras. Rev Argent Prod Anim. 2007;27(Supl 1):329–30.
19. Vancutsem PM, Babish JG, Schwark WS. The fluoroquinolone antimicrobials: structure, antimicrobial activity, pharmacokinetics, clinical use in domestic animals and toxicity. Cornell Vet. 1990;80:173–86.
20. López C, Fernández N, Sierra M, Diez MJ, Gonzalo JM, Sahagún AM, et al. Tissue distribution of enrofloxacin after intramammary and systemic administration in the isolated perfused sheep udder. Am J Vet Res. 2012;73:1728–34.
21. Manceau J, Gicquel M, Laurentie M, Sanders P. Simultaneous determination of enrofloxacin and ciprofloxacin in animal biological fluids by high-performance liquid chromatography. Application in pharmacokinetics studies in pig and rabbit. J Chromatogr. 1999;726:175–84.
22. Diaz D, Picco EJ, Encinas T, Rubio M, Litterio NJ, Boggio JC. Residuos tisulares de nicotinato de norfloxacina administrado por vía oral en cerdos. Arch Med Vet. 2001;33:37–42.
23. Ehinger AM, Kietzmann M. Pharmakokinetische aspekte der mastitistherapie. Berl Munch Tierarztl Wochenschr. 1998;9:337–43.
24. Ehinger AM, Kietzmann M. Tissue distribution of oxacillin and ampicillin in the isolated perfused bovine udder. J Vet Med. 2000;47:157–68.
25. Ehinger AM, Kietzmann M. Tissue distribution of benzylpenicillin after intramammary administration in the isolated perfused bovine udder. J Vet Pharmacol Ther. 2000;23:303–10.
26. Ehinger AM, Schmidt H, Kietzmann M. Tissue distribution of cefquinome after intramammary and systemic administration in the isolated perfused bovine udder. Vet J. 2006;172:147–53.
27. Kietzmann M, Niedorf F, Gossellin J. Tissue distribution of cloxacillin after intramammary administration in the isolated perfused bovine udder. BMC Vet Res. 2010;6:46.
28. Funke H. The distribution of 35S-labelled benzylpenicillin in normal and mastitic mammary glands of cows and goats after local and systemic administration. Acta Vet Scand. 1961;2 Suppl 1:11–88.
29. Moore GA, Heider LE. Treatment of mastitis. Vet Clin North Am Large Anim Pract. 1984;6:323–33.
30. Zeitlin IJ, Eshraghi HR. The release and vascular action of bradykinin in the isolated perfused bovine udder. J Physiol. 2002;543:221–31.
31. Goutalier J, Combeau S, Quillon JP, Goby L. Distribution of cephalexin and kanamycin in the mammary tissue following intramammary administration in lactating cow. J Vet Pharmacol Ther. 2012;36:95–8.
32. Clinical and Laboratory Standards Institute. Performance Standards for Antimicrobial Disk and Dilution Susceptibility Test for Bacteria Isolated from Animals. 3rd ed. Wayne, PA: Clinical and Laboratory Standards Institute; 2008.
33. De Garnica ML, Rosales RS, Gonzalo C, Santos JA, Nicholas RA. Isolation, molecular characterization and antimicrobial susceptibilities of isolates of Mycoplasma agalactiae from bulk tank milk in an endemic area of Spain. J Appl Microbiol. 2013;114:1575–81.
34. Bengtsson B, Ericsson H, Ekman T, Artursson K, Nilsson-Öst M, Persson K. Antimicrobial susceptibility of udder pathogens from cases of acute clinical mastitis in dairy cows. Vet Microbiol. 2009;136:142–9.
35. Blondeau JM, Borsos S, Blondeau LD, Blondeau BJ, Hesje CE. Comparative minimum inhibitory and mutant prevention drug concentrations of enrofloxacin, ceftiofur, florfenicol, tilmicosin and tulathromycin against

bovine clinical isolates of *Mannheimia haemolytica*. Vet Microbiol. 2012;160:85–90.

36. Feßler A, Scott C, Kadlec K, Ehricht R, Monecke S, Schwarz S. Characterization of methicillin-resistant Staphylococcus aureus ST398 from cases of bovine mastitis. J Antimicrob Chemother. 2010;65:619–25.

37. Rubin JE, Ball KR, Chirino-Trejo M. Antimicrobial susceptibility of *Staphylococcus aureus* and *Staphylococcus pseudintermedius* isolated from various animals. Can Vet J. 2011;52:153–7.

38. Baba K, Ishihara K, Ozawa M, Usui M, Hiki M, Tamura Y, et al. Prevalence and mechanism of antimicrobial resistance in *Staphylococcus* isolates from diseased cattle, swine and chickens in Japan. J Vet Med Sci. 2012;74:561–5.

39. Kaspar H. Results of the antimicrobial agent susceptibility study raised in a representative, cross-sectional monitoring study on a national basis. Int J Med Microbiol. 2006;296 Suppl 2:69–79.

40. McKellar QA, Sanchez SF, Jones DG. Pharmacokinetic/pharmadynamic relationships of antimicrobial drugs used in veterinary medicine. J Vet Pharmacol Ther. 2004;27:503–14.

41. Papich MG. Pharmacokinetic-pharmacodynamic (PK-PD) modelling and the rational selection of dosage regimes for the prudent use of antimicrobial drugs. Vet Microbiol. 2014;171:480–6.

3

Effects of dietary omega-3/omega-6 fatty acid ratios on reproduction in the young breeder rooster

Yun Feng[1†], Yu Ding[1†], Juan Liu[1], Ye Tian[1], Yanzhou Yang[2], Shuluan Guan[1] and Cheng Zhang[1*]

Abstract

Background: Polyunsaturated fatty acids (PUFAs) are necessary for the body's metabolism, growth and development. Although PUFAs play an important role in the regulation of reproduction, their role in testis development in the rooster is unknown. The present study was conducted to investigate the effects of omega-3/omega-6 (n-3/n-6, PUFAs) ratios on reproductive performance in young breeder roosters. Plasma levels of reproductive hormones, testis development, and reproductive hormone receptor and StAR mRNA expression were also assessed.

Results: Although PUFAs (n-3/n-6: 1/4.15) had no significant effect on the testis index ($P > 0.05$), the spermatogonial development and germ cell layers were increased. Moreover, serum levels of hormones (GnRH, FSH, LH and T) on day 35 were also significantly increased by PUFAs (n-3/n-6: 1/4.15). To investigate whether PUFAs regulate the expression of hormone receptors and StAR, real time-PCR was used to measure GnRHR, FSHR, LHR and StAR mRNA levels. PUFAs significantly increased the mRNA levels of all of these genes.

Conclusions: These results indicate that PUFAs enhance the reproductive performance of young roosters by increasing hormone secretion and function, the latter by up-regulating receptor expression. These findings provide a sound basis for a balanced n-3/n-6 PUFA ratio being beneficial to young rooster reproduction.

Keywords: PUFAs, Young breeder roosters, Reproductive hormones, Testis development, Reproductive hormone receptors, StAR mRNA

Background

Reproduction is a critical part of poultry production, especially the rooster's reproductive performance. The male gonads, testes secrete androgens and generate sperm, and are vital for males to maintain normal reproductive function. During testis development in the chicken, there is no significant increase in testicular weight from 2 to 15 weeks of age. However, the number of spermatogonia reaches more than one million [1,2]. Spermatogonia provide nutrients for sperm growth and development, and the number of spermatogonia is related to the capacity for testicular spermatogenesis. In addition, the early stage is the most important period for testicular development [3-6].

Polyunsaturated fatty acids (PUFAs) have 16 to 22 carbon atoms and more than one double bond. They have a great impact on reproduction, affecting prostaglandin (PG) synthesis, steroidogenesis, transcription factors and membrane properties [7]. Many studies showed that dietary supplementation with PUFAs, especially omega-3 (n-3) PUFAs, significantly increases sperm fertility in birds [8,9] and boars [10,11]. The long-chain n-3 PUFAs eicosapentaenoic acid (EPA; 20:5, n-3) and docosahexaenoic acid (DHA; 22:6, n-3) are especially abundant in natural sources such as fish oils and linseed oil [12]. Spermatogenesis and steroidogenesis of the avian testis depend on many gonadal hormones [13]. PUFAs such as arachidonic acid (AA) and its metabolites affect steroidogenesis through direct effects on steroid acute regulator (StAR) and cytochrome P450, which play a critical role in regulating steroid synthesis [7,14]. Meanwhile, 20-carbon PUFAs are the direct precursors of PGs [15], and participate in the regulation of reproductive endocrinology [16,17].

PUFAs influence the physical nature of cell membranes and are involved in membrane protein-mediated

* Correspondence: zhch8012@163.com
†Equal contributors
[1]College of Life Science, Capital Normal University, Beijing 100048, Peoples' Republic of China
Full list of author information is available at the end of the article

responses, lipid mediator generation, cell signaling and gene expression in many different cell types essential for brain and eye development and cardiac health [18]. It is reported that PUFAs may differentially affect cellular responses by changing membrane fluidity, receptor binding characteristics or their downstream activation [19-21]. Several reports suggest that the ratio of omega 6 to omega 3 fatty acids on man diet is approximately 1:1 [22,23]. Moreover, the appropriate ratio of omega6: omega3 fatty acids affect the reproductive performance of mature cockerels [8].

From 2 to 15 weeks, the growth and maturation of Sertoli and Leydig cells is an important step in early testicular development in the chicken [4]. Although n-3/n-6 (omega-3/omega-6) PUFAs are beneficial to male reproduction capacity, especially sperm quality, the appropriate ratio of n-3/n-6 PUFAs for young roosters' testicular development and reproductive hormones was not known. The present study aimed to evaluate the effects of n-3/n-6 PUFAs ratios on testis development in young cockerels (10 to 15 weeks of age), and to investigate the possible mechanism of testis development regulation.

Methods
Materials
All reagents were purchased from Sigma Chemical Co. (St. Louis, MO, USA) unless otherwise specified. The ELISA kit was obtained from Nanjing Jian Cheng Bioengineering Institute (Nanjing, Jiangsu, China). Trizol reagent was obtained from Takara Bio, Takara Holdings Inc. (Otsu, Shiga, Japan). The M-MLV Reverse Transcriptase kit was purchased from Omega Bio-Tek, Inc. (Norcross, GA, USA). Soybean oil (SO) and flaxseed oil (FO) were purchased from Xin Yuan (Beijing) Fragrance Technology Co., Ltd.

Animal treatment
Seventy-day-old Jing Hong breeder roosters (Beijing, China) were selected from the same batch and housed in cages individually under controlled environment conditions (light 13 h/dark 11 h, 22°C). The roosters were fed with dry powder feed and were given free access to feed and water. The present study was performed in accordance with the Guidelines for the Care and Use of Laboratory Animals and the China Council on Animal Care and was approved by the Institutional Animal Care and Use Committee of Capital Normal University.

The breeder roosters were randomly divided into five groups (six roosters per group at 0 days). All birds were fed diet 1 for 7 days and then received different ratios of n3/n6 PUFAs [1/18.39 (Treatment 1), 1/7.84 (Treatment 2), 1/5.04 (Treatment 3), 1/4.15 (Treatment 4) and 1/2.32 (Treatment 5)] from SO and FO. The basic formulations of the experimental diets contained n3/n6 PUFAs with different ratios from SO and FO: 2% SO/0% FO (Treatment

1), 1.5% SO/0.5% FO (Treatment 2), 1% SO/1% FO (Treatment 3), 0.5% SO/1.5% FO (Treatment 4) and 0% FO/2% SO (Treatment 5). The fatty acid compositions of the oils used in this study are presented in Table 1 and the fatty acid compositions of the diets are shown in Table 2.

Collection of blood and testis samples
Blood and testis samples were collected at 21 and 35 days after treatment. Blood samples were collected by cardiac puncture [24] and were centrifuged at 3000 rpm for 10 min at 4°C to isolate plasma. Plasma was stored at −20°C until assayed for reproductive hormones.

The birds were decapitated, and their body and testis weights were measured to determine the testis index (testis weight/body weight) [1]. One of the testes was fixed in formaldehyde and embedded in paraffin. The other was stored at −80°C for RT-PCR assay.

Histologic sections
Testes were fixed, dehydrated through a graded series of ethanol solutions and xylene, and embedded in paraffin. Testes embedded in paraffin were serially sectioned to a thickness of 3–5 μm and placed on slides coated with poly-L-lysine. The sections were stained with hematoxylin and eosin (HE) for morphological observation [1].

Table 1 Fatty acid composition of soybean oil and linseed oil (%)

Fatty acids	Soybean oil	Linseed oil
C14:0	0.11	0.04
C15:0	0.02	0.02
C16:0	11.86	5.87
C16:1	0.14	0.06
C18:0	4.74	4.49
C18:1	21.60	22.30
C18:3 n-6	52.58	16.67
C18:3 n-3	7.65	49.85
C20:0	0.25	0.12
C20:1	0.19	0.16
C20:3 n-6	—	—
C20:3 n-3	—	0.06
C22:0	0.36	0.10
C22:1	0.11	0.06
C24:0	0.07	0.03
Others	0.30	0.15
Total	100.00	100.00
n-3 PUFAs	7.65	49.91
n-6 PUFAs	52.58	16.67
n-3/n-6	1:7.34	1:0.33

The values were determined by feed analysis test.

Table 2 Fatty acid composition of diets (%)

Fatty acids	Treatment 1	Treatment 2	Treatment 3	Treatment 4	Treatment 5
C14:0	0.05	0.01	0.02	0.02	0.02
C15:0	0.03	0.03	0.03	0.03	0.03
C15:1	0.02	—	—	—	—
C16:0	14.48	14.67	13.74	13.03	13.15
C16:1	0.14	0.13	0.14	0.13	0.14
C18:0	3.12	3.34	2.99	3.35	3.26
C18:1	23.58	25.63	23.91	23.29	24.13
C18:2 n-6	53.93	48.53	48.19	47.40	40.38
C18:3 n-3	2.93	6.20	9.58	11.42	17.47
C20:0	0.43	0.44	0.38	0.37	0.37
C20:1	0.28	0.29	0.28	0.31	0.32
C20:3 n-6	0.04	0.04	0.06	0.09	0.14
C20:3 n-3	—	—	—	—	—
C22:0	0.27	0.24	0.20	0.19	0.18
C23:0	0.14	0.06	0.05	0.04	0.03
C22:1	0.15	0.10	0.18	0.14	0.16
C24:0	—	—	—	—	—
Others	0.42	0.29	0.25	0.19	0.22
Total	100.00	100.00	100.00	100.00	100.00
n-3 PUFAs	53.97	48.57	48.25	47.49	40.52
n-6 PUFAs	2.93	6.20	9.58	11.42	17.47
n-3/n-6	1:18.39	1:7.84	1:5.04	1:4.15	1:2.32

The values were determined by feed analysis test.

Measurement of reproductive hormones

The plasma concentrations of gonadotropin-releasing hormone (GnRH), luteinizing hormone (LH), follicle-stimulating hormone (FSH) and testosterone (T) were measured using an ELISA kit (Nanjing, Jiangsu, China) according to the manufacturer's instruction. All assays were performed in 96-well plates and the absorbance was measured at 450 nm (BioTek Instruments, Inc., Winooski, USA). A standard curve was used to determine hormone levels.

RNA extraction, cDNA synthesis, and real-time PCR analysis

Testes were ground in liquid nitrogen, and total RNA was extracted using Trizol reagent according to the manufacturer's instructions. Total RNA was reverse transcribed to cDNA using M-MLV Reverse Transcriptase. Briefly, 0.2 μg of total RNA was reverse transcribed in a 20-μl reaction containing 4 μl of 5× reaction buffer, 2 μl of 10 mM dNTPs, 20 U of RNase inhibitor, 200 U of RevertAid H Minus M-MULV RT enzyme, random decamer primers and RNase-free H_2O. Quantitative PCR analysis of GnRHR, FSHR, LHR, StAR and β-actin was performed using a LightCycler 2.0 System (Roche Diagnostics).

The GnRHR primers used for amplification were a 5' forward primer (5'- ACGAGCCATGCAGCAGAAG -3') and a 3'reverse primer (5'- CGAACAGTGGAAGGAACCC -3'). The FSHR primer sequences were 5'- CATGTCTCCGGCAAAGCAA -3' (5' forward primer) and 5'- AAAACGCGTGCCATAATGG -3'(3' reverse primer). The LHR primers used for amplification were a 5' forward primer (5' - ACTCCTGCGCAAACCCATTC -3') and a 3'reverse primer (5'- CTCGGCTCTTACAGCAACCT -3'). The StAR primer sequences used were a 5'forward primer (5'- TCAGCCGGCGGATTTAAGG -3') and a 3' reverse primer (5'- TGGTGGCTGCTACAAACACT-3'). β-actin primer sequences were 5'- AACACCCACACCCCTGTGAT -3' (5' forward primer) and 5'- TGAGTCAAGCGCCAAAAGAA -3'(3' reverse primer).

The reactions were incubated in a 96-well plate at 95 °C for 5 min, followed by 40 cycles at 95 °C for 15 s and 60 °C for 1 min. Relative mRNA abundance was determined using ABI PRISM 7500 software (Applied Biosystems, Grand Island, NY, USA). To avoid false-positive signals, dissociation-curve analyses were performed after the amplification and the PCR products were separated on a 1.5% agarose gel to confirm their sizes. Moreover, the PCR products were purified and sequenced to verify their identities. The results were normalized to the expression levels of β-actin, a housekeeping gene, by the 2-ΔΔCt method [25]. PCR reactions without reverse-transcribed cDNA were used as negative controls. The reactions were conducted in at least duplicate.

Statistical analysis

Results are presented as means ± SEM of at least three independent experiments, as detailed in the figure legends. All data were subjected to one way (repeated-measure) ANOVA (Prism 5.0 statistical software; GraphPad Software, Inc., San Diego, CA). Significant differences between treatment groups were determined by the Tukey's test. Statistical significance was defined at P < 0.05.

Results

Effects of n-3/n-6 PUFAs ratios on the testis index

To evaluate the effect of n-3/n-6 PUFAs on the testis index, various ratios of n-3/n-6 PUFAs were supplied in the diet. Body weight on day 21 tended to increase with increasing ratio of n-3/n-6 PUFAs (Table 3). There were significant differences among treatment 1/2 and treatment 3/4 (P < 0.05). However, weight was not significantly increased with the highest ratio compared with the control group. Although testis weight and testis index increased in a dose-dependent

Table 3 Effects of different ratios of N-3/N-6 PUFAs on the testes index

Time	Treatment	Body weight(kg)	Left testis weight(g)	Right testis weight(g)	Testis weight(g)	Testis index
21d	1	1.2157 ± 0.0779^a	0.2463 ± 0.0289	0.2610 ± 0.0291	0.5740 ± 0.1245	0.4185 ± 0.0432
	2	1.3115 ± 0.0542^a	0.2883 ± 0.0339	0.3030 ± 0.0325	0.4580 ± 0.1344	0.4483 ± 0.0315
	3	1.4752 ± 0.0139^b	0.3117 ± 0.0314	0.3223 ± 0.0364	0.6307 ± 0.0707	0.4304 ± 0.0483
	4	1.3922 ± 0.0161^b	0.3683 ± 0.0352	0.3807 ± 0.0349	0.9063 ± 0.1492	0.5382 ± 0.0508
	5	1.3055 ± 0.0610^a	0.3637 ± 0.0562	0.3807 ± 0.0544	0.7443 ± 0.1107	0.5648 ± 0.0622
35d	1	1.5703 ± 0.0504	0.8743 ± 0.0239	0.8904 ± 0.0211	1.7647 ± 0.0451	1.1276 ± 0.0610
	2	1.5948 ± 0.0431	0.8890 ± 0.0191	0.9103 ± 0.0136	1.7993 ± 0.0321	1.1294 ± 0.0298
	3	1.5680 ± 0.0264	0.8882 ± 0.0078	0.9025 ± 0.0134	1.7907 ± 0.0208	1.1428 ± 0.02678
	4	1.6027 ± 0.0440	0.9050 ± 0.0128	0.9317 ± 0.0093	1.8367 ± 0.0218	1.14789 ± 0.0371
	5	1.5797 ± 0.0170	0.8923 ± 0.0482	0.9167 ± 0.0673	1.8090 ± 0.0113	1.1423 ± 0.0058

Testis index = testis weight (g)/body weight (kg).
In the same column, values with different small letter superscripts mean significant difference (P < 0.05).

manner, there were no significant differences among treatments on day 35 (P > 0.05).

Effects of N-3/N-6 PUFAs ratios on testis morphology

Testis morphology in birds at 21 and 35 days are shown in Figure 1. The seminiferous tubule epithelium and spermatogonia of the underlying epithelial cells developed normally. Although no significant difference in testis morphology was found among treatments, 5–6 layers of germ cells were seen on day 21 in birds given treatment 4 (Figure 1D) and treatments 5 (Figure 1 E). There were 2–3 layers of germ cells with treatments 1 (Figure 1A) and 2 (Figure 1B) and 3–4 layers with treatments 3 (Figure 1C).

On day 35, 6–7 layers of germ cells were observed in the treatment 5 (Figure 1J). The formation speed of spermatogonial at day 35 was improved with an increase in the ratio of n-3/n-6 PUFAs.

Effects of n-3/n-6 PUFAs ratios on serum hormone levels

As shown in Table 4, the concentration of GnRH on day 21 and 35 increased with increasing n-3/n-6 PUFA ratio, but was lower at an n-3/n-6 PUFA ratio of 1/2.32 (treatment 5). The GnRH concentration at 21 and 35 days were significantly higher for treatment 4 compared with the other treatments (P < 0.05). The LH and T concentrations on days 21 and 35 and the FSH concentration on day 35 showed similar trends as that for GnRH concentration: the LH, FSH and T concentrations were significantly higher for treatment 4 than for other treatments (P < 0.05). There were no significant differences in FSH concentrations at 21 days.

Effects of n-3/n-6 PUFAs ratios on the mRNA levels of hormone receptor genes in the testis of breeder roosters

The relative mRNA levels of GnRH receptor (GnRHR), FSH receptor (FSHR) and LH receptor (LHR) in the chicken testis are shown in Figure 2. There were no differences among treatments in GnRHR mRNA expression on day 21

(Figure 2A). However, the mRNA level of GnRH was significantly increased by n3/n6 PUFAs, especially an n3/n6 ratio of 1/4.15 (Figure 2A).

FSHR expression on day 21 was significantly increased in a dose-dependent manner (P < 0.001) (Figure 2B) and was higher for treatment 4 compared with other treatments. Although treatment 3 significantly decreased FSHR expression on day 35 (P < 0.01), there were no differences among treatments 1, 2, 4 and 5 (P > 0.05) (Figure 2B).

The LHR mRNA level was lower for treatment 1 compared with the other treatments on day 21 (P < 0.001) (Figure 2C), and was highest for treatment 5 on day 35 (P < 0.01) (Figure 2C). There were no differences among treatments 1, 2, 3 and 4 (P > 0.05).

Effects of n-3/n-6 PUFAs ratios on the mRNA level of the StAR gene in the testis of breeder roosters

As show in Figure 2D, StAR mRNA expression in the rooster testis on day 21 was not significantly affected by the n-3/n-6 ratio, although treatments 4 and 5 increased the StAR mRNA level compared with treatment 1 (P > 0.05) (Figure 2D). At 35 days, treatments 3, 4 and 5 showed significant increases in StAR mRNA level (P < 0.001) (Figure 2D).

Discussion

The present study aimed to evaluate the effect of different n-3/n-6 PUFAs ratios on testicular development and reproductive hormones, and to provide the basis for determining the appropriate n-3/n-6 PUFA ratio for young chickens. Previous research on boars [10,11], rats [26] and birds [8,9] showed that consumption of an appropriate ratio of n-3/n-6 PUFAs was beneficial to male reproduction capacity, especially sperm quality. However, the appropriate ratio of n-3/n-6 PUFAs for testicular development and reproductive hormones in young roosters was not known.

Testes of chickens are located in the dorsal abdomen and are oval- or bean-shaped and milky white. Early testicular

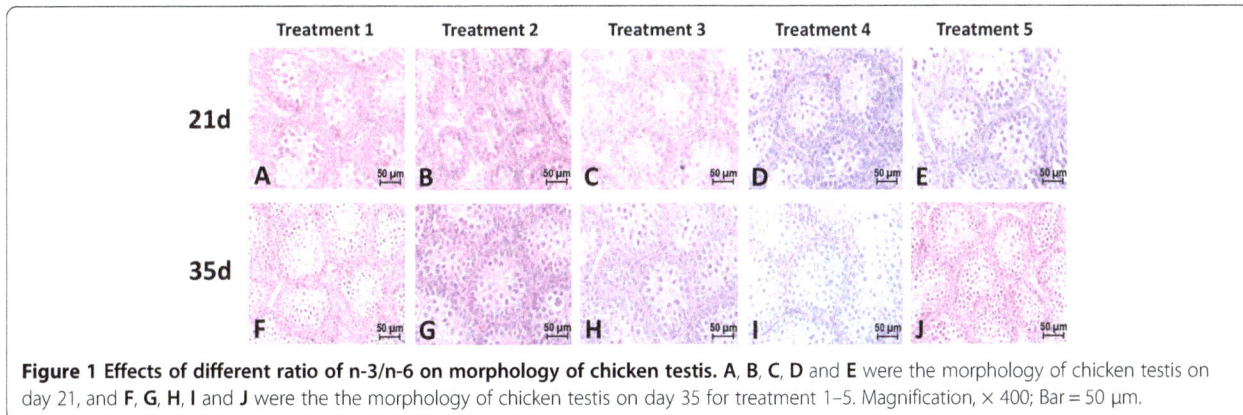

Figure 1 Effects of different ratio of n-3/n-6 on morphology of chicken testis. **A**, **B**, **C**, **D** and **E** were the morphology of chicken testis on day 21, and **F**, **G**, **H**, **I** and **J** were the the morphology of chicken testis on day 35 for treatment 1–5. Magnification, × 400; Bar = 50 μm.

development is crucial to improving the reproductive performance of roosters. From 2 to 15 weeks, the growth and maturation of Sertoli and Leydig cells is the important step in early testicular development in the chicken [4]. These cells facilitate the development of pluripotent PGCs into spermatogonia, which support the germinal cells throughout the life of the bird [27]. The period from 10 to 15 weeks is the key stage for later testicular development. Many studies have shown that testicular growth and development are delayed in underweight chicken [28,29]. The ratio of testis weight to total body weight can reflect testis growth. Yan et al. [26] found that a variety of ratios of n-3/n-6 PUFAs had no effect on the testis index in Sprague–Dawley rats. Our study had a similar result for the testis index, although the testis index tended to increase with increasing n-3/n-6 PUFA ratio.

Both n-6 and n-3 PUFAs affect reproduction. Many studies have shown the effects of n-3/n-6 PUFA ratio on male reproduction. GnRH, which is released by the hypothalamus, stimulates release of FSH and LH from the pituitary gland [30]. It is reported that a high-energy diet increased GnRH pulse frequency, testicular weight and sperm production [31]. The study indicated that spermatogenesis and steroidogenesis in the avian testis are dependent on FSH, LH and T [6]. FSH binds to its receptors in the membranes of Sertoli cells, and stimulates spermatogenesis. Testicular function is associated with FSH concentrations in male broiler breeders, and that testis weight is highly correlated with FSH [6]. On the other hand, FSH is necessary for initiation of spermatogenesis and maturation of spermatozoa. Meanwhile, the numbers of spermatogonia, spermatocytes and sperm cells would increase in male monkeys given recombinant human FSH [32]. FSH and LH regulate spermatogenesis via cyclic adenosine 3′, 5′-monophosphate (cAMP) [33]. LH binds to receptors in the membranes of Leydig cells, and stimulates the secretion of T. T levels determine the testicular development and behavior of roosters [26,31]. T may act on the Sertoli and peritubular cells of the seminiferous tubules and stimulate spermatogenesis [34]. In the present study, we showed that the concentrations of GnRH, FSH, LH and T were positively related to the quality and morphology of sperm. Similarly, Yan et al. [26] reported that the concentrations of GnRH, FSH, LH and T increased with increasing n-3/n-6 PUFA ratio, and that lower and higher n-3/n-6 ratios have opposite effects on reproduction. These results indicate that an appropriate n-3/n-6 PUFA ratio is important for the development of

Table 4 Effects of different ratios of N-3/N-6 PUFAs on the serum hormone levels

Time	Treatment	GnRH(ng/L)	LH(mIU/ml)	FSH(IU/L)	T(nmo/L)
21d	1	114.8510 ± 3.6500[a]	2.1117 ± 0.0816[b]	5.3316 ± 0.0935	9.4830 ± 0.2194[a]
	2	117.8113 ± 1.9410[a]	2.0503 ± 0.0245[ab]	5.3893 ± 0.1400	9.5000 ± 0.1830[ab]
	3	117.9606 ± 4.5833[a]	2.1187 ± 0.2904[b]	5.2857 ± 0.1560	9.5286 ± 0.5078[ab]
	4	128.3990 ± 4.2219[b]	2.3397 ± 0.1090[b]	5.5743 ± 0.2446	10.6810 ± 0.3215[b]
	5	118.7643 ± 5.0145[a]	1.6170 ± 0.0758[a]	5.3740 ± 0.1878	9.4426 ± 0.1897[ab]
35d	1	118.0626 ± 5.9451[a]	2.2897 ± 0.1448[a]	3.8223 ± 0.0789[a]	20.9670 ± 0.2361[a]
	2	124.7476 ± 1.7489[a]	2.8570 ± 0.1251[a]	4.2557 ± 0.1354[a]	20.8390 ± 0.4256[a]
	3	120.1923 ± 3.4892[a]	2.7343 ± 0.1044[a]	3.7997 ± 0.0837[a]	21.3133 ± 0.8362[ab]
	4	136.6667 ± 3.0792[b]	3.4170 ± 0.1306[b]	4.6900 ± 0.1718[b]	23.6027 ± 0.3857[b]
	5	122.5713 ± 2.0841[a]	2.7203 ± 0.1524[a]	4.3910 ± 0.3484[a]	20.2320 ± 1.3243[a]

In the same column, values with different small letter superscripts mean significant difference (P < 0.05).

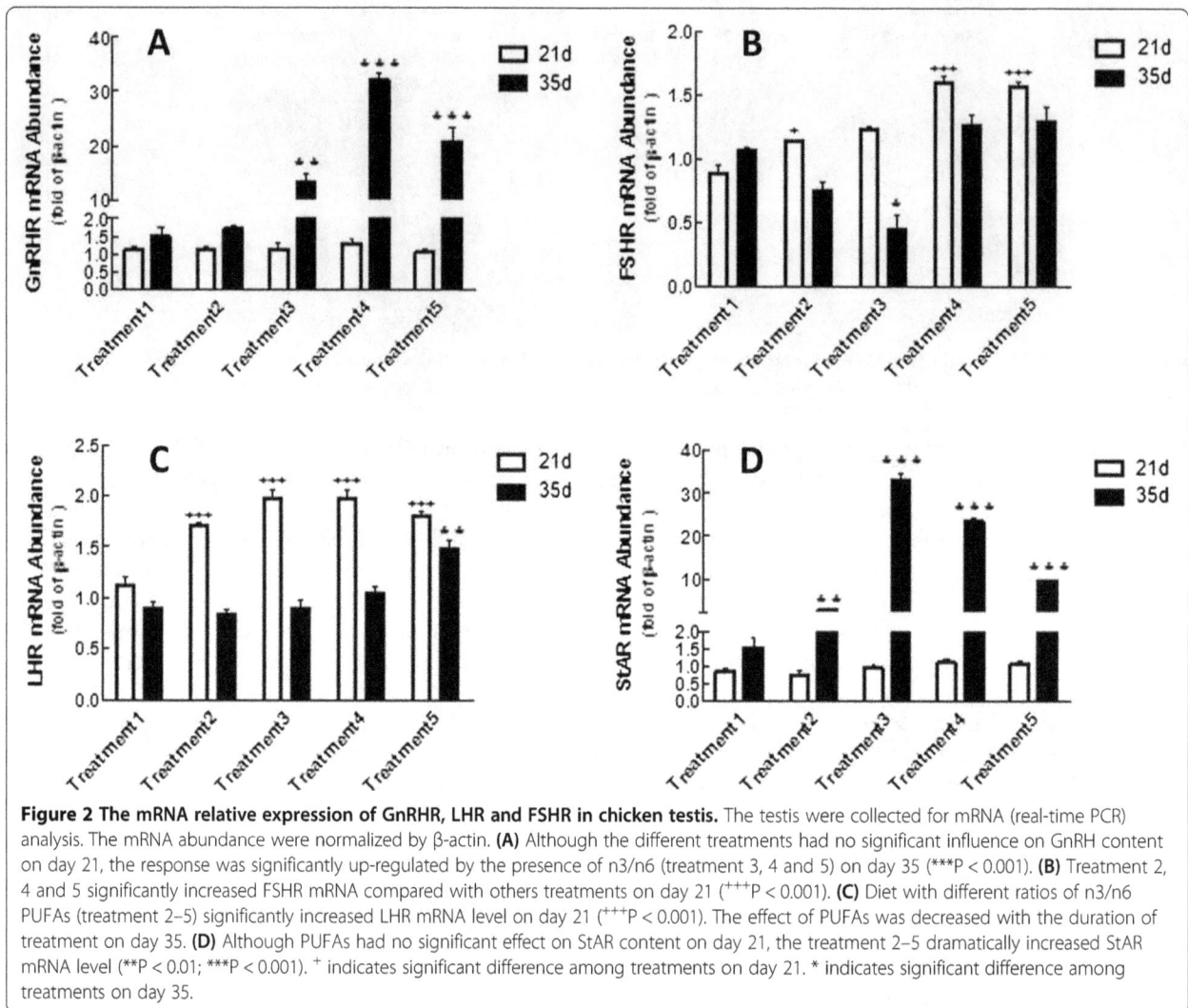

Figure 2 The mRNA relative expression of GnRHR, LHR and FSHR in chicken testis. The testis were collected for mRNA (real-time PCR) analysis. The mRNA abundance were normalized by β-actin. **(A)** Although the different treatments had no significant influence on GnRH content on day 21, the response was significantly up-regulated by the presence of n3/n6 (treatment 3, 4 and 5) on day 35 (***P < 0.001). **(B)** Treatment 2, 4 and 5 significantly increased FSHR mRNA compared with others treatments on day 21 (+++P < 0.001). **(C)** Diet with different ratios of n3/n6 PUFAs (treatment 2–5) significantly increased LHR mRNA level on day 21 (+++P < 0.001). The effect of PUFAs was decreased with the duration of treatment on day 35. **(D)** Although PUFAs had no significant effect on StAR content on day 21, the treatment 2–5 dramatically increased StAR mRNA level (**P < 0.01; ***P < 0.001). + indicates significant difference among treatments on day 21. * indicates significant difference among treatments on day 35.

spermatogonia in the rooster. From morphologic analyses of testes, treatments 4 and 5 yielded better histological changes. This suggests that the increased hormone levels improved testis development.

PUFAs act via cell surface and intracellular receptors/sensors that control cell signaling and gene expression patterns [35]. Some effects of n-3 PUFAs appear to be mediated by, or at least associated with, changes in the fatty acid composition of cell membranes. GnRHR, FSHR and LHR have important roles in the regulation of male reproduction [16,36,37]. In the present study, relative GnRHR, FSHR and LHR mRNA levels at 21 and 35 days differed significantly among ratios of n-3/n-6 PUFAs. This evidence suggests that PUFAs may affect cellular responses through changes in membrane fluidity, receptor binding characteristics or their downstream activation.

StAR promoter activity and StAR mRNA and protein levels in MA-10 Leydig cells were inhibited by inhibition of endogenous AA release, whereas addition of exogenous AA reversed these effects [16]. On the other hand, specific inhibition of PTGS2 was also associated with increased StAR expression [17]. We found that the relative StAR mRNA level on day 35 differed significantly among ratios of n-3/n-6 PUFAs.

Conclusions

In conclusion, dietary treatment of roosters with an appropriate n-3/n-6 PUFA ratio (treatment 4: 1/4.15) increased hormone secretion, thereby improving testis development. The treatment also increased reproductive performance, which may be related to changes in the mRNA levels of hormone receptors and StAR. These findings provide a sound basis for a balanced n-3/n-6 PUFA ratio being beneficial to young rooster reproduction.

Abbreviations
PUFAs: Polyunsaturated fatty acids; DHA: Docosahexaenoic; SO: Soybean oil; LO: Linseed oil; GnRH: Gonadotropin releasing hormone; FSH: Follicular

stimulating hormone; LH: Luteinizing hormone; T: Testosterone; StAR: Steroid acute regulator protein.

Competing interests
The authors declared that they have no competing interest.

Authors' contributions
CZ conceived and designed the experiments; YF, YD, JL performed the experiments; YD, YT, analyzed the data; SG contributed reagents/materials/analysis tool; YF, YD wrote the paper. CZ and YY revised the manuscript. All authors read and approved the final manuscript.

Acknowledgments
This work was supported by the grant (PXM2012_014207_0001666) from the Innovation team on Nutrition & Feedstuff in Poultry Beijing, China, Beijing Municipal Natural Science Foundation (No.5142003) and the National Natural Science Foundation of China (No. 31300958). And this project was also supported by Technology Foundation for Selected Overseas Chinese Scholar, Beijing Municipal Bureau of Personnel, China and Funding project for talent development of Beijing municipality (2013D005016000007). The funders had no role in study design, data collection and analysis, decision to publish, or preparation of the manuscript.

Author details
[1]College of Life Science, Capital Normal University, Beijing 100048, Peoples' Republic of China. [2]Key Laboratory of Fertility Preservation and Maintenance, Ministry of Education, Key Laboratory of Reproduction and Genetics in Ningxia, Department of Histology and Embryology, Ningxia Medical University, Ningxia 750004, Peoples' Republic of China.

References
1. Sarabia Fragoso J, Pizarro Diaz M, Abad Moreno JC, Casanovas Infesta P, Rodriguez-Bertos A, Barger K. Relationships between fertility and some parameters in male broiler breeders (body and testicular weight, histology and immunohistochemistry of testes, spermatogenesis and hormonal levels). Reprod Domest Anim. 2013;48(2):345–52.
2. Anastasiadou M, Theodoridis A, Avdi M, Michailidis G. Changes in the expression of Toll-like receptors in the chicken testis during sexual maturation and Salmonella infection. Anim Reprod Sci. 2011;128(1–4):93–9.
3. Huh MI, Jung JC. Expression of matrix metalloproteinase-13 (MMP-13) in the testes of growing and adult chicken. Acta Histochem. 2012;115(5):475–80.
4. Mucksova J, Brillard JP, Hejnar J, Poplstein M, Kalina J, Bakst M, et al. Identification of various testicular cell populations in pubertal and adult cockerels. Anim Reprod Sci. 2009;114(4):415–22.
5. Silversides FG, Robertson MC, Liu J. Growth of subcutaneous chicken testicular transplants. Poult Sci. 2013;92(7):1916–20.
6. Vizcarra JA, Kirby JD, Kreider DL. Testis development and gonadotropin secretion in broiler breeder males. Poult Sci. 2010;89(2):328–34.
7. Wathes DC, Abayasekara DR, Aitken RJ. Polyunsaturated fatty acids in male and female reproduction. Biol Reprod. 2007;77(2):190–201.
8. Zanini SF, Torres CA, Bragagnolo N, Turatti JM, Silva MG, Zanini MS. Evaluation of the ratio of omega6: omega3 fatty acids and vitamin E levels in the diet on the reproductive performance of cockerels. Arch Tierernahr. 2003;57(6):429–42.
9. Kelso KA, Cerolini S, Speake BK, Cavalchini LG, Noble RC. Effects of dietary supplementation with alpha-linolenic acid on the phospholipid fatty acid composition and quality of spermatozoa in cockerel from 24 to 72 weeks of age. J Reprod Fertil. 1997;110(1):53–9.
10. Estienne MJ, Harper AF, Crawford RJ. Dietary supplementation with a source of omega-3 fatty acids increases sperm number and the duration of ejaculation in boars. Theriogenology. 2008;70(1):70–6.
11. Strzezek J, Fraser L, Kuklinska M, Dziekonska A, Lecewicz M. Effects of dietary supplementation with polyunsaturated fatty acids and antioxidants on biochemical characteristics of boar semen. Reprod Biol. 2004;4(3):271–87.
12. Nettleton JA. Omega-3 fatty acids: comparison of plant and seafood sources in human nutrition. J Am Diet Assoc. 1991;91(3):331–7.
13. Sofikitis N, Giotitsas N, Tsounapi P, Baltogiannis D, Giannakis D, Pardalidis N. Hormonal regulation of spermatogenesis and spermiogenesis. J Steroid Biochem Mol Biol. 2008;109(3–5):323–30.
14. Stocco DM, Wang X, Jo Y, Manna PR. Multiple signaling pathways regulating steroidogenesis and steroidogenic acute regulatory protein expression: more complicated than we thought. Molecular endocrinology (Baltimore, Md. 2005;11:2647–59.
15. Needleman P, Turk J, Jakschik BA, Morrison AR, Lefkowith JB. Arachidonic acid metabolism. Annu Rev Biochem. 1986;55:69–102.
16. Wang XJ, Dyson MT, Jo Y, Eubank DW, Stocco DM. Involvement of 5-lipoxygenase metabolites of arachidonic acid in cyclic AMP-stimulated steroidogenesis and steroidogenic acute regulatory protein gene expression. J Steroid Biochem Mol Biol. 2003;85(2–5):159–66.
17. Fiedler EP, Plouffe Jr L, Hales DB, Hales KH, Khan I. Prostaglandin F(2alpha) induces a rapid decline in progesterone production and steroidogenic acute regulatory protein expression in isolated rat corpus luteum without altering messenger ribonucleic acid expression. Biol Reprod. 1999;61(3):643–50.
18. Calder PC, Yaqoob P. Understanding omega-3 polyunsaturated fatty acids. Postgrad Med. 2009;121(6):148–57.
19. Cheng Z, Abayasekara DR, Wathes DC. The effect of supplementation with n-6 polyunsaturated fatty acids on 1-, 2- and 3-series prostaglandin F production by ovine uterine epithelial cells. Biochim Biophys Acta. 2005;1736(2):128–35.
20. Jolly CA, Jiang YH, Chapkin RS, McMurray DN. Dietary (n-3) polyunsaturated fatty acids suppress murine lymphoproliferation, interleukin-2 secretion, and the formation of diacylglycerol and ceramide. J Nutr. 1997;127(1):37–43.
21. Fahrenholz F, Klein U, Gimpl G. Conversion of the myometrial oxytocin receptor from low to high affinity state by cholesterol. Adv Exp Med Biol. 1995;395:311–9.
22. Allen KG, Harris MA. The role of n-3 fatty acids in gestation and parturition. Experimental biology and medicine (Maywood, NJ. 2001;226(6):498–506.
23. Simopoulos AP. Omega-3 fatty acids in health and disease and in growth and development. Am J Clin Nutr. 1991;54(3):438–63.
24. Shang XG, Wang FL, Li DF, Yin JD, Li XJ, Yi GF. Effect of dietary conjugated linoleic acid on the fatty acid composition of egg yolk, plasma and liver as well as hepatic stearoyl-coenzyme A desaturase activity and gene expression in laying hens. Poult Sci. 2005;84(12):1886–92.
25. Livak KJ, Schmittgen TD. Analysis of relative gene expression data using real-time quantitative PCR and the 2(−Delta Delta C(T)) Method. Methods (San Diego, Calif. 2001;25(4):402–8.
26. Yan L, Bai XL, Fang ZF, Che LQ, Xu SY, Wu D. Effect of different dietary omega-3/omega-6 fatty acid ratios on reproduction in male rats. Lipids Health Dis. 2013;12:33.
27. Wilson HR, Waldroup PW, Jones JE, Duerre DJ, Harmds RH. Protein Levels in Growing Diets and Reproductive Performance of Cockerels. J Nutr. 1965;85:29–37.
28. Thurston RJ, Korn N. Spermiogenesis in commercial poultry species: anatomy and control. Poult Sci. 2000;79(11):1650–68.
29. Jones JE, Wilson HR, Harms RH, Simpson CF, Waldroup PW. Reproductive performance in male chickens fed protein deficient diets during the growing period. Poult Sci. 1967;46(6):1569–77.
30. de Kretser DM. Endocrinology of male infertility. Br Med Bull. 1979;35(2):187–92.
31. McGary Brougher S, Estevez I, Ottinger MA. Can testosterone and corticosterone predict the rate of display of male sexual behaviour, development of secondary sexual characters and fertility potential in primary broiler breeders? Br Poultry Sci. 2005;46(5):621–5.
32. Ramaswamy S, Plant TM. Operation of the follicle-stimulating hormone (FSH)-inhibin B feedback loop in the control of primate spermatogenesis. Mol Cell Endocrinol. 2001;180(1–2):93–101.
33. Huang HF, Li MT, Wang S, Pogach LM, Ottenweller JE. Alteration of cyclic adenosine 3',5'-monophosphate signaling in rat testicular cells after spinal cord injury. J Spinal Cord Med. 2003;26(1):69–78.
34. O'Donnell L, McLachlan RI, Wreford NG, Robertson DM. Testosterone promotes the conversion of round spermatids between stages VII and VIII of the rat spermatogenic cycle. Endocrinology. 1994;135(6):2608–14.
35. Calder PC. Mechanisms of action of (n-3) fatty acids. J Nutr. 2012;142(3):592S–9S.
36. Millar RP, Lu ZL, Pawson AJ, Flanagan CA, Morgan K, Maudsley SR. Gonadotropin-releasing hormone receptors. Endocr Rev. 2004;25(2):235–75.
37. Bortolussi M, Zanchetta R, Belvedere P, Colombo L. Sertoli and Leydig cell numbers and gonadotropin receptors in rat testis from birth to puberty. Cell Tissue Res. 1990;260(1):185–91.

4

Clinical features of idiopathic inflammatory polymyopathy in the Hungarian Vizsla

Anna Tauro[1*], Diane Addicott[2], Rob D Foale[3], Chloe Bowman[4], Caroline Hahn[5], Sam Long[4], Jonathan Massey[6], Allison C Haley[7], Susan P Knowler[9], Michael J Day[8], Lorna J Kennedy[6] and Clare Rusbridge[1,9]

Abstract

Background: A retrospective study of the clinicopathological features of presumed and confirmed cases of idiopathic inflammatory polymyopathy in the Hungarian Vizsla dog and guidelines for breeding.

Results: 369 medical records were reviewed (1992–2013) and 77 Hungarian Vizslas were identified with a case history consistent with idiopathic inflammatory polymyopathy. Inclusion criteria were: group 1 (confirmed diagnosis); histopathology and clinical findings compatible with an inflammatory polymyopathy and group 2 (probable diagnosis); clinical findings compatible with a polymyopathy including dysphagia, sialorrhea, temporal muscle atrophy, elevated serum creatine kinase (CK) activity, and sufficient clinical history to suggest that other neuromuscular disorders could be ruled out. Some group 2 dogs had muscle biopsy, which suggested muscle disease but did not reveal an inflammatory process. The mean age of onset was 2.4 years; male dogs were slightly overrepresented. Common presenting signs were dysphagia, sialorrhea, masticatory muscle atrophy, and regurgitation. Common muscle histopathological findings included degenerative and regenerative changes, with multifocal mononuclear cell infiltration with lymphoplasmacytic myositis of variable severity. A positive response to immunosuppressive treatment supported an immune-mediated aetiology. The mean age at death and survival time were 6.4 and 3.9 years, respectively. Recurrence of clinical signs and aspiration pneumonia were common reasons for euthanasia.

Conclusions: Diagnosis of Vizsla idiopathic inflammatory polymyopathy can be challenging due to lack of specific tests, however the presence of dysphagia, regurgitation and masticatory muscle atrophy in this breed with negative serological tests for masticatory muscle myositis and myasthenia gravis, along with muscle biopsies suggesting an inflammatory process, support the diagnosis. However, there is an urgent need for a more specific diagnostic test. The average of inbreeding coefficient (CoI) of 16.3% suggests an increased expression of a Dog Leukocyte Antigen Class II haplotype, leading to an increased disease risk. The prognosis remains guarded, as treatment can only manage the disease. Recurrence of clinical signs and perceived poor quality of life are the most common reasons for humane euthanasia.

Keywords: Regurgitation, Dysphagia, Canine, Dog Leukocyte Antigen, Familial polymyositis

Background

The immune-mediated inflammatory myopathies are acquired diseases, characterised by immunological processes primarily involving the skeletal muscle. In human medicine these disorders are divided into five major subsets: dermatomyositis, generalised polymyositis, focal myositis, necrotizing autoimmune myositis and inclusion-body myositis [1]. All but necrotising autoimmune myositis have been described in canine medicine. Dermatomyositis affects skin and muscle and is a complement-mediated microangiopathy in which complement deposition in small vessels leads to vascular damage and muscle ischaemia [2]. Canine dermatomyositis is an autosomal dominant condition with incomplete penetrance recognised in rough collies, Shetland sheepdogs and Pembrokeshire corgis [3,4]. In generalised polymyositis and inclusion-body myositis, muscle fibres expressing antigens of the major histocompatibility complex (MHC) are infiltrated by cytotoxic T cells, leading to myofibre necrosis [2,5,6]. In contrast to man, inclusion body myositis is recognised

* Correspondence: Annat@Fitzpatrickreferrals.co.uk
[1]Fitzpatrick Referrals, Halfway Lane, Eashing, Godalming GU7 2QQ, Surrey, UK
Full list of author information is available at the end of the article

infrequently in veterinary medicine [7]. Histopathology of inclusion body myositis is characterised by cytoplasmic filamentous inclusions, membranous structures and myeloid bodies, in addition to cellular infiltration and increased expression of MHC antigen [7].

Focal myositis is characterised by immune-mediated damage of specific muscle groups such as the masticatory muscles (e.g. temporalis, masseter, pterygoid, rostral portion of the digastricus) in masticatory muscle myositis (MMM) and the extraocular muscles in extraocular myositis. MMM is characterised by the presence of muscle-specific serum autoantibodies, most notably against masticatory myosin binding protein-C [8].

Polymyositis has been described previously in many breeds although large breed dogs are predisposed, especially Boxers, German shepherd dogs, Labrador and Golden retrievers, Doberman pinchers, and Newfoundlands [6,9-11]. A breed-specific idiopathic inflammatory polymyopathy has been described previously in dogs of the Hungarian Vizsla breed [12,13] and is characterised by cellular infiltration, particularly affecting masticatory and pharyngeal-oesophageal muscles.

The aim of this study was to describe the clinicopathological features of idiopathic inflammatory polymyopathy in the Hungarian Vizsla, in particular to emphasise the diagnostic approach, treatment, outcome, and to recommend guidelines for breeding practices.

Results

Signalment and clinical signs

Seventy-seven of the 369 Hungarian Vizsla dogs (Tables 1 and 2) were determined to have a case history consistent with Vizsla idiopathic inflammatory polymyopathy (VIP) (Group 1, n = 24 dogs; Group 2, n = 53 dogs including eight dogs with biopsy-confirmed non-inflammatory muscle disease). Two cases were shown to have acetylcholine receptor antibodies (consistent with myasthenia gravis) and they were excluded from the study. Eight of the 77 affected cases were from outside Europe: three were from USA, one was from New Zealand, and four were from Australia. The mean age of onset was 2.4 years (range 0.2–10.3 years). Male dogs were slightly overrepresented (entire male:neutered male:entire female:neutered female 26:24:9:17). In one case the gender was

Table 1 Clinical and diagnostic findings in Vizsla polymyopathy

Clinical and Diagnostic Findings in VIP		Number of dogs from Group 1	% of total Group 1 dogs (24)	Number of dogs from Group 2	% of total Group 2 (53)	Total number of CASES with this clinical signs or had this diagnostic test out of total 77 dogs	% of total cases (77)
Dysphagia (pharyngeal phase of deglutition)		20	83%	49	92%	69	90%
Drinking and eating difficulties (Oral phase of deglutition)		21	87%	48	91%	69	90%
Sialorrhea		21	87%	46	87%	67	87%
Masticatory muscle atrophy		20	83%	45	85%	65	84%
Regurgitation		19	79%	42	79%	61	79%
Trismus		3	12%	13	25%	16	21%
Masticatory myalgia		1	4%	8	15%	9	12%
Aspiration pneumonia		4	17%	13	25%	17	22%
Toxoplasma gondii serumantibody titre (tested for and negative)		14	58%	11	21%	25	32%
Neospora caninum serum antibody titre (tested for and negative)		15	62%	10	19%	25	32%
Elevated serum creatine kinase (>190 IU/L)		18	75%	23	43%	41	53%
Serum creatine kinase >1000		11	46%	14	26%	25	32%
Anti- 2 M antibody titre (Tested for and negative)		12	50%	17	32%	29	38%
Anti-acetylcholine receptor antibody titre (Tested for and negative)		16	67%	16	30%	32	42%
Electromyography (Performed and findings suggestive of myopathy)		15	62%	5	9%	20	26%
Electromyography (Performed and findings normal)		1	4%	2	4%	3	4%
Modality by which diagnosis Megaoesophagus was made	Radiographs	8	33%	18	34%	26	34%
	Barium	1	4%	9	17%	10	13%
	Fluoroscopy	4	17%	8	15%	12	16%

Table 2 Clinical signs of idiopathic inflammatory polymyopathy in the Vizsla – Percentage of dogs with this clinical sign is indicated (both Group 1 and 2 combined)

Clinical signs in VIP			
Most common		**Less common**	
Dysphagia (pharyngeal phase)	90%	Other muscle atrophy	43%
Drinking/Eating difficulty (oral phase)	90%	Exercise intolerance	35%
Sialorrhea	87%	Weakness	30%
Masticatory muscle atrophy	84%	Trismus	21%
Regurgitation	79%	Lameness	19%
		Masticatory myalgia	12%

unknown. The most common presenting signs in both groups (Tables 1 and 2) were dysphagia (i.e. pharyngeal phase of deglutition) (Additional file 1: Video 1) (90% of all dogs; group 1: 83% and group 2: 92%), difficulty in eating and drinking (i.e. oral phase of deglutition) (Additional file 2: Video 2) (90% combined; group 1: 87% and group 2: 91%), sialorrhea (87% of all dogs; group 1: 87% and group 2: 87%) (Figure 1) and regurgitation (79% of all dogs; group 1: 79% and group 2: 79%). Pain on opening the jaw was reported in 12% of all dogs (group 1: 4% and group 2: 15%). Masticatory muscle atrophy (i.e. masseter, temporalis and pterygoid muscles) (Figure 2) was present in 84% of all dogs (group 1: 83% and group 2: 85%), and 21% of all dogs had restricted jaw motility (group 1: 12% and group 2: 25%). Masticatory muscle atrophy either appeared early in the course of the disease, or had a more insidious onset, progressing slowly over several months or years (Figure 3). Enophthalmos, if present, was secondary to atrophy of the pterygoid muscle. Generalised muscle atrophy (43% of all dogs; group 1: 38% and Group 2: 45%), exercise intolerance (35% of all dogs; group 1: 46% and

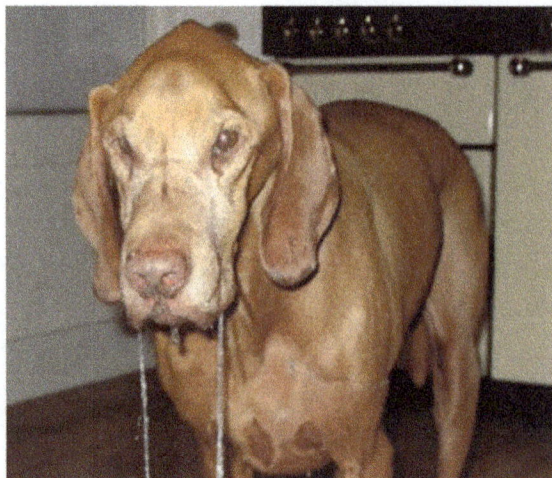

Figure 2 Masticatory muscle atrophy in VIP.

group 2: 30%), generalised weakness (30% of all dogs; group 1: 38% and group 2: 26%), and lameness (19% of all dogs; group 1: 21% and group 2: 19%) were less common signs. Three cases had dysuria (two in group 1 and one in group 2). The owners described a "stop-start flow" as if the dogs had difficulty maintaining a urine stream. The underlying pathophysiology for this was not ascertained.

In addition to clinical signs of neuromuscular disease, 25 dogs (seven in group 1, 18 in group 2) had other co-morbidities either concurrently or at some other stage in their life, including other inflammatory diseases (Table 3): 17 dogs with atopic dermatitis; two dogs with immune-mediated polyarthritis; nine dogs with inflammatory bowel disease; three dogs with keratoconjunctivitis sicca; one dog with sebaceous adenitis; one dog with steroid-responsive meningitis arteritis. There were also three dogs with idiopathic epilepsy, one dog with a fly-catching repetitive behavioural disorder and one dog with splenic haemangiosarcoma. Fourty dogs were dead at the time of writing and dysphagia and aspiration pneumonia were reported to be the main cause of death.

Laboratory findings

A summary of the diagnostic tests performed in each dog is detailed in Table 1 and more detailed results are available in Additional file 3. Serum CK activity was evaluated in 47/77 of cases and it was elevated (>190 IU/L) in 87% and above 1000 IU/L in 53%. In four cases the result was unknown. Serology for determination of antibodies against 2 M fibres for masticatory muscle myositis (MMM) or for antibodies against acetylcholine receptors for MG was

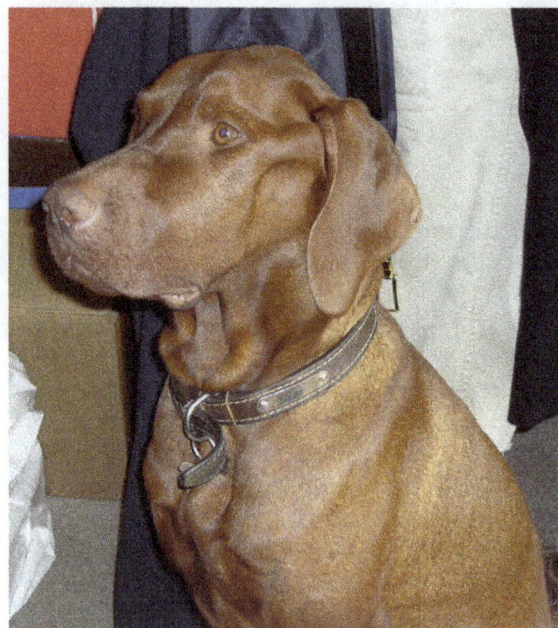

Figure 1 Sialorrhoea in VIP.

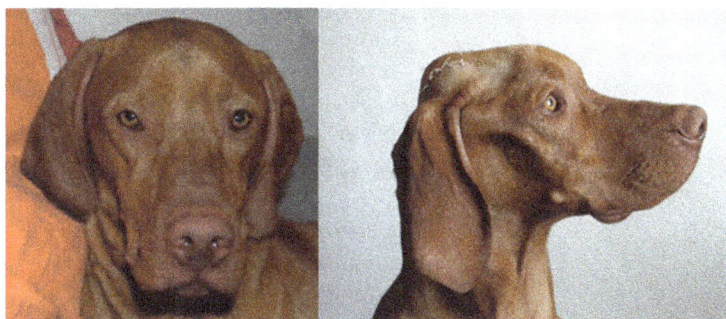

Figure 3 Hungarian Vizsla dog before and after VIP.

performed in 29 and 32 of 77 dogs, respectively. Serology for MMM was negative in all cases tested; two dogs were positive for MG and were excluded from this study. Serology for protozoal diseases causing inflammatory myopathy (*Toxoplasma gondii* and *Neospora caninum* serum antibody titres) was negative in 25 cases. Imaging techniques were performed in 52 cases. As part of the diagnostic work up for regurgitation, 28/77 of the dogs had oesophagogastroduodenoscopy. This investigation revealed the presence of *Helicobacter* spp. in two dogs and biopsy evidence suggestive of inflammatory bowel disease (IBD) in nine dogs. Thoracic radiographs confirmed megaoesophagus in 28 dogs (Figure 4) and aspiration pneumonia in 17 dogs (Figure 5). A barium study was performed in 10 cases; however, this test was not superior to plain radiography in proving oesophageal dysfunction. Fluoroscopy was performed in 12 cases where routine radiography with or without barium had not proved oesophageal dysfunction and in three dogs dysmotility, mainly involving the oral and pharyngeal phase, was demonstrated. Electromyography (EMG) of the appendicular and axial muscles including the masticatory muscles showed generalised abnormal spontaneous activity in 20 of 23 dogs, including positive sharp waves, fibrillation potentials, prolonged insertional activity, and occasional pseudomyotonia. EMG also confirmed tongue and pharyngeal involvement in 11 of 23 dogs. Magnetic Resonance Imaging (MRI) of the head was performed in five cases, and in two dogs it revealed changes within the masticatory muscle consistent with a multifocal inflammatory process. Identification of this change suggested a suitable biopsy site where clinical examination and other diagnostic tests such as EMG had not confirmed a diagnosis or the focal location of the pathology (Figure 6).

Muscle biopsy samples were taken in 36 of the 77 cases (37%) (Table 4); however, in seven cases the biopsy reports were not included in the case notes. In twenty-five of the 29 dogs for which histology was available, the biopsies were taken from the most accessible sites such as masseter, temporalis, lingual, triceps and cranial tibialis muscles, while in four cases the biopsy location was not reported. In 20 of the 25 dogs underwent biopsy following EMG or MRI identification of the most potentially useful sites. Post-mortem examinations were performed in four of the 40 deceased dogs and besides being a valuable aid towards confirming the diagnosis with multifocal lymphoplasmacytic and macrophagic cellular infiltrations having an endomysial and perimysial distribution with invasion of non-necrotic fibres being the most common histopathological finding in both ante and post mortem samples. In addition, in one case post-mortem examination revealed the presence of lymphoid cell infiltrate in the oesophageal

Table 3 Other idiopathic immune-mediated diseases seen in the dogs in this series

Concurrent immune-mediated diseases reported in the dogs in this series with VIP	Number of dogs
Atopic dermatitis	17
Immune-mediated polyarthritis (IMP)	2
Inflammatory bowel disease (IBD)	9
Keratoconjunctivitis sicca	3
Sebaceous adenitis (SA)	1
Steroid-responsive meningitis arteritis (SRMA)	1

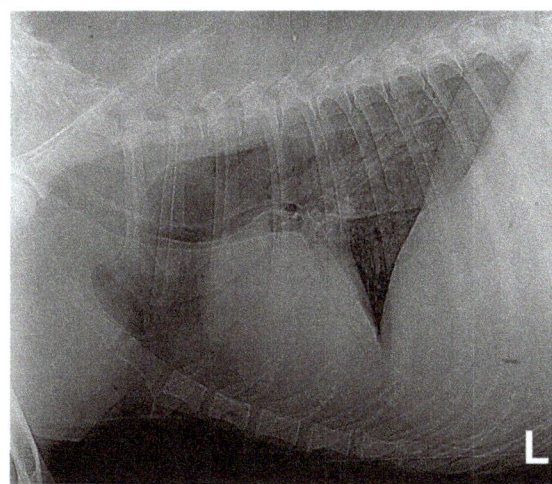

Figure 4 Left lateral thoracic view, showing megaoesophagus.

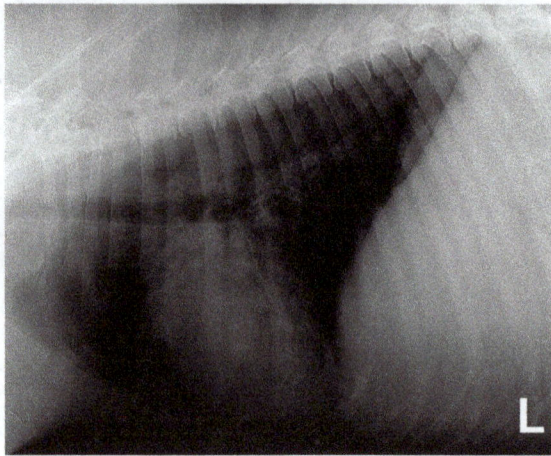

Figure 5 Left lateral thoracic view, showing aspiration pneumonia.

myenteric plexus with diminution in the number of ganglion cells (Table 3). Degenerative (e.g. variation in myofibre size, myofibre hyalinisation, necrosis, angular atrophy, nuclear internalisation, granular sarcoplasm, sarcolemmal fragmentation) and regenerative changes (e.g. cytoplasmic basophilia, nuclear rowing, presence of type 2C fibres, compensatory hypertrophy) were found variably (Figure 7). Myofibre loss, endomysial fibrosis and excessive perimysial fatty tissue were also found (Table 4). The presence of the adipose tissue was considered likely to be secondary to chronic injury as fat infiltration has been reported in chronically denervated muscles, but may also occur in severe chronic degenerative myopathy [14]. In 7/32 cases there was an absence of inflammatory changes. This was

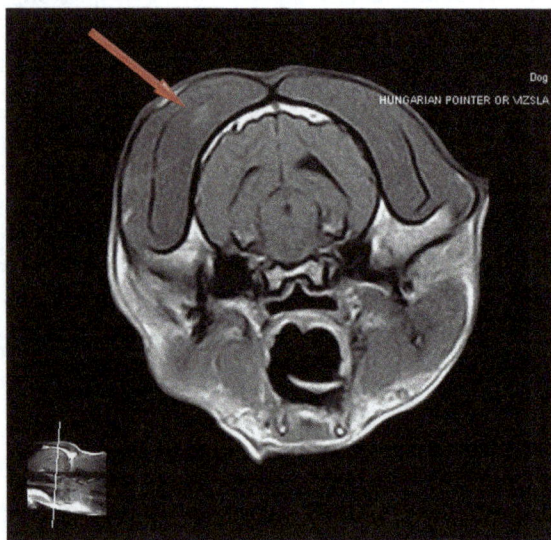

Figure 6 Transverse T1–weighted post-gadolinium contrast image at the level of the optic chiasm. Patchy up take of contrast is present within the right temporal muscle (arrow) suggesting an inflammatory process.

probably associated with recent steroid therapy (in two cases) or end-stage disease. However, in three dogs with recent onset disease that had not been treated, there was a degenerative and regenerative myopathy in the absence of obvious inflammatory change. In two cases antibodies against endplate proteins (SPA-HRPO) were identified.

Management

Sixty-one of 77 of the cases were treated with immune-suppressive doses of corticosteroids either as a monotherapy (32/61) or in combination with other immunosuppressive treatments (29/61). For the other 16 of 77 dogs, no treatment details were stated in the clinical record. A combination of immunosuppressive agents was considered preferable to reduce long-term corticosteroid side effects and/or when the clinical response to monotherapy was poor. The most common polypharmacy was prednisolone and azathioprine (25/29). Less commonly, ciclosporin was used in combination with prednisolone (2/29) or with both prednisolone and azathioprine (2/29). Leflunomide was used as an adjunct drug in one case in association with corticosteroids. Two cases were treated with methotrexate, either with corticosteroids or in combination with corticosteroids and azathioprine. The typical initial glucocorticoid dose was 1-2 mg/kg prednisolone twice a day, whilst azathioprine was used at 2 mg/kg or 50 mg/m^2 once a day. Leflunomide was used at 4 mg/kg once a day, while methotrexate was given at 2.5 mg/m^2 twice a week. The dosages were then tapered based on the response to treatment. Improvement of clinical signs especially sialorrhea, regurgitation, dysphagia was seen in 90% of the treated dogs. Unfortunately, we were unable to evaluate time frame to improvement due to lack of detailed temporal data, however the use of anti-inflammatory dose of corticosteroids or a rapid tapering regimen with withdrawal of drugs within a 1-year period appeared to be associated with earlier relapse and increased mortality in 23% of the treated cases. Two dogs treated with azathioprine had adverse gastrointestinal effects (i.e. profound vomiting and occasional diarrhoea) and exhibited marked elevation in serum hepatocellular enzymes resulting in cessation of therapy. Ciclosporin was discontinued in one case due to severe inappetence, while the other three cases in which this drug was used had undetermined clinical benefit. Corticosteroid side effects such polyphagia, polydipsia, polyuria, and iatrogenic hyperadrenocorticism were found in 15% of the treated cases. Supportive treatments including gastroprotectants and pro-kinetics were also commonly prescribed such as omeprazole, sucralfate, cimetidine, famotidine, ranitidine, maropitant, metoclopramide, erythromycin (as a pro-kinetic at a dose of 0.5-1 mg/kg three times a day), and cisapride. Three cases were treated with phenobarbital on the initial assumption that their

Table 4 Histological changes in the 32 Hungarian Vizslas with biopsy-confirmed polymyopathy

Histopathological changes (Total 32)	Group 1 25 total dogs (biopsies) (confirmed VIP diagnosis)	Group 2 7 dogs (3 biopsies, 1 biopsy and post-mortem/ 3 post-mortem) (myopathy diagnosis)
Inflammatory change e.g. Lymphohistiocytic inflammation	Variability in myofibres size with multifocal endomysial, interstitial and perivascular mononuclear cell infiltrations (lymphocytes & macrophages +/– plasma cells, eosinophils) of non-necrotic fibres. Underlying inflammatory process masked by corticosteroid treatment in one case. 25 dogs	0 dogs
Myopathic change	0 dogs	Variation in the myofibre size without inflammatory infiltration. 7 dogs
Adipose tissue	Small amount of adipose tissue associated with fibrosis. 2 dogs	Adipocytes present in some fascicles (endomysium and perimysium). 1 dogs
Fibrosis	None OR perimisial/endomysial fibrosis OR occasionally area of fibrosis with lack of myofibres with any significant inflammation (primary or secondary?) 3 dogs	0 dogs
Degenerative changes	Either any appreciable myofibre degeneration or active degenerative changes within the muscle fibres (variation in myofibre diameter, atrophy with round to polygonal/angular shape, hyalinisation, nuclear internalisation, sarcolemmal fragmentation). 19 dogs	Variation in muscle fibres, atrophy (occasionally smaller fibres grouped together, some angular but most round to polygonal profile), nuclear internalisation. 4 dogs
Regenerative changes	Nuclear rowing, centralisation/hyperthrophy of the nuclei increased cytoplasmic basophilia, type 2 fibres. 13 dogs	Occasional enlarged and round myofibres (compensatory hypertrophy), and nuclear rowing. 3 dogs
Necrotic fibres	Scattered to severe necrotic myofibres with some undergoing phagocytosis. 7 dogs	0 dogs
Fibrosis	Mild to moderate endomysial and perimysial fibrosis secondary to myofibre loss. 7 dogs	Increased endomysial and perimysial connective tissue secondary to myofibre loss. 2 dogs
Intramuscular nerve branches	Normal (25 dogs)	Normal (7 dogs)
Immunoreagent SPA-HRPO (Antibodies against endplate proteins)	Present in two cases	
Dystrophin protein		Decreased staining for carboxy terminus of the dystrophin protein was found in one case; however, the dog improved on immunosuppressive treatment and the suspicion for muscle dystrophy was abandoned.

diagnosis was phenobarbital-responsive hypersalivation, but there was no clinical benefit reported. In the dogs with dysuria, one dog was treated with 0.35 mg/kg diazepam three times a day and the other with 1 mg/kg dantrolene twice a day and 0.4 mg/kg phenoxybenzamine twice a day, and both showed clinical improvement; the third dog was treated with phenylpropanolamine at the dose of 0.8 mg/kg once a day and diazepam at the dose of 0.25 mg/kg twice a day with no improvements, while corticosteroid therapy was reported to be beneficial.

At the time of writing, 40 of 77 affected cases had died: thirty-seven dogs were euthanised due to the disease and three died of other causes including haemangiosarcoma, idiopathic epilepsy and reported natural causes. The mean age of death was 6.4 years (range 1.0 – 14.5 years), and the mean survival time following diagnosis was 3.9 years

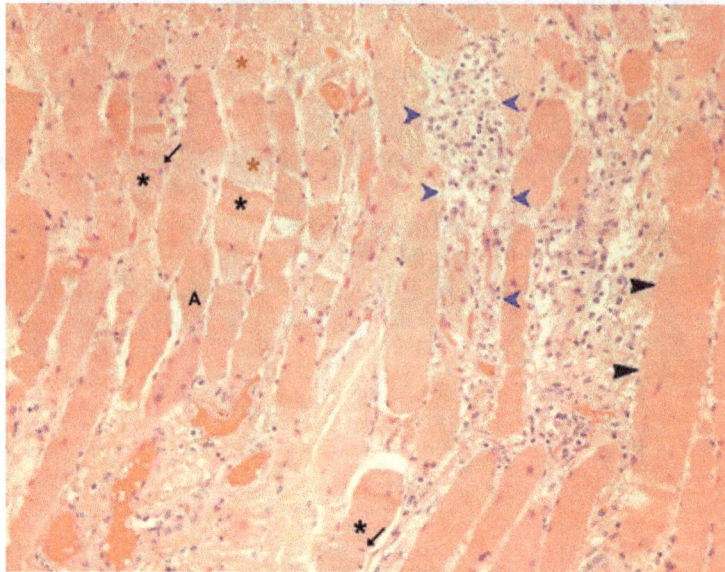

Figure 7 Histopathological section of temporal muscle (H&E stain, x100). Mild variation of myofibre size, with internal nuclei (black arrow) found along the plane of the fibre splitting (star), hypertrophied myofibres (black arrow head), granular sarcoplasm (yellow star), angular atrophy (A), and necrosis with infiltration of inflammatory cells (blue arrow head).

(range 0.1 – 12.5 years). Recurrent aspiration pneumonia and poor quality of life because of difficulty eating and drinking were common reasons cited for euthanasia.

Discussion

This paper describes a myopathy in the Hungarian Vizsla characterised by dysphagia, regurgitation, sialorrhea and masticatory muscle atrophy, which is responsive to immunosuppression in the majority of cases. Biopsy sampling in a proportion of cases suggested an idiopathic inflammatory polymyopathy. One of the authors (CR) first diagnosed idiopathic inflammatory polymyopathy in a Hungarian Vizsla in 1994, but anecdotal reporting by owners suggests that the disease has been a problem in the breed since the early 1980s or before. A serious shortcoming in this retrospective study was the inclusion of non-biopsy confirmed cases. However, group 2 dogs were included because excluding them might give the erroneous impression that this syndrome can be easily diagnosed by biopsy and exclusion of these cases would also lose clinical data that might be valuable to practising clinicians. Moreover, it is possible that this syndrome might actually represent a collection of immune-mediated diseases in the Hungarian Vizsla with a common theme of dysphagia, regurgitation and masticatory muscle atrophy; so although biopsy remains the gold standard for diagnosis, it was not always useful and in seven cases the muscle biopsies did not confirm an inflammatory process despite using EMG in two of these cases to direct biopsy and the dogs subsequently responding to immunosuppressive therapy. Postmortem was performed in four of these seven cases with

suspicion of VIP and in two of them the disease was confirmed. This finding, and the differences between VIP and the classical description of canine polymyositis [9] (in particular dysphagia), raises the question as to whether the pathogenesis is different. Diagnosis of typical myositis in man is dependent on the presence of inflammatory infiltrates and positive human leukocyte antigen (HLA – ABC) labelling of the sarcolemma. However, other immune-mediated myopathies exist, e.g. human necrotising myopathy has no inflammatory infiltrates which is associated with anti-signal recognition particle autoantibodies. Dysphagia is an important clinical feature of this disease and patients respond to immunosuppression [15]. A future goal to improve diagnosis of VIP is to investigate whether or not it is possible to identify myositis-specific autoantibodies. In the present study, incubation with staphylococcal protein A conjugated to horseradish peroxidase (SPA-HRPO) detected antibody (IgG) bound to the neuromuscular junction in two group 1 cases. This labelling was suggestive of an autoimmune polymyositis. In the present study, nine out of 29 muscle biopsies were subjected to labelling with SPA-HRPO (not used in three cases and not reported in the remainder) and further studies are necessary in order to better understand the pathophysiology of this disease and to aid the diagnosis. However, until this data is available, the following recommendations are offered to maximise the chance of successful diagnosis: (1) biopsy of end-stage muscles should be avoided as adipose or connective tissue replaces muscle tissue and diagnosis may be challenging, so clinicians should chose to biopsy muscles which are not severely atrophied); (2) our data suggests the most useful muscle biopsy site is the temporal muscle, which was sampled in 22/29 (76%) of the present cases and confirmed diagnosis in 19 cases; (3) lingual muscle biopsy was performed in five cases for which biopsy samples were collected and in two of these the procedure assisted in making a diagnosis, so this may also be useful biopsy site and this procedure is especially indicated when dogs are presented with oropharyngeal dysphagia; (4) EMG and MRI were valuable in helping identify the appropriate muscle to sample (Figure 6).

EMG has lower cost, but may not detect mild disease especially if there is minimal involvement of the appendicular muscle. MRI is generally more expensive to perform but where performed showed good association with the histopathology results. In people, whole-body MR imaging using rapidly acquired fat-suppressed Short TI Inversion Recovery (STIR) sequences has been recommended to facilitate a global overview of the extent and symmetry of muscle disease and to direct biopsy collection. STIR signal intensity has been documented to have a 97% specificity for identifying sites of inflammatory myopathy that have been confirmed at biopsy [16] [although, where previous corticosteroid treatment is used, post-contrast images may be more helpful. Inflammatory muscle lesions on MR images were characterised by diffuse and poorly marginated abnormal signal on T1- and T2-weighted images, with marked enhancement after contrast medium administration [16].

Other laboratory tests can be used to support a diagnosis of VIP and rule out other diseases, as when making a diagnosis of VIP, other causes of myopathy should be ruled out. The most important differential diagnoses are toxins [17], endocrine disease [18-20] and infectious causes of inflammatory myopathy, especially Toxoplasma gondii, Neospora caninum and in some geographical regions Leishmania, Ehrlichia canis, Sarcocystis neurona and Hepatozoon americanum. A limitation of our study was the lack of completeness of such laboratory tests for many cases. However it is noted that dysphagia and/or regurgitation are rarely reported as clinical signs of inflammatory myopathy associated with infectious diseases. In a comprehensive literature search [21-45] a single case report was found describing dysphagia and regurgitation in a puppy with neonatal neosporosis that also presented with neuromuscular paralysis [45]. It is not unusual for neospora tachyzoites to be found in the oesophagus on histological examination of post mortem material but more uncommon for there to be associated clinical signs and therefore the clinical significance is uncertain [35,38]. Therefore, although infectious diseases should be ruled out as an underlying cause in cases of suspected VIP, it is a rare differential for adult dogs presenting with dysphagia and regurgitation. Given the clinical presentation of VIP, the most important differential diagnoses are MMM and MG, which may also show similar clinical

features to VIP. Thus, serum titres for antibodies against type 2 M fibres and the acetylcholine receptor should be evaluated. Occasionally a dog may present with both myasthenia gravis and VIP [46]. In our study MMM was not diagnosed in any of the affected dogs, although it should be noted that only 38% of dogs were tested.

Marked elevation of CK is an indication of damage to skeletal muscles; however, only 25 of the 47 dogs tested had an elevation above 1000 IU/L. This may be because generalised muscle disease was not a feature. In most cases of VIP, the masticatory and pharyngeal muscles were most severely affected and constituted only a small volume of muscle mass compared with the whole body. Of the 25 dogs with marked elevation of CK, 18 had generalised muscle atrophy and/or exercise intolerance, but seven were considered to be normal in this regard.

The most consistent clinical signs of VIP are dysphagia and sialorrhea due to tongue, pharyngeal and oesophageal dysfunction, and masticatory muscle atrophy. The canine oesophageal anatomy differs from other species such as cats and people, especially in the musculature of the oesophageal body. In dogs the cranial oesophageal (cricopharyngeal) sphincter and the entire oesophageal body is composed of striated muscle, while the caudal oesophageal (gastroesophageal) sphincter is smooth muscle. Therefore the canine oesophagus is often involved in diseases that affect skeletal muscle [47]. However, in at least two of the present series of cases there were alternative explanations for the oesophageal involvement identified on postmortem examination: in one case there was no primary inflammatory process in oesophageal muscle, but there was invasion of inflammatory cells secondary to degeneration of myocytes and a second case revealed lymphoid cell infiltration of the oesophageal myenteric plexus with diminution in the number of ganglion cells, which may represent a ganglionopathy. The latter histopathological picture is similar to that observed in oesophageal achalasia in man [48]. Oesophageal achalasia is characterised by dysfunction of the lower oesophageal sphincter and derangement of oesophageal peristalsis. The cause is not fully known, but autoimmune processes appear to be involved in human patients with a genetic susceptibility to the disease [48].

The dysphagia reported in this case series may not be entirely due to oesophageal dysfunction, as masticatory, pharyngeal, and lingual muscle involvement could contribute to difficulty eating. In this case series, atrophy of the masticatory muscles was a common feature of the disease. Polymyositis with masticatory muscle atrophy and tongue involvement has been recognized previously in Pembroke corgi dogs in which end-stage lingual atrophy was a predominant feature [49]. In the present series, atrophy of the tongue was observed as an end-stage of disease in three untreated dogs and in one clinical history, the tongue was described as being shrivelled, soft, withered and dry with deficits of sensation as well as motor function. Sensory deficits could not be confirmed, however, the tongue is richly innervated and it is theoretically possible that end-stage fibrosis might interfere with nervous supply.

Perhaps surprisingly for a polymyopathy, exercise intolerance was not the most common clinical sign, with normal exercise ability being reported in 27 of 77 dogs and only 33 of 77 dogs developed generalised muscle atrophy. Others have described the clinical presentation of canine polymyositis being characterised by cervical ventroflexion and dysbasia (a stiff gait with short stride a.k.a. "walking on eggshells"); [9]. This was not a feature of VIP. The lack of appendicular muscle involvement coupled with an insidious onset of the disease may be a reason for delayed or incorrect diagnosis.

Dysuria was a surprising clinical sign associated with a skeletal muscle disease but was reported in three male dogs with biopsy-confirmed VIP. The detrusor is smooth muscle, so if detrusor myopathy was a cause of the dysuria then it would imply the presence of autoantibodies against smooth as well as skeletal muscle, which would be unlikely as in all human and laboratory animal models of myositis, autoantibodies are specific to striated muscle and correlate with distinct clinical phenotypes [50,51]. Additionally, an immune-mediated process targeting smooth muscle would reasonably be expected to result in intestinal and arterial smooth muscle disease too. Immune-mediated damage of the skeletal muscle of the external urethral sphincter is possible, although this might have been expected to result in clinical signs of sphincter mechanism incompetence. The possibility of a neurological cause of dysuria cannot be excluded; however, an anatomical difference exists between the urethra of female and male dogs, which may explain why dysuria was present only in male dogs. Female urethral smooth muscle occupies one-third of the volume of the vesical neck (both the bladder neck and the urethral smooth muscle constitute the internal urethral sphincter) and one fourth of the volume of the proximal urethra, while striated muscle is present in the distal half of the urethra [52]. In contrast, the male urethral smooth muscle is associated mainly with the trabeculae surrounding the prostate lobules and is fundamental for contraction of the lobules (i.e. the bladder neck acts as smooth muscle sphincter), while striated muscle is present caudal to the prostate (post-prostatic urethra), which also overlaps the caudal surface of the prostate gland [53]. Although we need to consider that in this study fifty of the 77 affected cases were male dogs, it can be speculated that the dysuria in male dogs with VIP may be associated with more extensive involvement of urethral striated muscle.

An easier and more reliable method of detecting canine oesophageal dysmotility would be of great benefit because complications associated with dysphagia and aspiration pneumonia are the main cause of death in VIP. Deglutition consists of three phases: the oral phase that occurs in the mouth and involves lips, tongue, teeth, and palate, and it is essential for the formation of the food bolus; the pharyngeal phase that is essential for the progression of the food bolus from the mouth to the oesophagus and preventing entry into the airway and the oesophageal phase that allows the food bolus to travel through the oesophagus towards the stomach. Plain or contrast thoracic radiographs may reveal megaoesophagus; however, if less severe or dynamic disease of the oesophagus is present, fluoroscopy may be more useful, especially in the detection of swallowing disorders that mainly involve the oral and pharyngeal phase. However difficulties in performing this test were reported either due to lack of equipment or to the difficultly in keeping the animal steady for the image intensifier. It is also advisable to perform these studies with great care in order to avoid barium aspiration pneumonia. In man, oesophageal manometry is considered the 'gold standard' for assessing oesophageal motor function and is used to measure the pressures and the pattern of muscle contractions in the oesophagus, and to detect abnormalities in the contractions and strength of the oesophageal muscle and its sphincter [54]. Over the last few years intraluminal oesophageal manometry has developed into high-resolution manometry, which improves acquisition of data, and the method of displaying and analysing the data using oesophageal pressure topography plots. This new technology is also patient-friendly as it allows for a shorter procedure time, and it is much easier to use and to interpret compared with conventional manometry [55]. High-resolution manometry could be useful in the detection of oesophageal disorders in animals, but further studies are required to confirm this. Previously the majority of the veterinary studies have used conventional manometry, and most of them used anaesthetised dogs [56-61].

The presence of *Helicobacter* spp. in two dogs and inflammatory bowel disease (IBD) in eight dogs that underwent oesophagogastroduodenoscopy was considered incidental to the primary diagnosis of VIP. *Helicobacter* spp. have been associated with chronic superficial gastritis in man and play a role in the pathogenesis of peptic ulcer disease, gastric carcinoma and lymphoma, but their clinical significance in companion animals is not clear [62]. The finding of IBD could be more significant, especially when the breed appears predisposed to other immune-mediated diseases including MG, MMM, atopy, sebaceous adenitis, keratoconjunctivitis sicca, steroid-responsive meningitis arteritis, and immune-mediated polyarthritis (Table 2). Vizslas have been also reported anecdotally to be predisposed to immune-mediated haemolytic anaemia [63] and immune-mediated thrombocytopenia [64]. There are occasional reports of human patients with both IBD and polymyositis [65]. The disruption of the tight junctions between enterocytes plays an important role in the pathophysiology of IBD, altering the intestinal epithelial barrier function and causing increased intestinal permeability. The 'leaky gut' may then lead to translocation of bacteria and endotoxin, which drives the intestinal inflammation. A normal response from the immune system should deal with the insult. However, in some individuals this normal response may be defective, increasing the risk of developing IBD, coeliac disease and possibly myositis [65]. When investigating VIP, we therefore recommend that comorbidities are looked for and treated if identified.

VIP is assumed to be an autoimmune disease because of the response to immunosuppressive treatment. The cornerstone of the treatment is glucocorticoid therapy due to its short-term tolerability, cost effectiveness, and clinical effectiveness [66]. Particular care however must be taken if there is a risk of aspiration pneumonia as the adverse effects of polydipsia, polyphagia and immunosuppression increases the likelihood of this potentially fatal complication. As the individual treatment plans for the dogs in this study varied, it was not possible to make firm conclusions regarding treatment, but the trends suggested the following: (1) early diagnosis improves the chance of successful treatment; (2) therapy should be tapered slowly with time of tapering depending on clinical signs. We do not have enough data to strongly determine the dosage and the length of the treatment protocol for the VIP, however inadequate corticosteroid dosage i.e. anti-inflammatory dose or a rapid tapering regimen with withdrawal of drugs within a 1-year period appeared to be associated with earlier relapse and increased mortality in 23% of the treated cases. The optimal glucocorticoid dosing regimen is not well defined [13]; however, as a general rule we would suggest the following: 2 mg/kg once a day for 2 weeks, then 1 mg/kg once a day for 4 weeks, then 0.5 mg/kg once a day for 10 weeks, then 0.25 mg/kg once a day for 16 weeks, then 0.25 mg/kg every other day for 16 weeks then continue to withdraw over a further 2–4 weeks; (3) close monitoring is required and the drugs are tapered on the basis of clinical signs and the concentration of serum CK, if this test had shown abnormal result prior treatment.

In four dogs, dysphagia and regurgitation prevented the use of oral therapy, but there was a good response to initial parenteral short-term corticosteroid therapy such as with dexamethasone and prednisone acetate. Other parental corticosteroids such as methylprednisolone seemed to be less effective (two cases), however the difficulty of comparing different treatments used is a limitation of this paper and further study is needed to establish the most effective therapeutic protocol for this disease. This study also suggested that a treatment based on a combination of immunosuppressive agents was preferable to reduce long-term corticosteroid side effects such polyphagia, polydipsia, polyuria, and iatrogenic hyperadrenocorticism, reduce the risk of aspiration pneumonia and/or when the clinical response to monotherapy was poor. The most common and successful drug used in addition to corticosteroids was azathioprine; however a well-designed prospective trial needs to be performed evaluating different treatments. The dosage of azathioprine used but we would suggest 2 mg/kg once a day for up to ten days, then 2 mg/kg every other day thereafter. Although our study cannot assess the most effective treatment protocol, we would advise that this dosage should be maintained for a month beyond the cessation of prednisolone. Again this regimen should be adjusted on the basis of assessment of both clinical response and serum CK levels. To reduce the risk of aspiration pneumonia and to aid swallowing dogs should be fed from a height and with small meals 4–6 times daily. Some foods are easier to swallow than others and our experience is that individually feeding small walnut-size balls of firm, but slippery-textured commercial food with a high protein and fat content is the most useful. This should be coupled with coupage after feeding in order to encourage belching and help to prevent aspiration. In some cases an anti-gulping bowl (Dogit® Go Slow Anti-Gulping Dog Bowl, Rolf C. Hagen Ltd., West Yorkshire, UK) can be useful, especially in dogs with polyphagia due to high dosage of corticosteroids. In cases where the megaoesophagus impedes the propulsion of the food bolus, we recommend the use of the Bailey chair in order to maintain a truly vertical oesophageal position and reduce the risk of aspiration pneumonia.

Immune-mediated diseases are thought to develop through a complex combination of genetic and environmental factors and have been associated with variants of MHC class I or II genes, which in the dog are referred to as the dog leukocyte antigen (DLA) system. The MHC molecules control the immune system's recognition of self and non-self-antigens. Class II molecules are involved in presenting antigens to CD4[+] T cells (T helper cells) [67]. CD4[+] T cells play a key role in regulating immune system function with a subset of immunoregulatory cells (CD25[+]CD4[+]) suppressing proliferation of other immune cells, especially CD25[−]CD4[+] T cells and CD8[+] T cells [68]. The basis of autoimmune reactions is the failure of this immunoregulatory T cell to properly control other immune cells and down-regulate the immune response. In polymyositis, inflammatory cells, including T cells and macrophages, are concentrated in the endomysium and surround and invade non-necrotic fibres [6]. Classically there are more CD8[+] T cells than CD4[+] T cells; however, Haley and others reported that cellular infiltrates in two dogs with VIP were composed predominantly of CD4[+]T cells with fewer CD8[+]T cells [13].

Labelling for MHC class I and class II antigens was increased on the sarcolemma and on the membrane of infiltrating cells in Haley and others study, however the assessment of this in our biopsies was not undertaken and needs to be considered in future studies to further help elucidate the pathogenesis of VIP.

Genes within the MHC are unusual because they are highly polymorphic, meaning that there are many allelic variations. This degree of variation most likely improves survival against infectious diseases. However in the dog, selective inbreeding has led to a restriction of DLA haplotypes in many breeds, which in turn influences susceptibility to infectious diseases and also to immune-mediated conditions [69]. Our group investigated DLA class II associations from 212 Hungarian Vizsla dogs, which were stratified both on disease status and degree of relatedness to an affected dog. One haplotype, DLA-DRB1*02001/DQA1*00401/DQB1*01303, had a significantly raised frequency in cases compared with controls. A single copy of the risk haplotype was sufficient to increase disease risk, with the risk substantially increasing for homozygotes. There was a trend of increasing frequency of this haplotype with degree of relatedness, indicating a low disease penetrance and suggesting involvement of other genetic and environmental factors [70]. Further genetic studies are required; however, our immediate advice to breeders wishing to reduce the risk of VIP is that a bitch should only be mated to a dog when the inbreeding coefficient (CoI) of the resulting puppies, as measured from a five generation pedigree, is less than 12.5% [71]. The CoI is the probability of homozygosity by descent, and it ranges from 0% to 100%. In other words, the lower the inbreeding coefficient, the lower the probability of homozygosity with a CoI of over 25% being the equivalent of a mother/son mating. The mean CoI in Vizsla Breed is 5.1% [72, 73]; however, the average CoI of 77 of the 79 dogs in our study of Vizslas was 16.3% (range: 2.5% - 40.7%). However it should be remembered that having a low CoI will not protect against VIP and breeding of dogs with immediate relatives with VIP should be avoided.

Conclusions

The Hungarian Vizsla has an inherited predisposition to a form of inflammatory polymyopathy. The most common clinical signs are dysphagia, sialorrhea, masticatory muscle atrophy, and regurgitation. The mainstay of treatment is immunosuppressive therapy in addition to feeding therapy designed to meet individual needs. Early diagnosis, careful monitoring and slow withdrawal of medication improves prognosis. To improve diagnosis the feasibility of other diagnostics techniques such as a high resolution manometry should be investigated. Further genetic and immunological studies will better define VIP; however, until then reducing inbreeding in order to minimise homozygosity of the risk haplotype is recommended.

Methods

Our retrospective cohort study was based on 369 medical records of Hungarian Vizsla dogs. The records were collected from dogs from which DNA had been submitted to the Centre for Integrated Genomic Medical Research (CIGMR, University of Manchester, UK) between 1992 and 2013. Cases had been recruited following a nationwide appeal for Hungarian Vizslas affected with polymyositis and their affected or unaffected relatives [74-76]. Details of the phenotype were generated for each case [77], stating Kennel Club registration number, pedigree name, common name, coat colour, gender, age, and weight. It also indicated clinical signs, diagnostic tests performed, and treatment. Based on certainty of diagnosis of VIP the cases were divided into two groups. Inclusion criteria for Group 1 were clinical signs and histopathology findings compatible with an inflammatory polymyopathy. Inclusion criteria for Group 2 was clinical signs of neuromuscular disease including presence of dysphagia, sialorrhea, temporal muscle atrophy, elevated serum creatine kinase (CK) activity, and sufficient clinical history to suggest that other neuromuscular disorders could be ruled out. This group also included dogs where muscle biopsy or post-mortem had been performed confirming a myopathy, but with no evidence of an inflammatory cell infiltrate. Pedigrees from dogs of all of the affected families were researched and collated, and a pedigree database was created. In order to investigate the genetic basis of this disorder, DNA was extracted from blood in excess of that required for diagnostic tests. Alternatively, oral swabs were submitted to the CIGMR in order to investigate the genetic basis of this disorder [70].

This is a non-experimental study based on a retrospective analysis of necessary diagnostic results and clinical history for which there was full owner written consent.

Additional files

Additional file 1: Video 1. Dysphagia.

Additional file 2: Video 2. Drinking difficulties.

Additional file 3: Detailed clinical and diagnostic features of the Hungarian Vizslas with idiopathic inflammatory polymyopathy.

Abbreviations

CIGMR: Centre for integrated genomic medical research; CK: Creatine kinase; Col: Inbreeding coefficient; DLA: Dog leukocyte antigen; EMG: Electromyography; IBD: Inflammatory bowel disease; MG: Myasthenia gravis; MHC: Major histocompatibility complex; MMM: Masticatory muscle myositis; MRI: Magnetic resonance image; STIR: Short time inversion recovery; VIP: Vizsla idiopathic inflammatory polymyopathy.

Competing interests
None of the authors of this article has financial or personal relationship with other people or organisations that could inappropriately influence or bias the content of the paper.

Authors' contributions
AT organised and interpreted the data, and wrote the paper; CR conceived, designed, coordinated the study, wrote the paper, provided support, and revised critically the manuscript; SPK coordinated the study, helped to draft and revise critically the manuscript, and provided technical and graphical support; DA substantial contribution to conceive the study, acquired the data, helped to draft, and revised critically the manuscript; RDF, JM, ACH, MJD, LJK, CH supported the study, provided clinical and pathology advice, and revised critically the manuscript; CB, SL provided additional data, and revised critically the manuscript. All authors read and approved the final manuscript.

Acknowledgements
The authors would like to thank the owners of the affected dogs in this study and also the Hungarian Vizsla club and Charity, UK for their outstanding commitment and contributions to this study. In addition, the authors thank the veterinary surgeons who kindly provided their support and case histories.

Author details
[1]Fitzpatrick Referrals, Halfway Lane, Eashing, Godalming GU7 2QQ, Surrey, UK. [2]Murrayfield, Lockerbie, UK. [3]Dick White Referrals, Six Mile Bottom, Suffolk, UK. [4]Adelaide Veterinary Specialist and Referral Centre (AVSARC), Norwood Adelaide, South Australia. [5]Royal (Dick) School of Veterinary Studies, University of Edinburgh, Roslin, UK. [6]CIGMR, The University of Manchester, Manchester, UK. [7]The University of Georgia, College of Veterinary Medicine, Athens, USA. [8]University of Bristol, Langford, Bristol, UK. [9]The University of Surrey, Guildford, Surrey, UK.

References
1. Dalakas MC. Pathogenesis and therapies of immune-mediated myopathies. Autoimmun Rev. 2012;11:203–6.
2. Dalakas MC, Hohlfeld R. Polymyositis and dermatomyositis. Lancet. 2003;362:971–82.
3. Clark LA, Credille KM, Murphy KE, Rees CA. Linkage of dermatomyositis in the Shetland Sheepdog to chromosome 35. Vet Dermatol. 2005;16:392–4.
4. Morris DO. Ischemic dermatopathies. Vet Clin North Am Small Anim Pract. 2013;43:99–111.
5. Morita T, Shimada A, Yashiro S, Takeuchi T, Hikasa Y, Okamoto Y, et al. Myofiber expression of class I major histocompatibility complex accompanied by CD8+ T-cell-associated myofiber injury in a case of canine polymyositis. Vet Pathol. 2002;39:512–5.
6. Pumarola M, Moore PF, Shelton GD. Canine inflammatory myopathy: analysis of cellular infiltrates. Muscle Nerve. 2004;29:782–9.
7. King J, LeCouteur RA, Aleman M, Williams DC, Moore PF, Guo LT, et al. Vacuolar myopathy in a dog resembling human sporadic inclusion body myositis. Acta Neuropathol. 2009;118:711–7.
8. Wu X, Li ZF, Brooks R, Komives EA, Torpey JW, Engvall E, et al. Autoantibodies in canine masticatory muscle myositis recognize a novel myosin binding protein-C family member. J Immunol. 2007;179:4939–44.
9. Podell M. Inflammatory myopathies. Vet Clin North Am Small Anim Pract. 2002;32:147–67.
10. Melmed C, Shelton GD, Bergman R, Barton C. Masticatory muscle myositis: pathogenesis, diagnosis, and treatment. In: Book masticatory muscle myositis: pathogenesis, diagnosis, and treatment. 2004. p. 590–604.
11. Evans J, Levesque D, Shelton GD. Canine inflammatory myopathies: a clinicopathologic review of 200 cases. J Vet Intern Med. 2004;18:679–91.
12. Foale RD, Whiting M, Wray JD. Myositis and pharyngeal dysphagia in Hungarian Vizsla. In: Proceedings of the 50th BSAVA Congress. Birmingham: Clinical research abstract; 2008. p. 462.
13. Haley AC, Platt SR, Kent M, Schatzberg SJ, Durham A, Cochrane S, et al. Breed-specific polymyositis in Hungarian Vizsla dogs. J Vet Intern Med. 2011;25:393–7.
14. McGavin MD, Zachary JF. Chronic myopathic change. In: McGavin MD, Zachary JF, editors. Textbook of pathologic basis of veterinary diseases. 4th ed. St. Louis, Missouri: Mosby Elsevier; 2006. p. 995–6.
15. Hengstman GJ, ter Laak HJ, Vree Egberts WT, Lundberg IE, Moutsopoulos HM, Vencovsky J, et al. Anti-signal recognition particle autoantibodies: marker of a necrotising myopathy. Ann Rheum Dis. 2006;65:1635–8.
16. Platt SR, McConnell JF, Garosi LS, Ladlow J, de Stefani A, Shelton GD. Magnetic resonance imaging in the diagnosis of canine inflammatory myopathies in three dogs. Vet Radiol Ultrasound. 2006;47:532–7.
17. Puschner B, Basso MM, Graham TW. Thallium toxicosis in a dog consequent to ingestion of Mycoplasma agar plates. J Vet Diagn Invest. 2012;24:227–30.
18. Fracassi F, Tamborini A. Reversible megaoesophagus associated with primary hypothyroidism in a dog. Vet Rec. 2011;168:329b.
19. Burgener IA, Gerold A, Tomek A, Konar M. Empty sella syndrome, hyperadrenocorticism and megaoesophagus in a dachshund. J Small Anim Pract. 2007;48:584–7.
20. Lifton SJ, King LG, Zerbe CA. Glucocorticoid deficient hypoadrenocorticism in dogs: 18 cases (1986–1995). J Am Vet Med Assoc. 1996;209:2076–81.
21. Parzefall B, Driver CJ, Benigni L, Davies E. Magnetic resonance imaging characteristics in four dogs with central nervous system neosporosis. Vet Radiol Ultrasound. 2014. doi:10.1111/vru.12160.
22. Ishigaki K, Noya M, Kagawa Y, Ike K, Orima H, Imai S. Detection of Neospora caninum-specific DNA from cerebrospinal fluid by polymerase chain reaction in a dog with confirmed neosporosis. J Vet Pharmacol Ther. 2012;74:1051–5.
23. Garosi L, Dawson A, Couturier J, Matiasek L, de Stefani A, Davies E, et al. Necrotizing cerebellitis and cerebellar atrophy caused by Neospora caninum infection: magnetic resonance imaging and clinicopathologic findings in seven dogs. J Vet Intern Med. 2010;24:571–8.
24. Paciello O, Oliva G, Gradoni L, Manna L, Foglia Manzillo V, Wojcik S, et al. Canine inflammatory myopathy associated with Leishmania Infantum infection. Neuromuscul Disord. 2009;19:124–30.
25. Dubey JP, Vianna MC, Kwok OC, Hill DE, Miska KB, Tuo W, et al. Neosporosis in Beagle dogs: clinical signs, diagnosis, treatment, isolation and genetic characterization of Neospora caninum. Vet Parasitol. 2007;149:158–66.
26. Crookshanks JL, Taylor SM, Haines DM, Shelton GD. Treatment of canine pediatric Neospora caninum myositis following immunohistochemical identification of tachyzoites in muscle biopsies. Can Vet J. 2007;48:506–8.
27. Dubey JP, Chapman JL, Rosenthal BM, Mense M, Schueler RL. Clinical Sarcocystis neurona, Sarcocystis canis, Toxoplasma gondii, and Neospora caninum infections in dogs. Vet Parasitol. 2006;137:36–49.
28. Webb JA, Keller SL, Southorn EP, Armstrong J, Allen DG, Peregrine AS, et al. Cutaneous manifestations of disseminated toxoplasmosis in an immunosuppressed dog. J Am Anim Hosp Assoc. 2005;41:198–202.
29. Cantile C, Arispici M. Necrotizing cerebellitis due to Neospora caninum infection in an old dog. J Vet Med A Physiol Pathol Clin Med. 2002;49:47–50.
30. Boydell P, Brogan N. Horner's syndrome associated with Neospora infection. J Small Anim Pract. 2000;41:571–2.
31. Peters M, Wagner F, Schares G. Canine neosporosis: clinical and pathological findings and first isolation of Neospora caninum in Germany. Parasitol Res. 2000;86:1–7.
32. Pasquali P, Mandara MT, Adamo F, Ricci G, Polidori GA, Dubey JP. Neosporosis in a dog in Italy. Vet Parasitol. 1998;77:297–9.
33. Dubey JP, Dorough KR, Jenkins MC, Liddell S, Speer CA, Kwok OC, et al. Canine neosporosis: clinical signs, diagnosis, treatment and isolation of Neospora caninum in mice and cell culture. Int J Parasitol. 1998;28:1293–304.
34. Dubey JP, Lindsay DS. A review of Neospora caninum and neosporosis. Vet Parasitol. 1996;67:1–59.
35. Barber JS, Payne-Johnson CE, Trees AJ. Distribution of Neospora caninum within the central nervous system and other tissues of six dogs with clinical neosporosis. J Small Anim Pract. 1996;37:568–74.
36. Barber JS, Trees AJ. Clinical aspects of 27 cases of neosporosis in dogs. Vet Rec. 1996;139:439–43.
37. Greig B, Rossow KD, Collins JE, Dubey JP. Neospora caninum pneumonia in an adult dog. J Am Vet Med Assoc. 1995;206:1000–1.
38. Knowler C, Wheeler SJ. Neospora caninum infection in three dogs. J Small Anim Pract. 1995;36:172–7.
39. Ruehlmann D, Podell M, Oglesbee M, Dubey JP. Canine neosporosis: a case report and literature review. J Am Anim Hosp Assoc. 1995;31:174–83.
40. Cuddon P, Lin DS, Bowman DD, Lindsay DS, Miller TK, Duncan ID, et al. Neospora caninum infection in English Springer Spaniel littermates.

Diagnostic evaluation and organism isolation. J Vet Intern Med. 1992;6:325–32.

41. Hay WH, Shell LG, Lindsay DS, Dubey JP. Diagnosis and treatment of Neospora caninum infection in a dog. J Am Vet Med Assoc. 1990;197:87–9.

42. Wolf M, Cachin M, Vandevelde M, Tipold A, Dubey JP. The clinical diagnosis of protozoal myositis syndrome (Neospora caninum) of puppies. Tierarztl Prax. 1991;19:302–6.

43. Hoskins JD, Bunge MM, Dubey JP, Duncan DE. Disseminated infection with Neospora caninum in a ten-year-old dog. Cornell Vet. 1991;81:329–34.

44. Odin M, Dubey JP. Sudden death associated with Neospora caninum myocarditis in a dog. J Am Vet Med Assoc. 1993;203:831–3.

45. Basso W, Venturini MC, Bacigalupe D, Kienast M, Unzaga JM, Larsen A, et al. Confirmed clinical Neospora caninum infection in a boxer puppy from Argentina. Vet Parasitol. 2005;131:299–303.

46. Clooten JK, Woods JP, Smith-Maxie LL. Myasthenia gravis and masticatory muscle myositis in a dog. Can Vet J. 2003;44:480–3.

47. Shaer M. Clinical medicine of the Dog and Cat. Philadelphia: Manson Publishing Lmt; 2010. p. 328–9.

48. Gockel I, Muller M, Schumacher J. Achalasia–a disease of unknown cause that is often diagnosed too late. Dtsch Arztebl Int. 2012;109:209–14.

49. Toyoda K, Uchida K, Matsuki N, Sakai H, Kitagawa M, Saito M, et al. Inflammatory myopathy with severe tongue atrophy in Pembroke Welsh Corgi dogs. J Vet Diagn Invest. 2010;22:876–85.

50. Fujimoto M. Myositis-specific autoantibodies. Brain Nerve. 2013;65:449–60.

51. Ernste FC, Reed AM. Idiopathic inflammatory myopathies: current trends in pathogenesis, clinical features, and up-to-date treatment recommendations. Mayo Clin Proc. 2013;88:83–105.

52. Cullen WC, Fletcher TF, Bradley WE. Histology of the canine urethra. I. Morphometry of the female urethra. Anat Rec. 1981;199:177–86.

53. Cullen WC, Fletcher TF, Bradley WE. Histology of the canine urethra II. Morphometry of the male pelvic urethra. Anat Rec. 1981;199:187–95.

54. Park MI. Recent concept in interpreting high-resolution manometry. J Neurogastroenterol Motil. 2010;16:90–3.

55. Pandolfino JE. High-resolution manometry: is it better for detecting esophageal disease? Gastroenterol Hepatol. 2010;6:632–4.

56. Rosin E, Galphin SP, Bowen JM. Intraluminal esophageal sphincter manometry in dogs immobilized with xylazine. Am J Vet Res. 1979;40:873–5.

57. Strombeck DR, Harrold D. Effects of atropine, acepromazine, meperidine, and xylazine on gastroesophageal sphincter pressure in the dog. Am J Vet Res. 1985;46:963–5.

58. Rosin E. Quantitation of the pharyngoesophageal sphincter in the dog. Am J Vet Res. 1986;47:660–2.

59. Jacob P, Kahrilas PJ, Herzon G, McLaughlin B. Determinants of upper esophageal sphincter pressure in dogs. Am J Physiol. 1990;259:G245–51.

60. Lang IM, Dantas RO, Cook IJ, Dodds WJ. Videoradiographic, manometric, and electromyographic analysis of canine upper esophageal sphincter. Am J Physiol. 1991;260:G911–9.

61. Mears EA, Jenkins C, Daniel G. The effect of cisapride and metoclopramide on esophageal motility in normal beagles. In: 14th American College of Veterinary Internal Medicine. San Antonio, Texas: ACVIM; 1996. Forum 738.

62. Wiinberg B, Spohr A, Dietz HH, Egelund T, Greiter-Wilke A, McDonough SP, et al. Quantitative analysis of inflammatory and immune responses in dogs with gastritis and their relationship to Helicobacter spp. infection. J Vet Intern Med. 2005;19:4–14.

63. McAlees TJ. Immune-mediated haemolytic anaemia in 110 dogs in Victoria, Australia. Aust Vet J. 2010;88:25–8.

64. Dodds WJ. Immune-mediated diseases of the blood. Adv Vet Sci Comp Med. 1983;27:163–96.

65. Ebert EC. Review article: the gastrointestinal complications of myositis. Aliment Pharmacol Ther. 2010;31:359–65.

66. Boumpas DT, Chrousos GP, Wilder RL, Cupps TR, Balow JE. Glucocorticoid therapy for immune-mediated diseases: basic and clinical correlates. Ann Intern Med. 1993;119:1198–208.

67. Harton JA, Ting JP. Class II transactivator: mastering the art of major histocompatibility complex expression. Mol Cell Biol. 2000;20:6185–94.

68. Takahashi T, Kuniyasu Y, Toda M, Sakaguchi N, Itoh M, Iwata M, et al. Immunologic self-tolerance maintained by CD25 + CD4+ naturally anergic and suppressive T cells: induction of autoimmune disease by breaking their anergic/suppressive state. Int Immunol. 1998;10:1969–80.

69. Wilbe M, Jokinen P, Truve K, Seppala EH, Karlsson EK, Biagi T, et al. Genome-wide association mapping identifies multiple loci for a canine SLE-related disease complex. Nat Genet. 2010;42:250–4.

70. Massey J, Rothwell S, Rusbridge C, Tauro A, Addicott D, Chinoy H, et al. Association of an MHC class II haplotype with increased risk of polymyositis in Hungarian Vizsla dogs. PLoS One. 2013;8, e56490.

71. Breeding standard. http://www.dogadvisorycouncil.com/resources/breeding-standard-final.pdf.

72. Mate select. http://www.thekennelclub.org.uk/services/public/mateselect/breed/Default.aspx.

73. Dog Breed Health: A Beginner's Guide to COI. http://www.dogbreedhealth.com/a-beginners-guide-to-coi/ (2011). Accessed 10 Dec 2014

74. Rusbridge C, Nicholas N, Addicott D. Polymyositis and DNA collection in the Hungarian vizsla dog. Vet Rec. 2011;168:85–6.

75. Vizsla Polymyositis: Instructions DNA collection. http://www.google.co.uk/url?sa=t&rct=j&q=&esrc=s&source=web&cd=11&ved=0CEoQFjAK&url=http%3A%2F%2Fwww.veterinary-neurologist.co.uk%2Fresources%2Fvizsla_dna-_collection_-pack2014.pdf&ei=TKo2VYK2FpLlaNOUgNAN&usg=AFQjCNFXpichPgmVD98j9zX39z1augl1XQ&bvm=bv.91071109,d.d2s.

76. Vizsla Myositis/Polymyositis. http://vizslamyositis.blogspot.co.uk/.

77. Vizsla Polymyositis. http://www.veterinary-neurologist.co.uk/Vizsla_Polymyosits.

5

Design and evaluation of a unique SYBR Green real-time RT-PCR assay for quantification of five major cytokines in cattle, sheep and goats

Carinne Puech[1,4*], Laurence Dedieu[2], Isabelle Chantal[3] and Valérie Rodrigues[1,4]

Abstract

Background: Today, when more than 60% of animal diseases are zoonotic, understanding their origin and development and identifying protective immune responses in ruminants are major challenges. Robust, efficient and cost-effective tools are preconditions to solve these challenges. Cytokines play a key role in the main mechanisms by which the immune system is balanced in response to infectious pathogens. The cytokine balance has thus become the focus of research to characterize immune response in ruminants. Currently, SYBR Green reverse transcriptase quantitative PCR (RT-qPCR) is the most widely method used to investigate cytokine gene expression in ruminants, but the conditions in which the many assays are carried out vary considerably and need to be properly evaluated. Accordingly, the quantification of gene expression by RT-qPCR requires normalization by multiple reference genes. The objective of the present study was thus to develop an RT-qPCR assay to simultaneously quantify the expression of several cytokines and reference genes in three ruminant species. In this paper, we detail each stage of the experimental protocol, check validation parameters and report assay performances, following MIQE guidelines.

Results: Ten novel primer sets were designed to quantify five cytokine genes (IL-4, IL-10, IL-12B, IFN-γ and TNF-α) and five reference genes (ACTB, GAPDH, H3F3A, PPIA and YWHAZ) in cattle, sheep, and goats. All the primer sets were designed to span exon-exon boundaries and use the same hybridization temperature. Each stage of the RT-qPCR method was detailed; their specificity and efficiency checked, proved and are reported here, demonstrating the reproducibility of our method, which is capable of detecting low levels of cytokine mRNA up to one copy whatever the species. Finally, we checked the stability of candidate reference gene expression, performed absolute quantification of cytokine and reference gene mRNA in whole blood samples and relative expression of cytokine mRNA in stimulated PBMC samples.

Conclusions: We have developed a novel RT-qPCR assay for the simultaneous relative quantification of five major cytokines in cattle, sheep and goats, and their accurate normalization by five reference genes. This accurate and easily reproducible tool can be used to investigate ruminant immune responses and is widely accessible to the veterinary research community.

Keywords: Cytokine expression, SYBR Green RT-qPCR, Cattle, Sheep, Goats, Immune response, Th1/Th2 response, Reference genes

* Correspondence: carinne.puech@cirad.fr
[1]INRA, UMR1309 CMAEE, Montpellier F-34398, France
[4]CIRAD, UMR CMAEE, Montpellier F-34398, France
Full list of author information is available at the end of the article

Background

Animal diseases have major economic, sanitary, health and environmental consequences worldwide. In 2013, the World Organization for Animal Health (OIE) calculated that more than 60% of animal diseases are zoonotic and that 75% of them are responsible for human emerging infections [1]. Infectious diseases are at the animal-human-ecosystem interface and are a major public health concern, particularly emerging infectious diseases [2]. The importance of ruminant livestock in sustainable agricultural systems [3] and the impact of major livestock diseases on food production is no longer the subject of debate [4]. However, developing efficient control strategies is a major challenge, and understanding disease pathogenesis and identifying protective immune responses are prerequisites, requiring robust, efficient, and cost-effective tools.

In response to pathogens, the immune system is regulated by complex mechanisms in which cytokines play a key role. They control the activation, proliferation and/or differentiation of different types of cells as well as in the secretion of antibodies and mediators [5]. Differential cytokine production and expression, in particular the Th1/Th2 balance, has thus become a widely used way to characterize disease pathogenesis in cattle [6,7], goats [8] and sheep [9,10].

The cytokine balance is routinely characterized either by quantification of secreted cytokine proteins or by the expression of cytokine messenger RNA (mRNA). A few optimized assays are currently available for the measurement of bovine and ovine cytokines secreted: ELISA kits, monoclonal antibodies and standards have been developed and marketed including interferon-gamma, (IFN-γ), tumor necrosis factor-alpha (TNF-α) [11], interleukin (IL)-10 [12], IL-12 [13] and IL-4 [14]. For the measurement of caprine cytokines secreted, most of the few specific tools available are based on cross-reactivity with other ruminants, but are not always sure [15]. Using the ELISA method for ruminants is costly and only a limited number of cytokines can be analyzed from a single sample. In addition, despite technological advances, veterinary immunologists working on ruminants lack tools to investigate host immunity [15-17]. Cost-effective tools able to quantify several cytokines in several species of ruminants would be a significant advance.

To achieve this objective, analyzing cytokine gene expression has become a widely used method to establish a cytokine profile in ruminants. Currently, reverse transcriptase quantitative polymerase chain reaction (RT-qPCR) is the routine method used to investigate gene expression. RT-qPCR makes it possible to simultaneously characterize different genes, using small quantities of sample with high specificity, sensitivity and accuracy [18,19]. Beside the specific probe strategy, the use of SYBR Green dye is also a sensitive, robust and reproducible method, provided that primer design and set up conditions are properly optimized. In addition, the SYBR Green method is cheaper than methods using probes, and is thus more widely and easily transferable. However, the wide range of published studies on ruminants cites many different procedures and conditions. Most of these assays are specific to only one species and some were even published without reporting all validation parameters.

The objective of our study was thus to develop an innovative and cost-effective RT-qPCR assay, to simultaneously quantify the expression of five major cytokines involved in Th1/Th2 responses, IL-4, IL-10, IL-12B, IFN-γ and TNF-α, using a single primer set and hybridization temperature for three species of ruminants, cattle, sheep and goats, in a single assay. Here we detail each stage of the experimental protocol used for the development of our SYBR Green RT-qPCR assay and offer a reliable and transferable tool. These stages range from template preparation, nucleic acid quality, reverse transcription (RT) strategy up to the PCR conditions and data reporting [20], and checking validation parameters and assay performances following the recommendations of the Minimum Information for publication of Quantitative real-time PCR Experiments (MIQE) guidelines [21]. We carefully selected five reference genes for accurate quantification of gene expression by RT-qPCR and checked the stability of their expression. The identification of internal controls to normalize gene expression is essential for relative gene expression [22], and normalization by multiple reference genes instead of one is recommended [23]. For that reason, we chose the reference genes most commonly used and/or described as stable in different types of samples. *Glyceraldehyde 3-phosphate dehydrogenase* (GAPDH) and *beta-actin* (ACTB) are the most commonly used reference genes. These genes have been described as optimal reference genes in bovine peripheral blood mononuclear cells (PBMC) [24] or whole blood [25] and thus can be used to normalize gene expression. Previous studies also showed that *Tyrosine 3-monooxygenase/tryptophan 5-monooxygenase activation protein, zeta polypeptide* (YWAHZ) [26,27], *Peptidylprolyl Isomerase A* (PPIA) [26,28] or *H3-histone family 3A* (H3F3A) [29] are the most stable genes in bovine peripheral lymphocytes and ovine whole blood.

The SYBR Green RT-qPCR assay we developed can be used for cattle, sheep and goats to quantify the expression of five major cytokine genes (IL-4, IL-10, IL-12B, IFN-γ and TNF-α) and five candidate reference genes (GAPDH, ACTB, YWHAZ, PPIA and H3F3A). Our SYBR Green RT-qPCR assay is based on an optimized and validated protocol and is an easily reproducible and reliable tool specifically designed to investigate immune response in ruminants.

Methods

In this paper, we use the nomenclature proposed by the Minimum Information for publication of quantitative real-time PCR experiments (MIQE) guidelines [19]. Candidate genes used for normalization are referred to as reference genes and the fractional PCR cycle used for quantification was Cq to quantification cycle.

Animals, blood collection and ethical considerations

Samples from healthy crossbreed cattle, Suffolk sheep and Saanen goats (three animals per species) were collected in an animal housing facility (Montpellier–France). Whole blood was collected from the jugular vein either with Tempus™ Blood RNA tubes (Applied Biosystems Ltd., Warrington, UK) or heparinized BD Vacutainer® tubes (Beckton Dickinson, New Jersey, USA) according to the manufacturer's instructions. Experimental procedures for animal maintenance and blood sampling were approved by the Languedoc-Roussillon regional ethics committee (French CE-LR #36) in the Authorised Project using animals for scientific purposes #12ANI01.

Tempus™ whole blood total RNA samples

Total RNA was extracted from whole blood of cattle, sheep and goats with Tempus™ Blood RNA System (Applied Biosystems®, Warrington, UK). After blood collection, RNA was immediately extracted using the Tempus™ Spin RNA Isolation Reagent Kit according to the manufacturer's instructions. All the samples were treated with DNAse, AbsoluteRNA Wash Solution, as recommended in the kit. RNA samples were stored at −80°C until conversion into cDNA. These samples are henceforth referred to as « Tempus™ total RNA ».

Isolation, stimulation and RNA extraction of PBMC

Peripheral blood mononuclear cells (PBMC) were isolated from heparinized whole blood by density gradient centrifugation. Briefly, PBMCs were collected after centrifugation on Histopaque®-1077 (Sigma Aldrich, France) for sheep and goats and on Histopaque®-1083 (Sigma Aldrich, France) for cattle, according to the manufacturer's instructions. Cell viability was assessed by Trypan blue exclusion. PBMCs were resuspended in RPMI 1640 Medium-glutaMAX™ (Life Technologies™, USA) supplemented with 5.10^{-5} M βmercaptoethanol (Life Technologies™, USA), 50 μg/ml gentamycin (Life Technologies™, USA) and 10% heat inactivated fetal calf serum (FCS; Eurobio AbCys, France) and were seeded in 12-well plates at 2.10^6 cells/ml. PBMCs were cultured in medium (unstimulated condition) or stimulated with 5 μg/ml of Concanavalin A (stimulated condition) for 36 h at 37°C and 5% CO_2. Total RNA was extracted using the RNeasy® Mini Kit (Qiagen Ltd., Crawley, UK) and treated with RNase-free DNase Set (Qiagen Ltd., Crawley, UK) for 30 min at room temperature. RNA samples were stored at −80°C until conversion into cDNA.

RNA quantification and quality control

The purity and quantity of RNA were assessed using a NanoDrop™ ND-1000 Spectrophotometer (Thermo Fisher Scientific, MA, USA). The A260:A280 ratio ranged from 2.1 to 2.2. RNA integrity was checked with the Agilent 2100 Bioanalyzer using the RNA 6000 Nano Assay Kit (Agilent Technologies, Inc. Santa Clara, USA). The RNA Integrity Number (RIN) ranged from 7 to 9.6.

Reverse transcription reaction

Two hundred nanograms of total RNA from each sample were reverse transcribed with the AffinityScript QPCR cDNA synthesis kit (Agilent Technologies, Inc. Santa Clara, USA) using oligo-dT strategy, and according to the manufacturer's instructions. cDNA samples were stored as multiple aliquots at −20°C for subsequent use. No-reverse transcription (no-RT) controls (assay without reverse transcriptase) were also prepared to check for non-specific amplification.

Cytokine and gene reference primers set design

All oligonucleotides were synthesized by Eurogentec (Seraing, Belgium).

Primers were designed by hand to span exon-exon boundaries and to fulfill the following criteria: located near the 3′ end, GC% between 40 and 70%, giving an approximately 200 bp amplicon and a melting temperature between 62 and 65°C. Exon spanning primers were designed by aligning *Bos taurus* gene sequences from National Center for Biotechnology Information (NCBI) GenBank database (btau 4.6.1) with mRNA-to-genomic alignment program, Spidey (www.ncbi.nlm.nih.gov/spidey). Species homologies and exon positions of ovine and caprine primers were checked *in silico*, respectively, with *Capra hircus* (chir_1.0) and *Ovis aries* (oar_V3.1) gene sequences from NCBI GenBank. The absence of primer-dimers and secondary structures was checked *in silico* using the OligoCalculator, an online oligonucleotide sequence calculator (Sigma Aldrich Co., St. Louis, USA).

Accession numbers and the exon location of each species are listed in Table 1 and primer sequences in Table 2.

Checking specificity with conventional PCR assays

The specificity of each primer pair was checked in preliminary conventional PCR assays with bovine, ovine and caprine cDNA synthesized from Tempus™ total RNA. All PCR reactions were performed with SureStart Taq DNA Polymerase (Agilent Technologies, Inc. Santa Clara, USA) following the manufacturer's instructions, with 10 ng of cDNA in 0.5 μM of each primer. PCR

Table 1 Accession number and exon locations of primers for bovine, caprine and ovine gene expression

Target gene	Species	Accession number[a]	Exon position	
			Primer F	Primer R
IL-4	*Bos taurus*	NM_173921	E2	E3-E4
	Capra hircus	NM_001285681	E2	E3-E4
	Ovis aries	NM_001009313	E2	E3-E4
IL-10	*Bos taurus*	NM_174088	E2-E3	E5
	Capra hircus	XM_005690416	E2-E3	E4-E5
	Ovis aries	NM_001009327	E2-E3	E4-E5
IL-12B	*Bos taurus*	NM_174356	E3-E4	E4-E5
	Capra hircus	NM_001285700	E3-E4	E4-E5
	Ovis aries	NM_001009438	E3-E4	E4-E5
INF-γ	*Bos taurus*	NM_174086	E3	E3-E4
	Capra hircus	NM_001285682	E2-E3	E3
	Ovis aries	NM_001009803	E2-E3	E3-E4
TNF-α	*Bos taurus*	NM_173966	E1-E2	E3-E4
	Capra hircus	NM_001286442	E1-E2	E3-E4
	Ovis aries	NM_001024860	E1-E2	E3-E4
GAPDH	*Bos taurus*	NM_001034034	E2-3	E4-5
	Capra hircus	XM_005680968	E2-E3	E4-5
	Ovis aries	NM_001190390	E2-E3	E4-5
H3F3A	*Bos taurus*	NM_00101489	E2	E2-E3
	Capra hircus	XM_005690530	E1	E1-E2
	Ovis aries	XM_004013633	E2	E2-E3
ACTB	*Bos taurus*	NM_173979	E4-E5	E5-E6
	Capra hircus	XM_005694067	E3-E4	E4-E5
	Ovis aries	NM_001009784	E4-E5	E5-E6
PPIA	*Bos taurus*	NM_178320	E4	E4-E5
	Capra hircus	XM_005679322	E3	E3-E4
	Ovis aries	XM_004013990	-	-
YWHAZ	*Bos taurus*	NM_174814	E3-E4	E4-E5
	Capra hircus	XM_005689196	E3-E4	E4-E5
	Ovis aries	NM_001267887	E2-E3	E3-E4

Abbreviations. F: forward; R: reverse; bp: base pair; IL, interleukin; IL12B, interleukin p40; TNF-α tumor necrosis factor-alpha; IFN-γ interferon-gamma; ACTB, beta-actin; GAPDH, Glyceraldehyde 3-phosphate dehydrogenase; H3F3A, H3-histone family 3A; PPIA, peptidylprolyl isomerase A; YWHAZ, tyrosine 3-monooxygenase/tryptophan 5-monooxygenase activation protein, zeta polypeptide;
[a]: GenBank accession number.

Table 2 Primer characteristics of cytokine and reference genes for bovine, caprine and ovine gene expression

Target gene	Primer sequence (5'-3')	Optimal primer concentration (nM)	Amplicon size (bp)
IL-4	F-CAGCATGGAGCTGCCT	300	177
	R-ACAGAACAGGTCTTGCTTGC	300	
IL-10	F-CTTTAAGGGTTACCTGGGTTGC	300	239
	R-CTCACTCATGGCTTTGTAGACAC	300	
IL-12B	F-CAGCAGAGGCTCCTCTGAC	600	237
	R-GTCTGGTTTGATGATGTCCCTG	600	
INF-γ	F-CAGAGCCAAATTGTCTCCTTC	300	167
	R-ATCCACCGGAATTTGAATCAG	300	
TNF-α	F-CCAGAGGGAAGAGCAGTCC	300	111
	R-GGCTACAACGTGGGCTACC	300	
GAPDH	F-ATCTCGCTCCTGGAAGATG	600	227
	R-TCGGAGTGAACGGATTCG	300	
H3F3A	F-GAGGTCTCTATACCATGGCTC	300	150
	R-GTACCAGGCCTGTAACGATG	300	
ACTB	F-TGGGCATGGAATCCTG	600	194
	R-GGCGCGATGATCTTGAT	600	
PPIA	F-TGACTTCACACGCCATAAT	300	180
	R-CTTGCCATCCAACCACTC	600	
YWHAZ	F-GAAAGGGATTGTGGACCAG	300	183
	R-GGCTTCATCAAATGCTGTCT	300	

Abbreviations. F: forward; R: reverse; bp: base pair; IL, interleukin; IL12B, interleukin p40; TNF-α tumor necrosis factor-alpha; IFN-γ interferon-gamma; ACTB, beta-actin; GAPDH, Glyceraldehyde 3-phosphate dehydrogenase; H3F3A, H3-histone family 3A; PPIA, peptidylprolyl isomerase A; YWHAZ, tyrosine 3-monooxygenase/tryptophan 5-monooxygenase activation protein, zeta polypeptide; Amplicon sizes were determinate in *Bos taurus*. Amplicon sizes in *Capra hircus* and *Ovis aries* were similar.

purified with QIAquick PCR Purification Kit (Qiagen Ltd., Crawley, UK), according to the manufacturer's instructions, (ii) quantified using a NanoDrop™ ND-1000 Spectrophotometer (Thermo Fisher Scientific, MA, USA), and (iii) sequenced (Beckman Coulter Genomics, Takeley, UK).

The absence of genomic DNA (gDNA) amplification was checked with bovine, ovine and caprine gDNA isolated from blood buffy coat, using the QIAamp DNA Mini Kit (Qiagen Ltd., Crawley, UK).

Quantitative PCR assays

Quantitative PCR (QPCR) reactions were conducted on Mx3005P QPCR Systems™ (Agilent Technologies, Santa Clara, USA). Amplifications were performed with Brilliant SYBR® II QPCR Master kit (Agilent Technologies, Santa Clara, USA). Following the manufacturer's instructions, reactions were carried out in a final volume of 25 μl with 1.5 μl of cDNA and 1 μl of each primer at the optimized concentration. Amplifications were performed as described above for conventional PCR assays. A dissociation

reactions were conducted on a SureCycler 8800 Thermal Cycler (Agilent Technologies, Santa Clara, USA). The PCR program consisted in an initial denaturation step of 10 min at 95°C, followed by 40 cycles of 30 sec at 95°C, 30 sec at 60°C, and 45 sec at 72°C, followed by a final elongation step of 10 min at 72°C. PCR products were analyzed on 2% agarose gel. Amplicon size was checked with agarose electrophoresis migration (amplicon sizes are listed in Table 2). Finally, PCR products were (i)

step was included for all reactions to confirm single specific PCR product amplification and define the Tm of each amplicon. A negative control (no-template control) was included in each primer assay to check for the formation of primer-dimers.

Linearity and efficiency of the qPCR reaction

QPCR reaction efficiency (E) was determined for each purified and quantified PCR product by performing a 10-fold serial dilution in eight points, in duplicate. Calibration curves were plotted; efficiencies and correlation coefficients were calculated by MxPro QPCR Software (Agilent Technologies, Santa Clara, USA).

Absolute quantification and relative expression genes in Tempus™ and PBMC samples

The RT-qPCR method was checked by amplification, in duplicate, of cDNA synthesized from (i) Tempus™ total RNA from three different animals (absolute quantification), and (ii) PBMC (ConcanavalinA-stimulated and unstimulated) total RNA from three independent experiments (relative expression).

Absolute quantification results are expressed as the mean number of copies (nc) from six amplification values with standard deviation. Nc was calculated using the following equation: Nc=(Relative amount of target (in ng) × 10^{-9})/(DNA length(dp) x 650) × 6.022×10^{23}. The relative amount of target (in ng) was calculated using the calibration curve and the following equation: Relative amount of target (in ng)=10 ((number of Cq-intercept)/slope).

Relative expression was calculated with efficiency correction using the relative expression software tool (REST) [30]. Multiple reference gene normalization was chosen.

Gene expression stability of the five candidate reference genes was determined in PBMC samples and calculated using the geNorm application in Microsoft Excel [23]. Stability values (M-value) and pairwise variations (V-score) were calculated and the optimal number of reference genes required for relative expression was determined. In addition, the best stable combination of reference genes was selected with NormFinder Excel Add-In [31]. The relative expression ratio (Er) of cytokine genes in ConcanavalinA-stimulated cells (n=3) compared to unstimulated cells (n=3) was calculated using the quantification of cytokine and reference gene as number of copies. Expression variation for each cytokine gene was provided by REST [30].

Stability of the five candidate reference genes using geNorm and NormFinder analysis

The gene expression stability of the five candidate reference genes was determined in Tempus™ and PBMC samples and calculated with two different reference gene selection algorithms. The geNorm application in

Microsoft Excel [23] and NormFinder Excell Add-In [31] calculate stability values (M-value in geNorm and ρ-value in NormFinder) and the reference gene with the lowest stability value is the most stable expression. NormFinder identify the best stable combination of reference genes.

As recommended by the authors of the geNorm method, an M-value <1.5 is the cut-off for suitability as reference genes for PBMC samples (heterogeneous samples) and M-value <0.5 for Tempus™ samples (homogeneous samples). In addition, using the geNorm application, we calculated the pairwise variation (V-score) to determine the optimal number of reference genes required using a V-value <0.25 as a cut-off for suitable reference genes in PBMC samples (heterogeneous samples) and V-value <0.15 in Tempus™ samples (homogeneous samples). All analyses were performed using the quantification of cytokine and reference genes as number of copies. Data were analyzed by NormFinder with groups identified (unstimulated and stimulated group).

Reproducibility and sensitivity of the RT-qPCR method

Inter-assay variability (R) is the variation in amplification results between different runs for each sample. R was determined by amplification of cDNA synthesized from the Tempus™ total RNA, in duplicate, repeated in three independent runs. R is expressed as Cq and as the mean number of copies (nc) with standard deviation.

The limit of detection (LOD) was the highest to the lowest quantifiable number of copies performed after serial dilutions of the cDNA pool synthesized from the Tempus™ total RNA. LOD is expressed as nc.

Results
Primer design and control of primer specificity

Cytokine and reference gene primer sets were designed jointly for the three ruminant species, cattle, sheep and goats, according to the predefined parameters described in "Methods". The characteristics of the primer sets are listed in Table 2. All primer sets allowed specific hybridization and amplification at 60°C. Products were checked by electrophoresis migration and led to a single specific amplicon of the expected size. Also, the absence of amplification with bovine genomic DNA was confirmed.

In addition, similarities between the sequenced PCR products and the corresponding target on the mRNA reference sequences (*Bos taurus*, *Capra hircus*, *Ovis aries*) from the NCBI GenBank database were checked using the standard nucleotide BLAST program [32]. To sum up, all qPCR amplifications led to a single specific peak and confirmed the amplification of a single specific product.

Linearity and efficiency

The optimal concentration of each primer was determined as the lowest concentration of the reverse and forward PCR primers that resulted in the lowest Cq with no formation of primer-dimer. The absence of no-specific products and primer-dimers was confirmed. Concentrations of primers are listed in Table 2. Single-peak melting curves of the PCR products defined the melting temperatures of PCR products (see Table 3 and Table 4). No amplification was detected in no-RT controls and no-template controls.

All calibration curves produced a linear standard curve and efficiency (E) ranged from 91% (for bovine TNF-α) to 102% (bovine IL-4, ovine and caprine GAPDH, caprine ACTB). All correlation coefficients were higher than 0.998 and confirmed the reaction linearity of all primer sets. PCR efficiency, the slopes and intercepts of calibration curves are listed in Table 3 (cytokine genes) and Table 4 (reference genes). Representative dissociation and calibration curves for the three species are presented in Additional file 1 (cytokine genes) and in Additional file 2 (reference genes).

Reproducibility and sensitivity

To evaluate the reproducibility of our qPCR assays, we performed amplification of Tempus™ samples (whole blood samples). All genes were correctly amplified whatever the species and led to single specific product amplification at the expected Tm. Inter-assay variability was calculated using the standard deviation of the six amplification values (Cq and copy values). Variability of cytokine gene amplifications ranged between 0.0 Cq (bovine INF-γ, corresponding to 2 copies) and 0.4 Cq (bovine IL-12B, corresponding to 8 copies). Variability of reference gene amplifications ranged between 0.1 Cq (caprine YWHAZ, corresponding to 33 copies) and 0.4 Cq (bovine ACTB, corresponding to 5.1 10^4 copies). Inter-assay variability is listed in Table 3 (cytokine genes) and Table 4 (reference genes).

Finally, we evaluated the lowest number of correctly amplified and quantified copies that led to single specific product amplification at the expected Tm (LOD) with our assay. In bovine samples, the lowest quantifiable number of copies was one copy both cytokine genes (IL-12B) and reference genes (GAPDH). In caprine samples, the lowest quantifiable number of copies was two copies for cytokine genes (IL-12B) and one copy for reference genes (GAPDH and ACTB). In ovine samples, the lowest quantifiable number of copies was one copy for cytokine genes (TNF-α) and two copies for reference genes (GAPDH). LOD are listed in Table 3 (cytokine genes) and Table 4 (reference genes).

Table 3 Assay performances for five cytokine genes for bovine, caprine and ovine gene expression

Target gene	Species	Tm (°C)	Intercept	Slope	E (%)	Inter-assay variability				LOD nc
						Mean Cq	SD Cq	Mean nc	SD nc	
IL-4	cattle		2.02	−3.372	102	28.5	0.2	25	3	9
	goat	83.9	1.37	−3.276	99	28.6	0.2	30	4	11
	sheep		1.39	−3.283	99	28.1	0.1	38	2	5
IL-10	cattle		0.27	−3.50	95	27.6	0.2	104	16	6
	goat	86.6	0.91	−3.33	97	28.9	0.2	30	4	7
	sheep		1.12	−3.34	101	29.2	0.2	17	2	5
IL-12B	cattle		0.8	−3.32	97	27.3	0.4	95	8	1
	goat	86.5	1.70	−3.28	95	35	0.6	<1	-	2
	sheep		1.59	−3.31	95	33	0.5	2	0.6	5
INF-γ	cattle		1.27	−3.449	95	27.8	0.0	79	2	5
	goat	80.2	1.63	−3.309	95	28.3	0.1	68	5	6
	sheep		1.02	−3.409	96	27.2	0.2	128	18	2
TNF-α	cattle		2.18	−3.417	91	25.0	0.3	837	192	2
	goat	84.5	0.38	−3.350	99	25.1	0.1	387	35	3
	sheep		0.04	−3.350	97	25.7	0.2	307	35	1

Abbreviations. E, reaction efficiency; Tm, melting temperature; SD: Standard deviation; LOD, limit of detection; nc: number of copies. Abbreviations for cytokine genes see Table 1.

Inter-assay variability (R) is the variation in amplification results between different runs for each sample. R was determined with amplification of cDNA synthesized from Tempus™ whole blood total RNA, in duplicate, repeated in three independent runs. R is expressed in Cq and mean number of copies (nc) with standard deviation (SD).

Limit of detection (LOD) is the lowest number of copies correctly amplified, quantified that led to single specific product amplification at the expected Tm after serial dilutions of cDNA pool synthesized from the Tempus™ total RNA. Nc was calculated using the following equation: Nc=(Relative amount of target (in ng) × 10^{-9})/(DNA length (dp) x 650) × 6.022×10^{23}. Relative amount of target (in ng) was calculated using the calibration curve and the following equation: Relative amount of target (in ng)=10 ((number of Cq-intercept)/slope).

Table 4 Assay performances for reference genes for bovine, caprine and ovine gene expression

Target gene	Species	Tm (°C)	Intercept	Slope	E (%)	Inter-assay variability				LOD nc
						Mean Cq	SD Cq	Mean nc	SD nc	
GAPDH	cattle		2.02	−3.372	98	18.3	0.2	$6.2\ 10^4$	$0.7\ 10^4$	1
	goat	84.5	1.37	−3.276	102	19.6	0.2	$1.1\ 10^4$	$0.2\ 10^4$	1
	sheep		1.39	−3.283	102	24.9	0.1	285	12	2
H3F3A	cattle		0.27	−3.50	93	16.8	0.1	$11.4\ 10^4$	$0.5\ 10^4$	20
	goat	85	0.91	−3.33	100	16.4	0.1	$14.2\ 10^4$	$0.7\ 10^4$	11
	sheep		1.12	−3.34	99	16.5	0.1	$15.4\ 10^4$	$1.1\ 10^4$	14
ACTB	cattle		0.8	−3.32	100	15.4	0.4	$19.4\ 10^4$	$5.1\ 10^4$	8
	goat	85.7	1.70	−3.28	102	15.7	0.2	$25.6\ 10^4$	$3.8\ 10^4$	1
	sheep		1.59	−3.31	101	15.6	0.3	$27.8\ 10^4$	$0.5\ 10^4$	6
PPIA	cattle		1.27	−3.449	95	17.9	0.1	$7.7\ 10^4$	$0.5\ 10^4$	6
	goat	82.3	1.63	−3.309	100	17.5	0.1	$8.3\ 10^4$	$0.6\ 10^4$	3
	sheep		1.02	−3.409	96	17.4	0.1	$8.2\ 10^4$	$0.5\ 10^4$	8
YWHAZ	cattle		2.18	−3.417	96	18.7	0.1	$7.2\ 10^4$	$0.7\ 10^4$	9
	goat	81.3	0.38	−3.350	99	23.8	0.1	506	33	4
	sheep		0.04	−3.350	99	23.5	0.1	506	24	3

Abbreviations and notes, see Table 3.

Validation of the RT-qPCR method: absolute quantification of cytokine and reference gene expression

Absolute quantification was checked by amplification, in duplicate, of cDNA synthesized from Tempus™ total RNA (whole blood samples) from three different animals of each species. All genes were correctly amplified whatever the species, and led to a single specific product amplification at the expected Tm. The mean number of copies and Cq with SD from the six amplification values are listed in Table 5.

In bovine samples, the number of cytokine gene copies detected was between 24 +/−5 copies (IL-4, corresponding to 28.7 +/−0.3 Cq) and 965 +/−199 copies (TNF-α, corresponding to 24.7 +/−0.3 Cq). In ovine and caprine samples, the number of cytokine gene copies detected was similar: between 2 +/−0.7 copies (ovine IL-12B, corresponding 33.3 +/−0.5 Cq) and 798 +/−34 copies (caprine TNF-α, corresponding to 24.0 +/−0.1 Cq).

GAPDH was the most weakly expressed reference gene with 264 +/−38 copies (ovine GAPDH, corresponding to 25.0 +/−0.2 Cq) and PPIA was the most strongly expressed reference gene with $75.6\ 10^4$ +/−$0.8\ 10^4$ copies (caprine PPIA, corresponding to 17.7 +/−0.2 Cq). H3F3A and ACTB were expressed almost identically in the three species with, for example, respectively $12.5\ 10^4$ +/−$0.7\ 10^4$ copies in bovine samples (corresponding to 16.7 +/−0.1 Cq) and $30.2\ 10^4$ +/−$4.6\ 10^4$ copies in ovine samples (corresponding to 15.5 +/−0.2 Cq). Surprisingly, the level of GAPDH and YWHAZ was differently expressed in the three species. GAPDH was weakly expressed in ovine samples with 264 +/−38 copies (corresponding to 25.0 +/−0.2 Cq) but strongly expressed in bovine and caprine samples with $7.6\ 10^4$ +/−$1.2\ 10^4$ copies (corresponding to 18.0 +/−0.3 Cq). YWHAZ was weakly expressed in ovine and caprine samples with 482 +/−81 copies (ovine, corresponding to 23.6 +/−0.2 Cq) but strongly expressed in bovine samples with $70.9\ 10^4$ +/−$1.9\ 10^4$ copies (corresponding to 18.8 +/−0.5 Cq). These differences in expression gene levels are consistent with the levels observed in unstimulated PBMC assays (see Additional file 3).

Validation of the RT-qPCR method: relative expression of cytokine genes in stimulated PBMC samples

The relative expression of ConcanavalinA-stimulated PBMC samples compared with unstimulated PBMC samples in three independent experiments for each species was calculated using the expression level of cytokine and reference genes. The stability results are presented in Figure 1. Quantification of cytokine and reference genes in unstimulated and ConcanavalinA-stimulated PBMC samples are presented in Additional file 3.

First, the optimal number of reference genes required for relative expression was determined using the geNorm application. Based on the cut-off pairwise variation of 0.25 (V-score), in our study, the use of two reference genes was sufficient for accurate normalization whatever the species, with a V-score of between 0.12 (pairwise variation V2/3 in ovine PBMC samples) and 0.24 (pairwise variation V2/3 in caprine PBMC samples). Second, the best stable combination of two reference genes was identified by Norm-Finder analysis: PPIA/H3F3A genes for bovine samples

Table 5 Absolute quantification of cytokine and reference gene expression in whole blood samples

Target gene	Species	Cq values		Copie number values	
		Mean Cq	SD Cq	Mean nc	SD nc
IL-4	cattle	28.7	0.3	24	5
	goat	28.5	0.2	31	3
	sheep	28.1	0.5	39	12
IL-10	cattle	27.2	0.6	156	54
	goat	28.2	0.5	48	17
	sheep	28.5	0.1	28	1
IL-12B	cattle	27.9	0.6	62	21
	goat	34.9	1.2	2	0.4
	sheep	33.3	0.5	2	0.7
INF-γ	cattle	27.4	0.4	106	28
	goat	27.7	0.3	103	21
	sheep	26.3	0.3	241	52
TNF-α	cattle	24.7	0.4	965	199
	goat	24.0	0.1	978	34
	sheep	24.4	0.1	728	34
GAPDH	cattle	18.0	0.3	$7.6\ 10^4$	$1.2\ 10^4$
	goat	19.1	0.1	$1.6\ 10^4$	$0.1\ 10^4$
	sheep	25.0	0.2	264	38
H3F3A	cattle	16.7	0.1	$12.5\ 10^4$	$0.7\ 10^4$
	goat	16.3	0.2	$14.9\ 10^4$	$2.3\ 10^4$
	sheep	16.2	0.1	$19.4\ 10^4$	$1.6\ 10^4$
ACTB	cattle	15.1	0.3	$24.5\ 10^4$	$4.3\ 10^4$
	goat	15.4	0.1	$32.9\ 10^4$	$2.8\ 10^4$
	sheep	15.5	0.2	$30.2\ 10^4$	$4.6\ 10^4$
PPIA	cattle	18.4	0.2	$58.0\ 10^4$	$0.6\ 10^4$
	goat	17.7	0.2	$75.6\ 10^4$	$0.8\ 10^4$
	sheep	17.7	0.1	$65.8\ 10^4$	$0.4\ 10^4$
YWHAZ	cattle	18.8	0.5	$70.9\ 10^4$	$1.9\ 10^4$
	goat	23.5	0.3	647	120
	sheep	23.6	0.2	482	81

Abbreviations for cytokine and reference genes, see Table 1.
Absolute quantification was checked by amplification of cDNA synthesized from Tempus™ total RNA from three different animals of each species. Absolute quantification used the standard curve method and is expressed as the number of copies (nc) and Cq with standard deviation (SD) from six amplification values.

(with a stability value of 0.024), GAPDH/H3F3A genes for caprine samples (with a stability value of 0.072) and PPIA/H3F3A genes for ovine samples (with a stability value of 0.064). Each combination of reference genes was used to calculate the relative expression of cytokine genes.

Finally, a qPCR assay enabled the relative expression of cytokine to be determined in all samples, whatever the species, even in cases of strong up-regulation of cytokine mRNA expression (i.e. caprine INF-γ) or in cases of decreased expression of cytokine mRNA (i.e. bovine IL-10). Cytokine expression results are presented in the whisker-box plots provided by REST [30] (see Figure 2).

Stability of the five reference genes and comparison between geNorm and NormFinder analyses and samples

The expression of the five selected reference genes (GAPDH, ACTB, YWHAZ, PPIA and H3F3A) was determined in all samples, in both PBMC and Tempus™ (whole blood) samples, using two statistical approaches, geNorm application [23] and NormFinder software [31]. Figure 1 shows the ranked lists of genes and pairwise variations for the PBMC samples and Figure 3, for the whole blood samples.

In the PBMC samples, M-values were lower than 1.5 and between 0.455 (bovine ACTB) and 0.999 (ovine H3F3A), and V-values were lower than 0.25 and between 0.12 (caprine V2/3) and 0.24 (ovine V2/3). In whole blood samples, M-values were lower than 0.5 and between 0.152 (caprine PPIA) and 0.374 (ovine H3F3A), and V-values were lower than 0.15 and between 0.039 (caprine V2/3) and 0.062 (ovine V2/3).

In bovine samples, the most stable reference gene in both whole blood and PBMC samples was ACTB, whatever the analysis. Also, the ranked list of reference genes, provided by both software, was the same for PBMC and for whole blood samples.

In ovine samples, stability results were very similar. For PBMC samples, the ranked lists of reference genes, produced by geNorm and NormFinder were the same and the most stable reference gene was ACTB. In whole blood samples, the three most stable genes were GAPDH, ACTB and PPIA, with very similar stability values (0.209 < M-value < 0.220).

In caprine samples, the ranked lists of reference genes for samples and analyses differed. In PBMC samples, ACTB and YWHAZ were the two most stable reference genes according to both geNorm and NormFinder analyses. In the whole blood samples, PPIA was the most stable reference gene and the three most stable genes were the same, with very close stability values (0.152 < M-value < 0.176).

Discussion

We developed a novel SYBR Green RT-qPCR assay for the simultaneous relative quantification of five major cytokines (IL-4, IL-10, IL-12B, IFN-γ and TNF-α) in cattle, sheep and goats, and accurate normalization with five candidate reference genes (GAPDH, ACTB, H3F3A, PPIA and YWHAZ). The main advantage of this original work is the design of an optimal primer set for three ruminant species with the same hybridization temperature. To our knowledge, this is the first SYBR Green assay

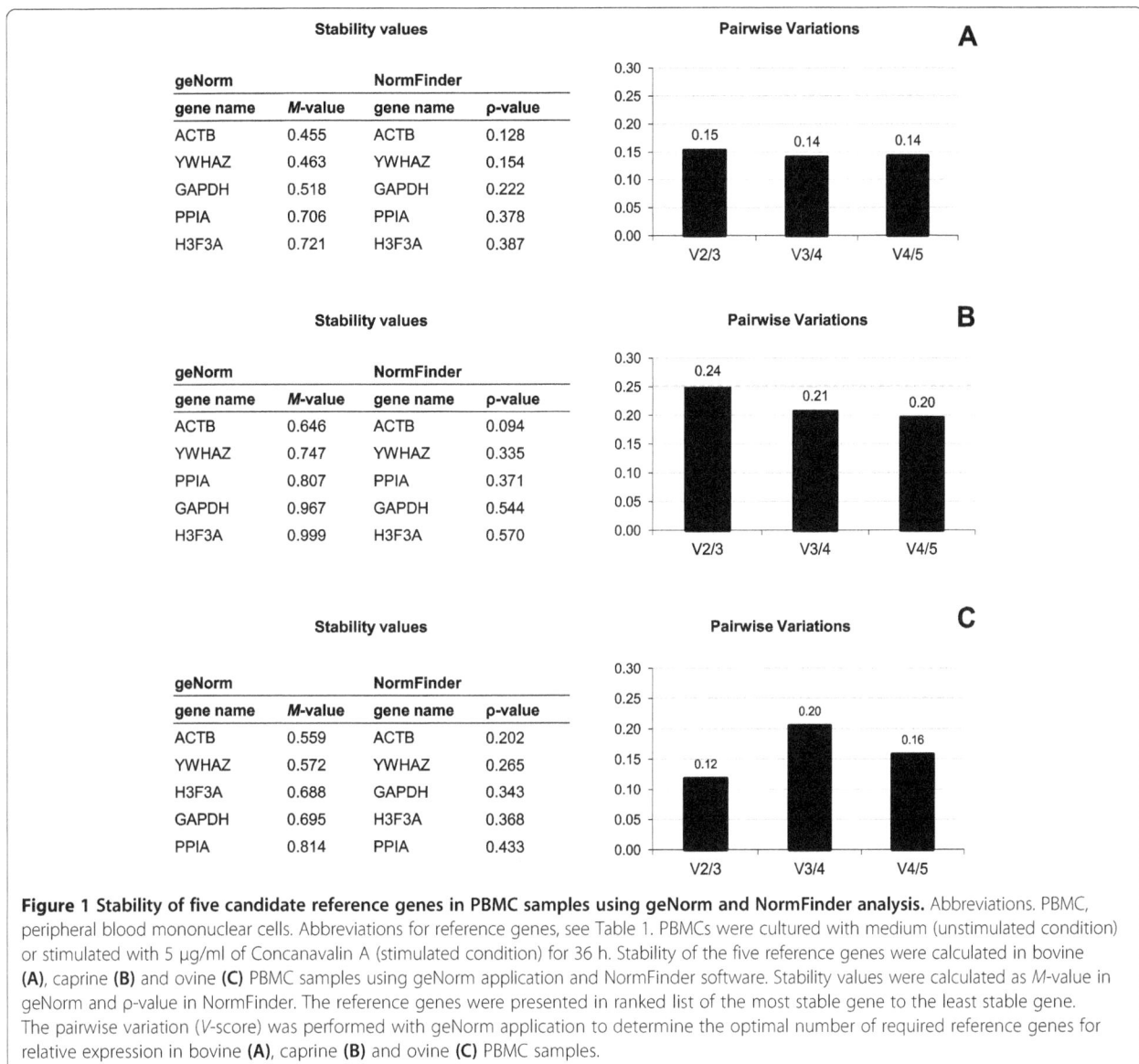

Figure 1 Stability of five candidate reference genes in PBMC samples using geNorm and NormFinder analysis. Abbreviations. PBMC, peripheral blood mononuclear cells. Abbreviations for reference genes, see Table 1. PBMCs were cultured with medium (unstimulated condition) or stimulated with 5 µg/ml of Concanavalin A (stimulated condition) for 36 h. Stability of the five reference genes were calculated in bovine **(A)**, caprine **(B)** and ovine **(C)** PBMC samples using geNorm application and NormFinder software. Stability values were calculated as *M*-value in geNorm and ρ-value in NormFinder. The reference genes were presented in ranked list of the most stable gene to the least stable gene. The pairwise variation (*V*-score) was performed with geNorm application to determine the optimal number of required reference genes for relative expression in bovine **(A)**, caprine **(B)** and ovine **(C)** PBMC samples.

that enables quantification of bovine, ovine and caprine cytokines with a single set of reagents using the same protocol. Due to the lack of tools to investigate host immunity by quantification of secreted cytokines, analysis of cytokine gene expression has become a widely used method to establish a cytokine profile in ruminants. Many infectious diseases (for example Johne's disease) affect many animal species and threaten livestock especially in the case of multi-species grazing. Our assay could thus greatly improve research by scientists involved in ruminant diseases, particularly to characterize the immune response to pathogens affecting cattle, sheep, and goats.

RT-qPCR is one of the most widely used methods to investigate cytokine gene expression in ruminants thanks to its high specificity, sensitivity and accuracy. It is also the most suitable for expression analysis of miscellaneous

cytokines from a single sample and a small quantity of template material. However, to ensure accurate reproducible quantitative data, strict standard operating procedures have to be followed and many reviews have demonstrated the importance of the RT-qPCR workflow [21,33,34].

For that reason, we developed the novel SYBR Green RT-qPCR assay presented here taking particular care to maximize the assay, detailing each step of the experimental protocol, from primer design, sample preparation or reverse transcription to the choice and normalization by reference genes, and reporting on the performance of the assays.

We first focused our attention on the criteria needed for primer design, particularly primer location straddling exons, and the choice of a single hybridization

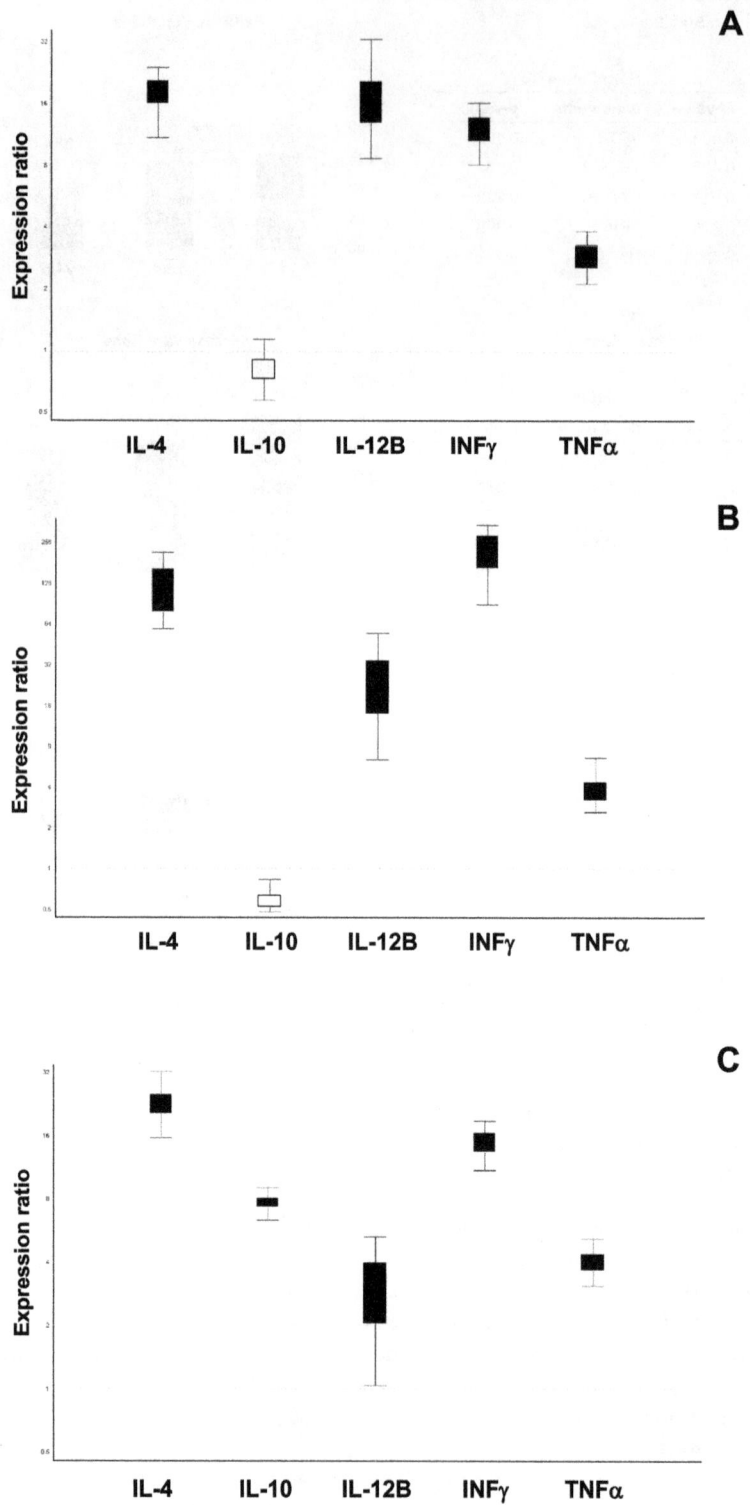

Figure 2 Cytokine relative expression in bovine, caprine and ovine stimulated PBMC samples. Abbreviations. PBMC, peripheral blood mononuclear cells. Abbreviations for reference genes, see Table 1. PBMCs were cultured with medium (unstimulated condition) or stimulated with 5 μg/ml of Concanavalin A (stimulated condition) for 36 h. The relative expression ratio (Er) of cytokine genes in Concanavalin A-stimulated cells compared to unstimulated cells was calculated (amplification of three independent experiments in duplicate) in bovine **(A)**, caprine **(B)** and ovine **(C)** samples using the relative expression software tool (REST) with the most stable combination of two reference genes identified with NormFinder software. REST Software uses randomization technique and error bars represents distribution of permutated expression data. Black boxes represent up-regulated cytokine expression and white boxes down-regulated cytokine expression.

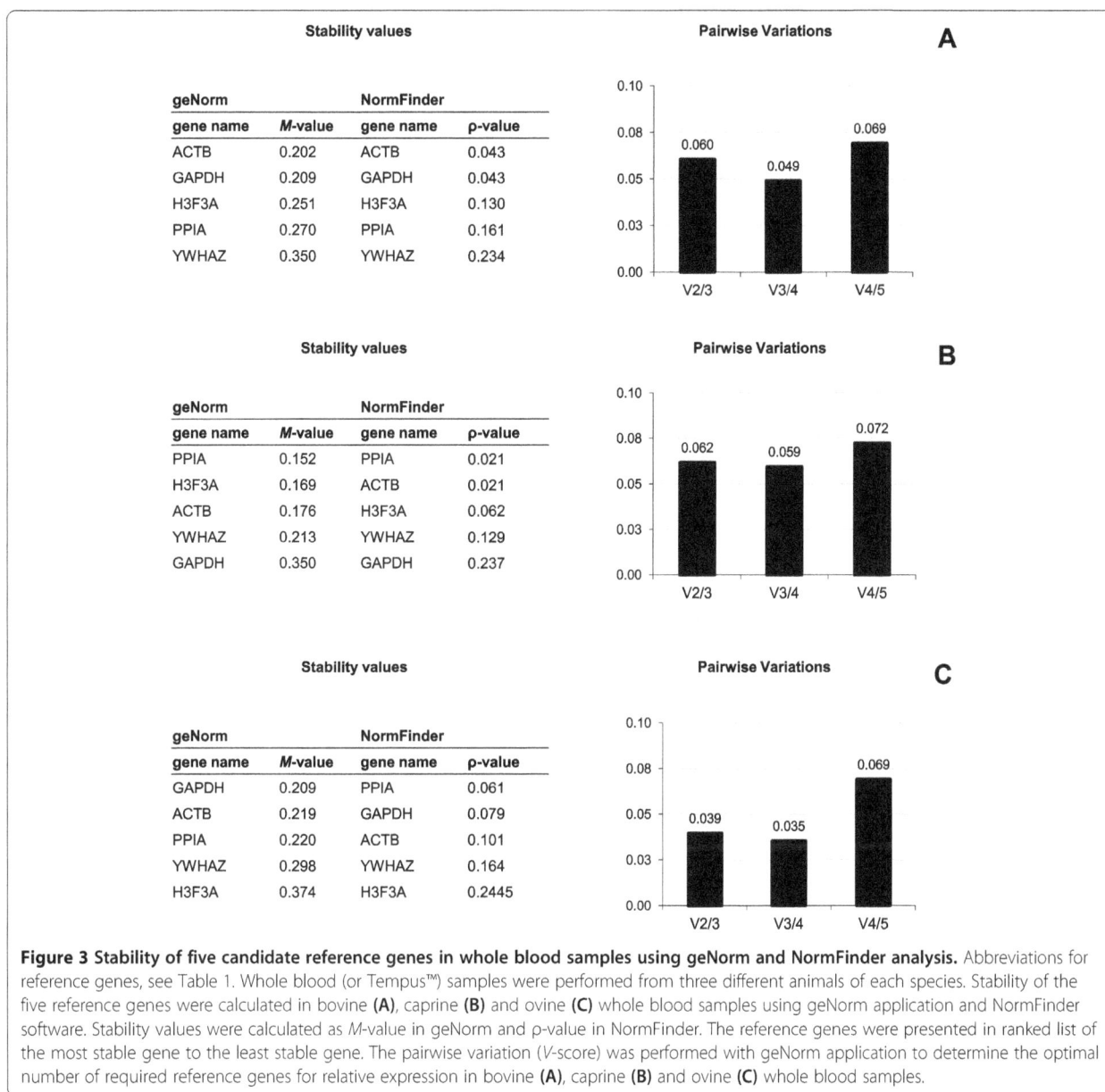

Figure 3 Stability of five candidate reference genes in whole blood samples using geNorm and NormFinder analysis. Abbreviations for reference genes, see Table 1. Whole blood (or Tempus™) samples were performed from three different animals of each species. Stability of the five reference genes were calculated in bovine **(A)**, caprine **(B)** and ovine **(C)** whole blood samples using geNorm application and NormFinder software. Stability values were calculated as *M*-value in geNorm and ρ-value in NormFinder. The reference genes were presented in ranked list of the most stable gene to the least stable gene. The pairwise variation (*V*-score) was performed with geNorm application to determine the optimal number of required reference genes for relative expression in bovine **(A)**, caprine **(B)** and ovine **(C)** whole blood samples.

temperature. S. Taylor [33] underlines the importance of primer design and the choice of target sequence to ensure specific efficient amplification of the products. Indeed, a design that spans exon-exon boundaries of at least one of the two primers, in addition to the DNAse treatment, prevents amplification of the target from contaminating gDNA. In our study, all primers were carried out fulfilling our criteria-with the exception of five primers that could not be designed to span exon-exon boundaries-to achieve a GC% of between 40% and 70% and a melting temperature of between 62°C and 65°C. This was the case for forward primers of H3F3A, PPIA, IL-4, and INF-γ genes, and for the reverse primer of the IL-10 gene. In these cases, the

second primer was then designed to span exon-exon boundaries. Thus, absence of amplification in no-RT controls and with genomic DNA, reaction linearity higher than 0.998 and high PCR efficiencies of all primer sets helped design sound primers and ensured that contaminating gDNA amplification did not occur.

Using the same hybridization temperature made it possible to analyze many samples in the same run, to compare the level of expression of a particular gene between different samples and to perform simultaneous normalization. With the common primer design, the same hybridization temperature had the additional advantage of enabling different samples of three ruminant species to be analyzed in the same run. This reduced the time and cost of the analysis, and also improved reproducibility, as demonstrated by our low run-to-run variation.

We then carefully selected five reference genes, the most widely used (GAPDH and ACTB) and/or those reported to be the most stable, for accurate normalization in both different types of samples and in the three target species. Accurate normalization is essential to eliminate sample-to-sample variations and to obtain reliable results, particularly in relative gene expression studies [21] for which multiple normalization genes with three to five reference genes could be required [23].

Before selecting suitable reference genes for normalization, the stability of the candidate reference genes (GAPDH, ACTB, H3F3A, PPIA and YWHAZ) has to be confirmed and the optimal number of reference genes required for an accurate relative expression has to be determined. In fact, there is no consensus on which method should be used to examine reference gene expression stability. We chose to evaluate the gene expression stability of the five reference genes using geNorm application [23] and NormFinder software [31] as two complementary statistical approaches. We showed that the most stable genes were similar or very close with the geNorm application and NormFinder software. In whole blood and PBMC assays, stability analyses allowed confirmation of the stability of the five candidate reference genes, which two were sufficient for an accurate normalization of our assays. While many studies recommend multiple normalization genes with three to five reference genes [33], we performed new REST analyses and compared the results of cytokine expression using the best combination genes selected by NormFinder software and the two or three most stable genes selected by geNorm application. Our results showed that gene expression was similar whatever the combination of genes selected (see results in Additional file 4), suggesting that a panel of five reference genes could be sufficient and underlining the importance of selecting adequate reference genes and checking their stability. In addition, differences and similarities in the expression stability of the reference genes were compiled. In our ovine PBMC assay, ACTB, YWHAZ and PPIA were the three most stable genes. These results were confirmed in our whole blood assay, where ACTB and PPIA were two of the three most stable reference genes. Several studies reported YWHAZ to be the most stable reference gene in ovine samples [27,35-37]. In addition to the above mentioned results, in our study, ACTB was also the most stable reference genes in bovine PBMC and whole blood samples, followed by YWHAZ and GAPDH. These results are partially in agree with Sheridan's results using whole blood samples and with Spalenza and Robinson's results using PBMC samples [24-26]. Our results emphasize the importance of following strict standard operating procedures and maximizing the assay to prevent technical variations. Finally, our results demonstrate the advantages of our RT-qPCR workflow, especially in the case of limited sample availability and funds.

In addition, we revealed an original difference in the expression level of GAPDH and YWHAZ genes among the three species, in both unstimulated PBMC and in whole blood samples. GAPDH and YWHAZ are involved in two different biological processes and have sophisticated functions in organisms in which their expression profile might fluctuate. GAPDH is an important enzyme for energy metabolism while YWHAZ plays a role in protein folding. The absence of any correlation between them in the variations we observed could exclude a GAPDH/YWHAZ co-regulation.

Our results emphasize the need to select different reference genes for accurate normalization, i.e. the most stable gene, or better yet, the most stable gene combination.

We demonstrated the sensitivity of the method and the correct cytokine gene expression quantification. In the case of low level mRNA, up-regulation, or a decrease in expression genes, an efficient RT-qPCR must be able to assess the cytokine profile regardless of the status of the animal or of the experimental conditions. Our assay ensured the detection of low levels of cytokine mRNA up to one or two copies. This was the case, for example, for IL-12B expression. We observed a low level of IL-12B expression in bovine and ovine unstimulated PBMC samples, as previously reported by Weiss in bovine macrophages and by Budhia in ovine PBMC [38]. Also, despite the low levels of IL-12B expression, 3 +/−1 copies and 8 +/−2 copies were obtained in bovine and ovine unstimulated PBMC samples respectively, up-regulation was determined relative to bovine and ovine stimulated PBMC samples by REST.

Relative expression results showed that IL-10 is up-regulated in ovine stimulated PBMC and not or only weakly down-regulated in bovine and caprine stimulated PBMC. We are unable to explain this difference in expression genes between species but we can compare with IL-12 expression, which was more strongly up-regulated in bovine and caprine stimulated PBMC.

Our SYBR Green RT-qPCR assay and the method we used to develop it, from primer design, through sample preparation and including validation, could be used to develop new cytokine primer sets and to increase the panel of cytokines and reference genes. These reference genes will also be useful for any gene expression studies whatever the species of ruminant.

Conclusions

We developed a novel SYBR Green RT-qPCR assay for the simultaneous relative quantification of five major cytokines (IL-4, IL-10, IL-12B, IFN-γ and TNF-α) in cattle, sheep and goats, and their accurate normalization with five candidate reference genes. This novel SYBR Green RT-qPCR assay, which we validated in whole blood and PBMC samples, carries out accurate and reproducible quantitative data and ensures the detection of low levels of cytokine mRNA. This original assay is a robust, efficient, cost-effective, widely accessible tool to identify immunological markers for infections in three species of ruminants, cattle, sheep and goats.

Additional files

Additional file 1: Representative dissociation and calibration curves of qPCR for reference genes. Dissociation curves were plotted by MxPro QPCR Software. Single-peak melting curves defined the melting temperatures of PCR products and confirmed the amplification of a single specific product. QPCR reaction efficiency was determined for each purified and quantified PCR product by performing a 10-fold serial dilution in eight points, in duplicate. Calibration curves were plotted by MxPro QPCR Software.

Additional file 2: Representative dissociation and calibration curves of qPCR for cytokine genes. Dissociation curves were plotted by MxPro QPCR Software. Single-peak melting curves defined the melting temperatures of PCR products and confirmed the amplification of a single specific product. QPCR reaction efficiency was determined for each purified and quantified PCR product by performing a 10-fold serial dilution in eight points, in duplicate. Calibration curves were plotted by MxPro QPCR Software.

Additional file 3: Quantification of cytokine and reference gene expression in unstimulated/stimulated PBMC assays. Abbreviations for cytokine and reference genes, see Table 1. Quantification of cytokine and reference gene expression was checked by amplification of cDNA synthesized from ConcanavalinA-stimulated and unstimulated PBMC total RNA from three independent experiments for each species. Quantification of gene expression used the standard curve method and is expressed as the number of copies (nc) and Cq with standard deviation (SD) from three amplification values.

Additional file 4: Cytokine gene expression using three combinations of reference genes selected by NormFinder and geNorm analyses. Abbreviations for cytokine and reference genes, see Table 1. The relative expression ratio of cytokine genes in Concanavalin A-stimulated cells compared to unstimulated cells was calculated (amplification of three independent experiments in duplicate) in bovine (A), caprine (B) and ovine (C) samples using the relative expression software tool (REST) using three different combinations of reference genes selected by geNorm application an NormFinder software.

Abbreviations
RT-qPCR: Reverse transcriptase quantitative polymerase chain reaction; IL: Interleukin; IL-12B: Interleukin p40; TNF-α: Tumor necrosis factor-alpha; IFN-γ: Interferon-gamma; ACTB: Beta-actin; GAPDH: Glyceraldehyde 3-phosphate dehydrogenase; H3F3A: H3-histone family 3A; PPIA: Peptidylprolyl Isomerase A; YWHAZ: Tyrosine 3-monooxygenase/tryptophan 5-monooxygenase activation protein, zeta polypeptide; MIQE: Minimum Information for publication of Quantitative Real-time PCR Experiments; E: Reaction efficiency; PBMC: Peripheral blood mononuclear cells; REST: Relative expression software tool; Er: Relative expression ratio.

Competing interests
The authors declare that they have no competing interests.

Authors' contributions
CP conceived the study, designed the experiments, performed all the experiments, analyzed the data and drafted the manuscript. LD participated in writing the manuscript. IC participated in developing the proposal. VR conceived the study and corrected the manuscript. All the authors have read and approved the final manuscript.

Acknowledgements
The authors would like to thank Virginie Dupuy for helpful discussions and her critical review of this paper. We thank also Noël Richard and Thierry Maccota for their technical assistance in animal care and sampling.

Author details
[1]INRA, UMR1309 CMAEE, Montpellier F-34398, France. [2]CIRAD, DGD-RS-Dist, Montpellier F-34398, France. [3]CIRAD, UMR Intertryp, Montpellier F-34398, France. [4]CIRAD, UMR CMAEE, Montpellier F-34398, France.

References
1. OIE. 2012. Animal health: a multifaceted challenge. [http://www.oie.int/fileadmin/Home/eng/Media_Center/docs/pdf/Key_Documents/ANIMAL-HEALTH-EN-FINAL.pdf]
2. Lefrançois T, Pineau T. Public health and livestock: emerging diseases in food animals. Animal Frontiers. 2014;4:4–6.
3. Hackmann TJ, Spain JN. Invited review: ruminant ecology and evolution: perspectives useful to ruminant livestock research and production. J Dairy Sci. 2010;93:1320–34.
4. Grace D, Mutua F, Ochungo P, Kruska R, Jones K, Brierley L, et al. Mapping of Poverty and Likely Zoonoses Hotspots. 2012.
5. Mosmann TR, Coffman RL. TH1 and TH2 cells: different patterns of lymphokine secretion lead to different functional properties. Annu Rev Immunol. 1989;7:145–73.
6. Boddu-Jasmine HC, Witchell J, Vordermeier M, Wangoo A, Goyal M. Cytokine mRNA expression in cattle infected with different dosages of Mycobacterium bovis. Tuberculosis. 2008;88:610–5.
7. Coussens PM, Verman N, Coussens MA, Elftman MD, McNulty AM. Cytokine gene expression in peripheral blood mononuclear cells and tissues of cattle infected with mycobacterium avium subsp. paratuberculosis: evidence for an inherent proinflammatory gene expression pattern. Infect Immun. 2004;72:1409–22.
8. Singh PK, Singh SV, Saxena VK, Singh MK, Singh AV, Sohal JS. Expression profiles of different cytokine genes in peripheral blood mononuclear cells of goats infected experimentally with native strain of Mycobacterium avium subsp. paratuberculosis. Anim Biotechnol. 2013;24:187–97.
9. Smeed JA, Watkins CA, Rhind SM, Hopkins J. Differential cytokine gene expression profiles in the three pathological forms of sheep paratuberculosis. BMC Vet Res. 2007;3:18.
10. Channappanavar R, Singh KP, Singh R, Umeshappa CS, Ingale SL, Pandey AB. Enhanced proinflammatory cytokine activity during experimental bluetongue virus-1 infection in Indian native sheep. Vet Immunol Immunopathol. 2012;145:485–92.
11. Kwong LS, Thom M, Sopp P, Rocchi M, Wattegedera S, Entrican G, et al. Production and characterization of two monoclonal antibodies to bovine tumour necrosis factor alpha (TNF-alpha) and their cross-reactivity with ovine TNF-alpha. Vet Immunol Immunopathol. 2010;135:320–4.
12. Kwong LS, Hope JC, Thom ML, Sopp P, Duggan S, Bembridge GP, et al. Development of an ELISA for bovine IL-10. Vet Immunol Immunopathol. 2002;85:213–23.
13. Hope JC, Kwong LS, Entrican G, Wattegedera S, Vordermeier HM, Sopp P, et al. Development of detection methods for ruminant interleukin (IL)-12. J Immunol Methods. 2002;266:117–26.
14. Hope JC, Kwong LS, Thom M, Sopp P, Mwangi W, Brown WC, et al. Development of detection methods for ruminant interleukin (IL)-4. J Immunol Methods. 2005;301:114–23.
15. Hope JC, Sopp P, Wattegedera S, Entrican G. Tools and reagents for caprine immunology. Small Rumin Res. 2012;103:23–7.
16. Entrican G, Lunney JK, Rutten VP, Baldwin CL. A current perspective on availability of tools, resources and networks for veterinary immunology. Vet Immunol Immunopathol. 2009;128:24–9.
17. Entrican G. New technologies for studying immune regulation in ruminants. Vet Immunol Immunopathol. 2002;87:485–90.
18. Giulietti A, Overbergh L, Valckx D, Decallonne B, Bouillon R, Mathieu C. An overview of real-time quantitative PCR: applications to quantify cytokine gene expression. Methods. 2001;25:386–401.
19. Bustin SA. Absolute quantification of mRNA using real-time reverse transcription polymerase chain reaction assays. J Mol Endocrinol. 2000;25:169–93.

20. Bustin SA, Nolan T. Pitfalls of quantitative real-time reverse-transcription polymerase chain reaction. J Biomol Tech. 2004;15:155–66.

21. Bustin SA, Benes V, Garson JA, Hellemans J, Huggett J, Kubista M, et al. The MIQE guidelines: minimum information for publication of quantitative real-time PCR experiments. Clin Chem. 2009;55:611–22.

22. Livak KJ, Schmittgen TD. Analysis of relative gene expression data using real-time quantitative PCR and the $2=\Delta\Delta CT$ method. Methods. 2001;25:402–8.

23. Vandesompele J, Preter KD, Pattyn F, Poppe B, Roy NV, Paepe AD, et al. Accurate normalization of real-time quantitative RT-PCR data by geometric averaging of multiple internal control genes. Genome Biol. 2002;3: research0034.

24. Robinson TL, Sutherland IA, Sutherland J. Validation of candidate bovine reference genes for use with real-time PCR. Vet Immunol Immunopathol. 2007;115:160–5.

25. Sheridan MP, Browne JA, MacHugh DE, Costello E, Gormley E. Impact of delayed processing of bovine peripheral blood on differential gene expression. Vet Immunol Immunopathol. 2012;145:199–205.

26. Spalenza V, Girolami F, Bevilacqua C, Riondato F, Rasero R, Nebbia C, et al. Identification of internal control genes for quantitative expression analysis by real-time PCR in bovine peripheral lymphocytes. Vet J. 2011;189:278–83.

27. Peletto S, Bertuzzi S, Campanella C, Modesto P, Maniaci MG, Bellino C, et al. Evaluation of internal reference genes for quantitative expression analysis by real-time PCR in ovine whole blood. Int J Mol Sci. 2011;12:7732–47.

28. Taraktsoglou M, Szalabska U, Magee DA, Browne JA, Sweeney T, Gormley E, et al. Transcriptional profiling of immune genes in bovine monocyte-derived macrophages exposed to bacterial antigens. Vet Immunol Immunopathol. 2011;140:130–9.

29. Meade KG, Gormley E, Doyle MB, Fitzsimons T, O'Farrelly C, Costello E, et al. Innate gene repression associated with Mycobacterium bovis infection in cattle: toward a gene signature of disease. BMC Genomics. 2007;8:400.

30. Pfaffl MW, Horgan GW, Dempfle L. Relative expression software tool (REST©) for group-wise comparison and statistical analysis of relative expression results in real-time PCR. Nucleic Acids Res. 2002;30:e36.

31. Andersen CL, Jensen JL, Ørntoft TF. Normalization of real-time quantitative reverse transcription-PCR data: a model-based variance estimation approach to identify genes suited for normalization, applied to bladder and colon cancer data sets. Cancer Res. 2004;64:5245–50.

32. Altschul SF, Gish W, Miller W, Myers EW, Lipman DJ. Basic local alignment search tool. J Mol Biol. 1990;215:403–10.

33. Taylor S, Wakem M, Dijkman G, Alsarraj M, Nguyen M. A practical approach to RT-qPCR-publishing data that conform to the MIQE guidelines. Methods. 2010;50:S1–5.

34. Derveaux S, Vandesompele J, Hellemans J. How to do successful gene expression analysis using real-time PCR. Methods. 2010;50:227–30 [The Ongoing Evolution of qPCR].

35. Jarczak J, Kaba J, Bagnicka E. The validation of housekeeping genes as a reference in quantitative Real Time PCR analysis: application in the milk somatic cells and frozen whole blood of goats infected with caprine arthritis encephalitis virus. Gene. 2014;549:280–5.

36. Vorachek WR, Hugejiletu, Bobe G, Hall JA. Reference gene selection for quantitative PCR studies in sheep neutrophils. Int J Mol Sci. 2013;14:11484–95.

37. Zang R, Bai J, Xu H, Zhang L, Yang J, Yang L, et al. Selection of suitable reference genes for real-time quantitative PCR studies in Lanzhou Fat-tailed Sheep (Ovis aries). Asian J Animal Vet Adv. 2011;6:789–804.

38. Budhia S, Haring LF, McConnell I, Blacklaws BA. Quantitation of ovine cytokine mRNA by real-time RT–PCR. J Immunol Methods. 2006;309:160–72.

6

DNA-based diagnosis of rare diseases in veterinary medicine: a 4.4 kb deletion of ITGB4 is associated with epidermolysis bullosa in Charolais cattle

Martin Peters[1], Irene Reber[2], Vidhya Jagannathan[2], Barbara Raddatz[3], Peter Wohlsein[3] and Cord Drögemüller[2*]

Abstract

Background: Rare diseases in livestock animals are traditionally poorly diagnosed. Other than clinical description and pathological examination, the underlying causes have, for the most part, remained unknown. A single case of congenital skin fragility in cattle was observed, necropsy, histological and ultrastructural examinations were carried out and whole genome sequencing was utilized to identify the causative mutation.

Results: A single purebred female Charolais calf with severe skin lesions was delivered full-term and died spontaneously after birth. The clinical and pathological findings exactly matched the gross description given by previous reports on epitheliogenesis imperfecta and epidermolysis bullosa (EB) in cattle. Histological and ultrastructural changes were consistent with EB junctionalis (EBJ). Genetic analysis revealed a previously unpublished ITGB4 loss-of-function mutation; the affected calf was homozygous for a 4.4 kb deletion involving exons 17 to 22, and the dam carried a single copy of the deletion indicating recessive inheritance. The homozygous mutant genotype did not occur in healthy controls of various breeds but some heterozygous carriers were found among Charolais cattle belonging to the affected herd. The mutant allele was absent in a representative sample of unrelated sires of the German Charolais population.

Conclusion: This is the first time in which a recessively inherited ITGB4 associated EBJ has been reported in cattle. The identification of heterozygous carriers is of importance in avoiding the transmission of this defect in future. Current DNA sequencing methods offer a powerful tool for understanding the genetic background of rare diseases in domestic animals having a reference genome sequence available.

Keywords: Cattle, Rare genetic disease, Skin fragility, Junctional epidermolysis bullosa, Whole genome sequencing, Integrin beta 4, ITGB4

Background

Rare or so-called orphan diseases, which affect only a very small number of individuals, have been identified in both humans and domestic animal species. The majority of rare diseases are caused by altered functions of single genes. Although the individual diseases are rare, collectively they are common, affecting millions of people worldwide [1]. In non-laboratory animals, the number of rare genetic diseases is unknown, but Online Mendelian Inheritance in Animals (OMIA), a catalogue of inherited disorders and associated genes in animals, reports more than 2500 phenotypes in eleven domestic animal species [2]. Currently, the gene mutation responsible for approximately 20% of rare diseases in domestic animals has been determined [2]. This has been accomplished over the past 25 years either by the targeted analysis of individual candidate genes or labor- and resource-intensive positional cloning approaches, such as linkage mapping or genome-wide association studies [3]. For this purpose, a series of cases showing an identical phenotype was needed [4]. The advent of next-generation sequencing technology, in combination with the establishment of a reference genome sequence for domestic animal species, such as for the bovine genome in 2009 [5], have changed the prospects enormously [6]. Today, studying the molecular aetiology of single cases is also feasible, e.g., in cattle [6,7], as has been successfully carried out in humans for approximately five years now [1].

* Correspondence: cord.droegemueller@vetsuisse.unibe.ch
[2]Institute of Genetics, Vetsuisse Faculty, University of Bern, Bremgartenstrasse 109a, 3001 Bern, Switzerland
Full list of author information is available at the end of the article

Congenital skin fragility, also called epidermolysis bullosa (EB), represents a heterogeneous group of rare diseases reported in different species, including livestock animals. In the majority of cases it is genetically determined and, in humans, 18 EB-associated genes have currently been identified which encode the structural proteins involved in epidermal and dermal adhesion [8]. Various EB forms have been described in cattle [9-16], but the associated genes (KRT5 and COL7A1) have been identified for only two outbreaks of recessively inherited EB forms (OMIA 000340–9913 and OMIA 000341–9913) [13,16]. As is known for EB in other domestic animals, these two bovine EB diseases were genetically characterised by analysing well-known EB candidate genes [16,17].

A single case of severe congenital EB was observed in Charolais cattle. The purpose of this study was to characterise the phenotype in comparison to the known EB forms of different species. In parallel, a whole genome sequencing-based mutation analysis was carried out focusing on known EB candidates, and an associated loss-of-function mutation in the integrin beta 4 (ITGB4) gene was detected.

Results
Phenotype description
A single purebred, female Charolais calf of 22.4 kg was delivered full-term and died immediately after birth. The calf underwent post-mortem examination at the Chemisches und Veterinäruntersuchungsamt Westfalen (Northrhine Westphalia, Germany). The calf exhibited multifocally extensive alopecia, erosions and ulcers on the rump, head, and external surfaces of the pinnae, eyelids, nose, muzzle, lips and distal extremities with onychomadesis of all four feet (Figure 1A). Parts of the small intestine protruded through the navel. The hairless skin showed crusts and multiple small vesicles at the border with the haired skin (Figure 1B). There were severe oral lesions with focally missing cutaneous mucous membranes of the gingiva, hard palate, and on the back (Figure 1C) and ventral aspect of the tongue. There were linear skin defects at the anal- and vulvocutaneous junctions. No other gross lesions were detected.

Histopathological and ultrastructural findings
Histological examination of the affected skin lesions or oral mucous membranes multifocally confirmed a complete loss of the epidermis or the epithelium which was covered by serocellular crusts. The underlying dermis or submucosa multifocally showed mild to moderate, acute, diffuse haemorrhages and a mild infiltration of neutrophils and mononuclear cells. The adjacent skin or mucous membranes displayed severe, subepidermal or subepithelial cleft formations of various lengths occasionally filled

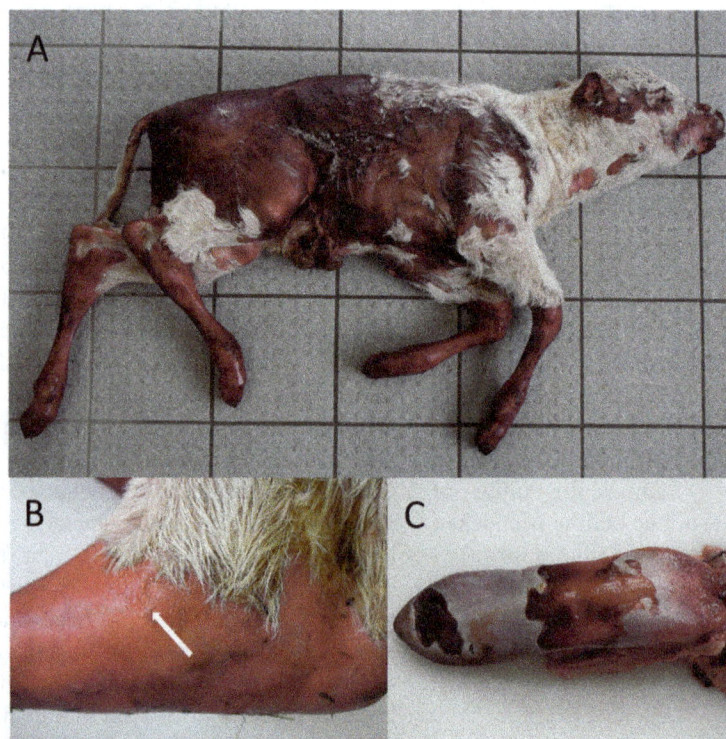

Figure 1 Epidermolysis bullosa in a female Charolais calf. (A) Note the extensive epidermal loss at the trunk, ears, distal limbs and muzzle as well as exungulation of the claws. **(B)** Multiple cutaneous vesicles (arrow) at the transition area between alopecic and haired skin. **(C)** Extensive mucosal defects of the tongue.

with eosinophilic, proteinaceous fluid, cellular debris, haemorrhage and single neutrophils. The cleft formation extended around the hair follicles in varying degrees (Figure 2). periodic acid-Schiff (PAS)-reaction identified the basement membrane associated with the floor of the cleft. Consequently, the cleft formation was located between the basal layers of the epithelial cells and the basement membrane. Ultrastructurally, the cleft formation was located in the lamina lucida of the basement membrane. The lamina densa was attached to the dermis (Figure 3).

Mutation analysis

The dam of the affected calf showed no clinically visible skin anomalies. In addition, the owner did not observe any similar congenitally malformed newborns in his herd. Unfortunately, the identity of the sire could not be determined as the farmer keeps more than 200 cows and some natural service sires which were used simultaneously had already been slaughtered. Since it was difficult to predict whether the disease was dominantly or recessively inherited without family information, we hypothesised two different possible scenarios: either a fully penetrant dominant acting *de novo* mutation which occurred in a single parental gamete or happened during early embryonic development of the calf, or a recessively inherited mutation present in the homozygous state transmitted by both parents due to inbreeding.

First, a recent dominant *de novo* mutation was hypothesised and the entire genome of the affected animal was therefore sequenced in order to detect all the variants in the known EB comparative candidate genes. A total of 203,557,590 100 bp paired-end reads were collected from

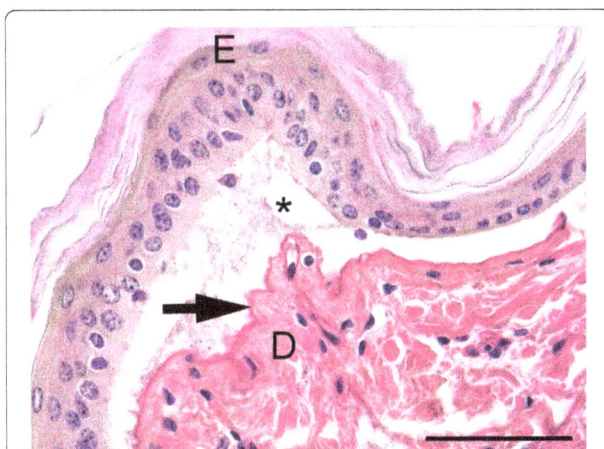

Figure 3 Transmission electron microscopy of the skin. Macroscopically unaffected skin from the left hind leg with a severe subepidermal cleft formation (asterisk) located in the lamina lucida of the basement membrane. The lamina densa (arrow) is attached to the dermis. E = epidermis; D = dermis. Bar = 250 nm.

a shotgun fragment library corresponding roughly to a 14.3 fold coverage of the genome. The single nucleotide variants, and short insertions or deletions were called and compared to the reference genome and 68,729 high quality variants across the entire exome, including untranslated regions and 10 bp of flanking introns, were detected. The variants were additionally compared with 50 cow genomes of various breeds which had been sequenced in our laboratory in the course of other ongoing studies. Assuming that the causative variant would be completely absent in these controls but present in the affected calf, a total of 981 variants, of which 955 were coding variants, occurred privately only in the EB-affected calf and were not present in any control. For these variants, a total of 1458 effects on annotated genes and loci were predicted (Additional file 1). Of the 955 coding variants, 745 were present in the heterozygous state and 322 in the homozygous state. This analysis revealed no exomic sequence variants located within one of the 18 EB candidate genes. In addition, larger deletions in the sequenced case and in 10 control cow genomes with a genome-wide coverage of more than 10 fold were searched for. A total of 890 deletions were private deletions occurring only in the genome of the affected Charolais animal in which a single 4.8 kb deletion was detected in the region of one of the comparative candidate genes (ITGB4), starting at position 56,488,275 on cattle chromosome 19 (UMD3.1/bosTau6 assembly). Visual inspection of the mapped sequence reads confirmed the presence of a large (4809 bp) deletion in the ITGB4 gene affecting six coding exons (c.1,765-1,863_2,613-2,636del) with breakpoints in intron 16 and intron 22 (Figure 4). The presence of the genomic deletion in the homozygous

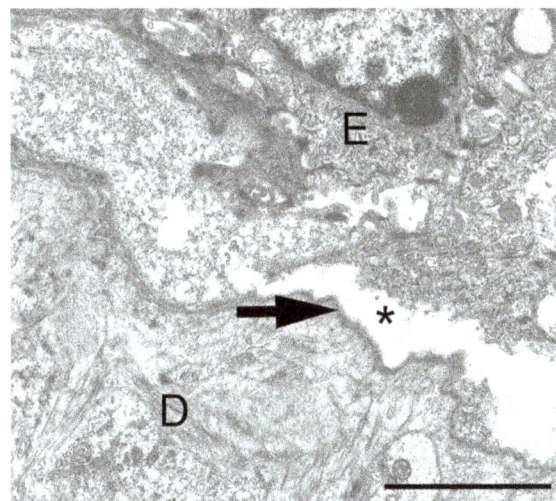

Figure 2 Micrograph of the affected skin. Macroscopically unaffected skin from the left hind leg of a Charolais calf having a subepidermal cleft formation with acellular, proteinaceous fluid (asterisk): the PAS-positive basement membrane (arrow) is located at the floor of the cleft attached to the adjacent dermis. E = epidermis; D = dermis. Periodic acid-Schiff (PAS)-reaction. Bar = 25 μm.

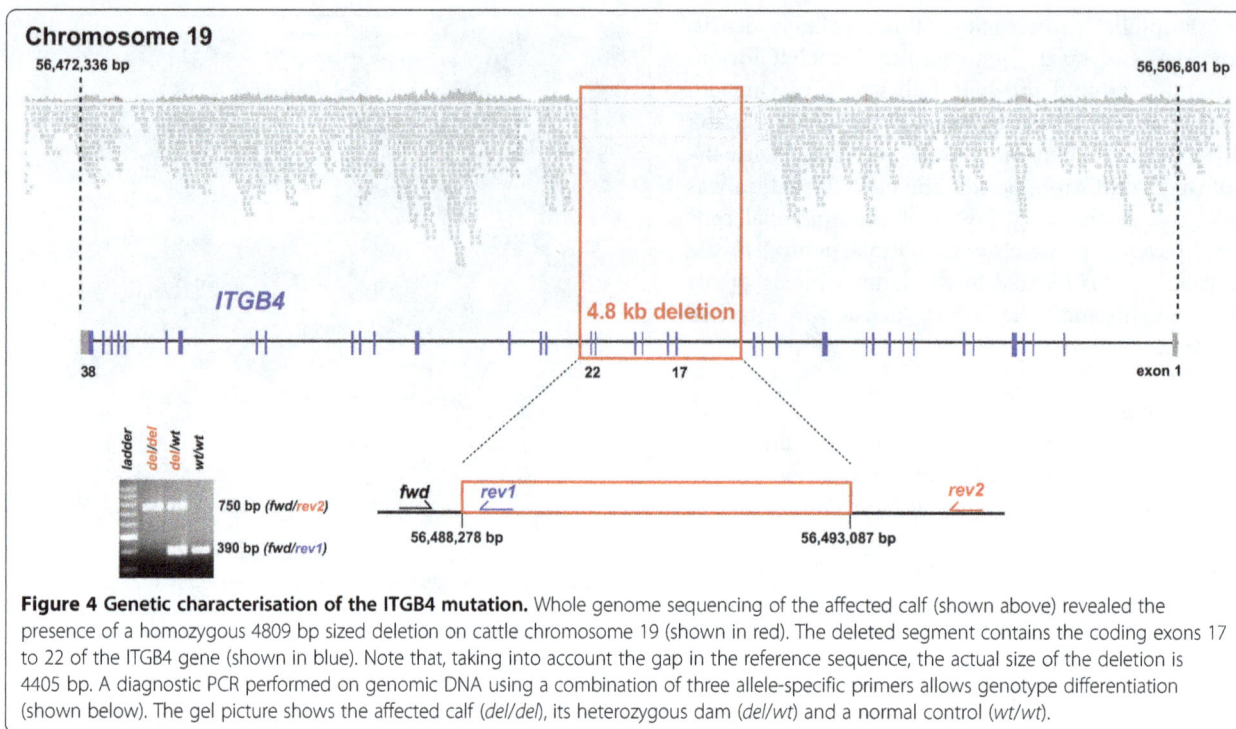

Figure 4 Genetic characterisation of the ITGB4 mutation. Whole genome sequencing of the affected calf (shown above) revealed the presence of a homozygous 4809 bp sized deletion on cattle chromosome 19 (shown in red). The deleted segment contains the coding exons 17 to 22 of the ITGB4 gene (shown in blue). Note that, taking into account the gap in the reference sequence, the actual size of the deletion is 4405 bp. A diagnostic PCR performed on genomic DNA using a combination of three allele-specific primers allows genotype differentiation (shown below). The gel picture shows the affected calf (del/del), its heterozygous dam (del/wt) and a normal control (wt/wt).

state was confirmed by polymerase chain reaction (PCR) and agarose gel electrophoresis (Figure 4). To prove and define the precise breakpoints of this deletion, the obtained PCR products were sequenced. In this way, it was possible to sequence a previously uncharacterised sequence gap in the bovine reference sequence which was present in intron 16, revealing that this region is 404 bp shorter than presented in the reference sequence (Additional file 2). This detailed analysis finally showed that the exact size of the deletion on chromosome 19 was 4405 bp (4809 bp minus 404 bp).

In addition, under the assumption of a possible recessive mutation, it was decided to apply a homozygosity mapping approach to determine the homozygous regions in the genome of the affected calf. It was hypothesised that the affected animal would be identical by descent for the causative mutation and flanking chromosomal segments due to parents which shared a common ancestor. The genotypes of 777,962 single nucleotide polymorphisms (SNPs) were analysed and the genotypes were checked for extended regions of homozygosity. A total of 80 genomic regions larger than 1 Mb were located on different cattle chromosomes (Figure 5). The largest homozygous region by far was located on cattle chromosome 19, containing 16,393 SNP markers and corresponding to a 54.7 Mb interval from 7.6 to 62.3 Mb (Figure 5). Within this genomic segment, 4 of the 18 known EB comparative candidate genes were located in the bovine genome including the ITGB4 gene which contains the above mentioned large genomic deletion. To

experimentally prove the inheritance of this deletion, a diagnostic PCR was designed (Figure 4). This analysis confirmed the homozygous genotype of the affected calf and showed that the dam was carrying a single copy of the deletion (Figure 4). As expected, normal controls showed a single band of 390 bp, the homozygous affected calf showed a single band of 750 bp and the heterozygous dam showed both PCR products. Genotyping was carried out on a total of 162 Charolais cattle belonging to the herd into which the affected calf was born. This revealed that the homozygous mutant genotype was absent in all animals but we identified a total of 15 heterozygous carriers including the maternal grandmother of the affected calf. Due to missing detailed pedigree records we were not able to identify a possible common ancestor among the disease allele carriers. Finally, a total of 88 unrelated Charolais sires which were used for artificial insemination in Germany and 50 controls from various breeds were tested negatively for the presence of the ITGB4 deletion.

Discussion

The skin fragility phenotype observed in a Charolais calf resembles previous reports of epidermolysis bullosa and epitheliogenesis imperfecta in calves [9-16]. Since epitheliogenesis imperfecta is not genetically defined and an in-depth pathological examination is necessary for distinction, both conditions might have been confused in the past and recorded in veterinary literature. Epidermolysis bullosa is a mechanobullous disorder and is classified into three groups according to the ultrastructural location of

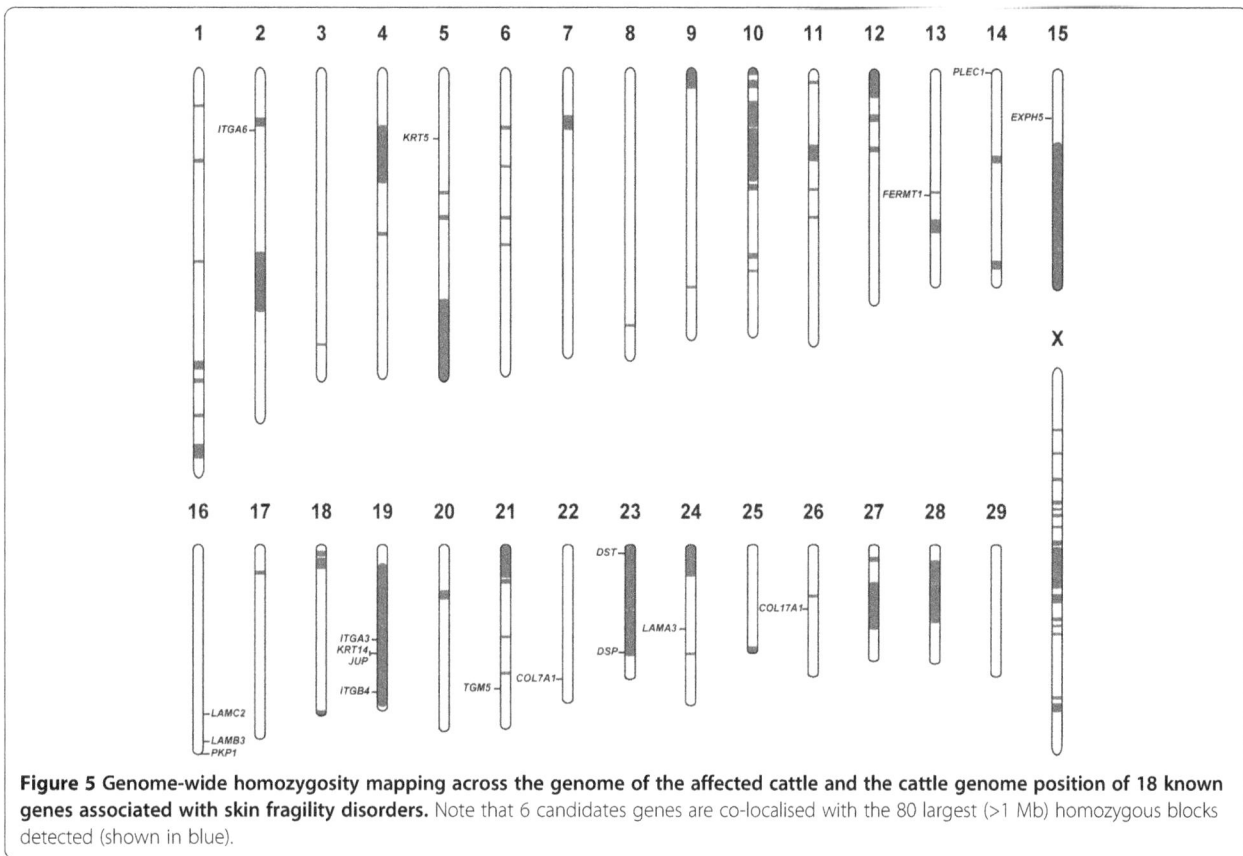

Figure 5 Genome-wide homozygosity mapping across the genome of the affected cattle and the cattle genome position of 18 known genes associated with skin fragility disorders. Note that 6 candidates genes are co-localised with the 80 largest (>1 Mb) homozygous blocks detected (shown in blue).

the blistering between the epidermis and the dermis. In EB simplex, the blister formation tissue separation occurs within the epidermal basal keratinocytes adjacent to the basal lamina. In junctional EB, the blister formation arises within the lamina lucida of the basal lamina. In dystrophic EB, the blister formation takes place at the dermal side of the basal lamina below the lamina densa. Which subtype of EB develops and how severe the lesions are depend on the functional defects of particular proteins. All three types of EB have been reported in cattle [17]. Ultrastructurally, the case reported in a Charolais calf could clearly be identified as EB junctionalis (EBJ). There is high morphologically agreement with another case of EBJ in this breed [18] in which, based on immuno-histological examination, a deficient expression of integrin α6β4 was hypothesised as being a possible cause. The identification of a loss-of-function mutation in the bovine ITGB4 gene could finally confirm this suspicion since the current case belongs to the same breed. In regard to the recessive inheritance of the deletion identified one can hypothesise that the mutation was possibly already present more than ten years ago in the French Charolais population. A likely scenario could be that, due to the importation of semen or living sires which were heterozygous for the mutation, the defective allele was introgressed into the German Charolais population. Alternatively, it could be that the formerly

reported French case was caused by an independent ITGB4 mutation.

Mutations in ITGB4 are known to cause EBJ in humans [8]. The integrins are cell membrane receptors composed of alpha and beta subunits which orchestrate adhesive events in all tissues of the body. In the skin, they play an essential role in the architecture of the hemidesmosomes which mediate the stable attachment of the basal epithelial cells to the underlying basement membrane [19]. Due to the severity of EBJ in this case, a very likely causative mutation in the coding region of one of the well-characterised candidate genes was hypothesised. The approach of whole genome sequencing allowed the consideration of two possible scenarios: a recent dominant acting *de novo* mutation or a recessively inherited mutation which had already occurred some generations ago. That the EBJ phenotype could be explained by a recessive ITGB4 deletion which was very likely responsible for a similar case already one decade ago was able to be shown [18]. The transcript of the mutant allele lacked information regarding a significant part of the encoded protein since the deletion led to a frameshift and a premature stop codon. It was therefore assumed that the mutant transcripts probably underwent nonsense mediated decay so that, in the final analysis, the deletion represented a loss-of-function mutation with a non-existing integrin protein in the epidermis of the affected animal. In humans, a broad spectrum of clinical and morphological EBJ manifestations exists associated with ITGB4 mutations [8]. They range from non-lethal forms with very mild skin features to severe lethal phenotypes [20]. To date, at least 69 different mutations in human ITGB4 have been reported [21]. Pyloric atresia, which found regularly in humans suffering from the altered synthesis of integrin α6β4, was not detected in either of the affected Charolais calves [8,18].

Conclusions

This study presents a recessively inherited ITGB4 associated EBJ form in cattle. Selection against this candidate causative mutation can now be used to eliminate this genetic disorder from Charolais cattle in production systems. The results obtained showed that current DNA sequencing methods offer a powerful tool for understanding the genetic background of rare diseases in domestic animals with a reference genome sequence available.

Methods

Ethics statement

The study was conducted according to national and international guidelines for animal welfare. Permission was obtained from the cattle owner agreed for the samples to be used in the study. The data were obtained during diagnostic procedures which would have been carried out regardless. This is a very special situation in veterinary medicine. Since the data were from client-owned cattle which underwent veterinary exams, according to the legal definitions in Germany, no "animal experiment" took place.

Histopathological examination

Samples of various locations of the skin, oral mucosa, tongue, brain, lung, heart, muscle, liver, spleen, kidney and intestine were fixed in 10% neutral buffered formalin, embedded in paraffin wax, sectioned at 3 μm, and stained with haematoxylin/eosin according to routine methods. Selected sections were stained with PAS-reaction

Ultrastructural examinantion

For transmission electron microscopy skin and oral mucosa tissue were fixed in 2.5% glutaraldehyde/cacodylate buffer for 24 h, post-fixed in 1% osmium tetroxide, dehydrated in a graded series of alcohol and embedded in epon (Serva, Heidelberg, Germany). Sixty nm thick ultra-thin sections were contrasted with 2% aqueous uranyl acetate and lead citrate and examined with a Zeiss EM 10C electron microscope (Zeiss, Oberkochen, Germany).

Animals and genotyping

Blood samples were taken from the affected animal and from a total of 162 animals belonging to the herd into which the affected calf was born. Genomic DNA was isolated using the DNeasy Blood & Tissue Kit (Qiagen, Hilden, Germany) according to the manufacturer's protocol. In addition, archived DNA samples of 81 Charolais bulls and 50 animals from different cattle breeds were used for genotyping the ITGB4 deletion.

The genotyping of the affected animal was carried out using the BovineHD BeadChip (illumina, San Diego, USA), including 777,961 evenly distributed SNPs and standard protocols as recommended by the manufacturer.

Whole genome sequencing and variant calling

A fragment library with 300 bp insert size was prepared and one lane of illumina HiSeq2000 paired-end reads (2 × 100 bp) were collected. The reads were mapped to the cow reference genome UMD3.1/bosTau6 and aligned using Burrows-Wheeler Aligner (BWA) version 0.5.9-r16 [22] with default settings. The SAM file generated by BWA was then converted to BAM and the reads were sorted by chromosome using samtools [23]. The PCR duplicates were marked using Picard tools [24]. The Genome Analysis Tool Kit (GATK version 2.4.9) [25], was used to carry out local realignment and to produce a cleaned BAM file. Variant calls were then made with the unified genotyper module of GATK. The variant data for each sample were obtained in variant call format (version 4.0) as raw calls for all samples and sites flagged using the variant filtration module of GATK. Variant filtration was performed, following the best practice documentation of GATK version 4. The snpEFF software [26] together with the UMD3.1/bosTau Ensembl annotation was used to predict the functional effects of the variants detected. The pindel package using split-read approaches to identify large deletions and medium-size insertions in pair-end reads was used to detect structural variants in cleaned BAM files [27]. Hence, in order to avoid missing large inserts, deletions and false positives of all the variants detected in the region of EB genes (Additional file 3) were also manually inspected using the Integrative Genomics Viewer (IGV) [28].

The variants of a total of 50 genomes from various cattle breeds (14× Holstein, 6× Simmental, 5× Angler, 4× Brown Swiss, 3× Hinterwalder, 3× Vorderwalder, 2× Galloway, 2× Eringer, 2× Romagnola, 2× Scotish Highland Cattle, 2× Tyrolean Grey Cattle, 1× Hereford, 1× Limousin, 1× Pezzata Rossa Italiana, 2× crossbred), which had been sequenced in our laboratory in the course of other ongoing studies, were used as controls during filtering.

Genetic testing

Primers for the amplification of the deletion were designed using the Primer3 software [29] after masking repetitive sequences with RepeatMasker [30]. The positions of the three primers used for genotyping (fwd

GTGAGGGCTTCGTATGGGTA; rev 1 TGAACGAG GTGTACCGACAA; rev 2 AGTCGCTCTACACGGA CACC) are displayed in Figure 4. Sanger sequencing was used to confirm the illumina sequencing results. For these experiments, PCR products using AmpliTaqGold360 Mastermix (Life Technologies, Darmstadt, Germany) were amplified. The PCR products were loaded on 2% agarose gels for visual inspection of band size. The PCR products were directly sequenced on an ABI3730 capillary sequencer (Life Technologies) after treatment with exonuclease I and shrimp alkaline phosphatase. The sequence data were analysed using Sequencher 5.1 software (GeneCodes, Ann Arbor, USA).

Availability and requirements

The genome data were made available freely at the European Nucleotide Archive [ENA:PRJEB7528] [31]. Further supporting data are included as additional files.

Additional files

Additional file 1: Private exome variants of the affected calf. A list of 981 DNA variants with 1471 predicted effects on annotated genes and loci.

Additional file 2: Sequence details of the disease-associated deletion in the bovine ITGB4 gene. The genomic sequence of the wild-type sequence surrounding the detected mutation on chromosome 19 is displayed. The upper line corresponds to the reference sequence of the UMD3.1 assembly and the lower line to the experimentally verified, shorter sequence. The 4405 bp deletion is indicated by a frame showing the precise breakpoints.

Additional file 3: Candidate genes for epidermolysis bullosa (EB). A list of 18 genes and their annotated position in the bovine genome.

Abbreviations

COL7A1: Collagen 7A1; EB: Epidermolysis bullosa; EBJ: Epidermolysis bullosa junctionalis; ITGB4: Integrin beta 4; KRT5: Keratin 5; OMIA: Online Mendelian Inheritance in Animals; SNP: Single nucleotide polymorphism.

Competing interests

The authors declare that they have no conflicting interests.

Authors' contributions

MP, IR and CD did the experimental work and drafted the manuscript. VJ performed the bioinformatics analysis. BR and PW carried out the histopathology and electron microscopy. IR established the diagnostic gene test. MP and CD supervised the study and carried out the manuscript editing. All authors read and approved the final manuscript.

Acknowledgements

The authors wish to thank Michèle Ackermann and Muriel Fragnière for their invaluable technical assistance. We would like to express our appreciation to the University of Bern for the use of the Next Generation Sequencing Platform in performing the whole genome re-sequencing experiment and the Vital-IT high-performance computing centre of the Swiss Institute of Bioinformatics for carrying out computationally intensive tasks (http://www.vital-it.ch/). We are grateful to the Institute of Veterinary Medicine, University of Göttingen, Germany for providing DNA samples.

Author details

[1]Chemisches und Veterinäruntersuchungsamt Westfalen, Zur Taubeneiche 10-12, 59821 Arnsberg, Germany. [2]Institute of Genetics, Vetsuisse Faculty, University of Bern, Bremgartenstrasse 109a, 3001 Bern, Switzerland. [3]Department of Pathology, University of Veterinary Medicine Hannover, Bünteweg 17, 30559 Hannover, Germany.

References

1. Boycott KM, Vanstone MR, Bulman DE, MacKenzie AE. Rare-disease genetics in the era of next-generation sequencing: discovery to translation. Nat Rev Genet. 2013;14:681–91.
2. Online Mendelian Inheritance in Animals, OMIA. Faculty of Veterinary Science, University of Sydney, World Wide Web URL: http://omia.angis.org.au/
3. Nicolas FW, Hobbs M. Mutation discovery for Mendelian traits in non-laboratory animals: a review of achievements up to 2012. Anim Genet. 2014;45:157–70.
4. Charlier C, Coppieters W, Rollin F, Desmecht D, Agerholm JS, Cambisano N, et al. Highly effective SNP-based association mapping and management of recessive defects in livestock. Nat Genet. 2008;40:449–54.
5. Bovine Genome Sequencing and Analysis Consortium, Elsik CG, Tellam RL, Worley KC, Gibbs RA, Muzny DM, et al. The genome sequence of taurine cattle: a window to ruminant biology and evolution. Science. 2009;324:522–8.
6. Daetwyler HD, Capitan A, Pausch H, Stothard P, van Binsbergen R, Brøndum RF, et al. Whole-genome sequencing of 234 bulls facilitates mapping of monogenic and complex traits in cattle. Nat Genet. 2014;46:858–65.
7. Murgiano L, Jagannathan V, Benazzi C, Bolcato M, Brunetti B, Muscatello LV, et al. Deletion in the EVC2 gene causes chondrodysplastic dwarfism in Tyrolean Grey cattle. PLoS ONE. 2014;9:e94861.
8. Has C, Bruckner-Tuderman L. The genetics of skin fragility. Annu Rev Genomics Hum Genet. 2014;15:245–68.
9. Thompson KG, Crandell RA, Rugeley WW, Sutherland RJ. A mechanobullous disease with sub-basilar separation in Brangus calves. Vet Pathol. 1985;22:283–5.
10. Agerholm JS. Congenital generalized epidermolysis bullosa in a calf. Zentralbl Veterinarmed A. 1994;41:139–42.
11. Stocker H, Lott G, Straumann U, Rüsch P. Epidermolysis bullosa in a calf (German). Tierarztl Prax. 1995;23:123–6.
12. Bähr C, Drögemüller C, Distl O. Epitheliogenesis imperfecta in German Holstein calves (German). Tierarztl Prax. 2004;32:205–11.
13. Ford CA, Stanfield AM, Spelman RJ, Smits B, Ankersmidt-Udy AE, Cottier K, et al. A mutation in bovine keratin 5 causing epidermolysis bullosa simplex, transmitted by a mosaic sire. J Invest Dermatol. 2005;124:1170–6.
14. Foster AP, Skuse AM, Higgins RJ, Barrett DC, Philbey AW, Thomson JR, et al. Epidermolysis bullosa in calves in the United Kingdom. Science Direct. 2010;142:336–40.
15. Medeiros GX, Riet-Correa F, Armién AG, Dantas AF, de Galiza GJ, Simões SV. Junctional epidermolysis bullosa in a calf. J Vet Diagn Invest. 2012;24:231–4.
16. Menoud A, Welle M, Tetens J, Lichtner P, Drögemüller C. A COL7A1 mutation causes dystrophic epidermolysis bullosa in Rotes Höhenvieh cattle. PLoS ONE. 2012;7:e38823.
17. Bruckner-Tuderman L, McGrath JA, Robinson EC, Uitto J. Animal models of epidermolysis bullosa: update 2010. J Invest Dermatol. 2010;130:1485–8.
18. Guaguere E, Berg K, Degorce-Rubioales F, Spadafora A, Meneguzzi G. FC-26 junctional epidermolysis bullosa in a Charolais calf with deficient expression of integrin α6β4. Vet Derm. 2004;15:28.
19. de Pereda JM, Ortega E, Alonso-García N, Gómez-Hernández M, Sonnenberg A. Advances and perspectives of the architecture of hemidesmosomes: lessons from structural biology. Cell Adh Migr. 2009;3:361–4.
20. Schumann H, Kiritsi D, Pigors M, Hausser I, Kohlhase J, Peters J, et al. Phenotypic spectrum of epidermolysis bullosa associated with α6β4 integrin mutations. Br J Dermatol. 2013;169:115–24.
21. Homepage OMIM. [http://omim.org/entry/147557 Accessed 17 October 2014].
22. Li H, Durbin R. Fast and accurate long-read alignment with Burrows-Wheeler transform. Bioinformatics. 2010;26:589–95.
23. Li H, Handsaker B, Wysoker A, Fennell T, Ruan J, Homer N, et al. Durbin R; 1000 Genome Project Data Processing Subgroup. The Sequence Alignment/Map format and SAMtools. Bioinformatics. 2009;25:2078–9.
24. McKenna A, Hanna M, Banks E, Sivachenko A, Cibulskis K, Kernytsky A, et al. The Genome Analysis Toolkit: a MapReduce framework for analyzing next-generation DNA sequencing data. Genome Res. 2010;20:1297–303.
25. Homepage Picard. [http://sourceforge.net/projects/picard/ Accessed 17 October 2014].

26. Cingolani P, Platts A, le Wang L, Coon M, Nguyen T, Wang L, et al. A program for annotating and predicting the effects of single nucleotide polymorphisms, SnpEff: SNPs in the genome of Drosophila melanogaster strain w1118; iso-2; iso-3. Fly (Austin). 2012;6:80–92.

27. Ye K, Schulz MH, Long Q, Apweiler R, Ning Z. Pindel: a pattern growth approach to detect break points of large deletions and medium sized insertions from paired-end short reads. Bioinformatics. 2009;25:2865–71.

28. Thorvaldsdóttir H, Robinson JT, Mesirov JP. Integrative Genomics Viewer (IGV): high-performance genomics data visualization and exploration. Brief Bioinform. 2013;14:178–92.

29. Homepage Primer3. [http://primer3.sourceforge.net. Accessed 17 October 2014].

30. Homepage Repeatmasker. [http://repeatmasker.genome.washington.edu. Accessed 17 October 2014].

31. Homepage European Nucleotide Archive. [http://www.ebi.ac.uk/ena/data/view/PRJEB7528. Accessed 17 October 2014].

7

Livestock trade networks for guiding animal health surveillance

Jo L Hardstaff[1*], Barbara Häsler[2] and Jonathan R Rushton[3]

Abstract

Background: Trade in live animals can contribute to the introduction of exotic diseases, the maintenance and spread endemic diseases. Annually millions of animals are moved across Europe for the purposes of breeding, fattening and slaughter. Data on the number of animals moved were obtained from the Directorate General Sanco (DG Sanco) for 2011. These were converted to livestock units to enable direct comparison across species and their movements were mapped, used to calculate the indegrees and outdegrees of 27 European countries and the density and transitivity of movements within Europe. This provided the opportunity to discuss surveillance of European livestock movement taking into account stopping points en-route.

Results: High density and transitivity of movement for registered equines, breeding and fattening cattle, breeding poultry and pigs for breeding, fattening and slaughter indicates that hazards have the potential to spread quickly within these populations. This is of concern to highly connected countries particularly those where imported animals constitute a large proportion of their national livestock populations, and have a high indegree. The transport of poultry (older than 72 hours) and unweaned animals would require more rest breaks than the movement of weaned animals, which may provide more opportunities for disease transmission. Transitivity is greatest for animals transported for breeding purposes with cattle, pigs and poultry having values of over 50%.

Conclusions: This paper demonstrated that some species (pigs and poultry) are traded much more frequently and at a larger scale than species such as goats. Some countries are more vulnerable than others due to importing animals from many countries, having imported animals requiring rest-breaks and importing large proportions of their national herd or flock. Such knowledge about the vulnerability of different livestock systems related to trade movements can be used to inform the design of animal health surveillance systems to facilitate the trade in animals between European member states.

Keywords: Livestock, European Union, Transport, Surveillance

Background

Animal trade is an effective way of introducing, maintaining and spreading animal diseases, as observed with the spread of different strains of foot and mouth disease (FMD) in Africa, the Middle-East and Asia [1] and the spread of bovine spongiform encephalopathy (BSE), for example into Oman and Canada through the importation of infected cattle [2,3]. Within a year, millions of live animals of many different species are transported between countries within Europe for breeding, fattening,

sports, companionship, conservation and slaughter. This creates opportunities for communicable diseases to be spread across the European Union (EU), which is the focus of this study, even though animals must be in a fit state to be transported i.e. healthy animals without clinical signs of illness [4]. However, animals with sub-clinical infections may go unnoticed, providing an opportunity to transport disease to different regions. Live animal trade complicates tracing the origin of any disease outbreak that may occur due to an infected animal being displaced. For this reason, the EU has established a Trade Control and Expert System (TRACES) to monitor imports, exports and trade in animals and animal products across the EU and to ensure traceability within the food chain [5], in addition to livestock movements recorded by the Food

---

* Correspondence: J.Hardstaff@Liverpool.ac.uk
[1]University of Liverpool- Institute of Infection and Global Health, The Farr Institute@HeRC, 2nd Floor - Block F, Waterhouse building, Liverpool L69 3GL, UK
Full list of author information is available at the end of the article

and Agricultural Organisation of the United Nations (FAO). TRACES records the number of animals and consignments entering and leaving EU countries. Despite the availability of this comprehensive database, animal health surveillance systems are rarely based on international live animal movements. To understand better livestock trade within Europe with a view to inform disease surveillance we analysed trade networks across the EU for all major livestock species and purposes of movements.

Animal health surveillance includes the systematic, continuous or repeated, measurement, collection, collation, analysis, interpretation and timely dissemination of animal health and welfare related data from defined populations, essential for describing health hazard occurrence and to contribute to the planning, implementation and evaluation of risk mitigation measures [6]. Recent outbreaks and spread of exotic or emerging diseases such as avian influenza (AI), Schmallenberg virus (SBV) and bluetongue virus (BTV) in previously unaffected territories of the EU have emphasised the need for well-developed and adequately resourced health systems, including surveillance, to ensure early detection and rapid containment, the complexities of which are highlighted by Braks et al. (2011) [7]. At the same time investment is being constrained due to significant financial budget reductions in many European countries. Livestock disease is important economically with regards to a loss of productivity, its potential impact on human and animal health, and the mitigation activities implemented when disease occurs (for example trade or movement bans, testing and culling). For example, the economic cost of BSE in the UK accrued from the value loss in infected carcasses, disposal costs, and, most importantly, the sharp drop in domestic beef demand due to consumer scares (sales of beef products declined by 40% once the possible link between BSE and new variant Creutzfeldt-Jakob disease (CJD) was announced, but the costs were partly offset by an increase in consumption of substitute meat), and a complete loss in export markets [8]. Further costs accrued from operating various public schemes, establishment and enforcement of new legislation and the adjustment of the industry to the new structure and markets [8]. Livestock disease can be spread directly for example the introduction of FMD from Irish calves imported to the Netherlands that were also held responsible for the infection of a farm near to the port of introduction to mainland Europe [9]. It can be spread by infected equipment, crates or transporter vehicles which can be contaminated by microbes. For example *Escherichia coli* (*E. coli*) bacteria were detected on the sides and floors of lorries [10] and contaminated transporters were found to be responsible for spreading classical swine fever to different farms in Lithuania [11]. By moving animals with latent or asymptomatic infections this enables disease to spread to wherever the animal travels or where the

necessary vectors may be present. Particularly in the case of epidemic diseases where the reduction of time from introduction of a hazard to its detection can enable early response and thereby lead to a reduction in intervention costs to contain an outbreak [12], effective surveillance is critical. Few surveillance systems however, are designed based on international livestock movement data, even though such data can provide information on the quantity and seasonality of livestock movements, the types of movement (for example flows from production of point of lay birds to laying units), the route the animals take and associated stopover or resting points. Surveillance for many livestock species occurs at the farm where it is the responsibility of the farmer (and veterinarian) to report notifiable diseases or at the abattoir where it is the role of the official veterinarian to inspect livestock according to Council Regulation (EC) 854/2004 [13] and report notifiable diseases to the national authorities, which in the UK is the Department of the Environment, Food and Rural Affairs (DEFRA), which in turn must inform the European Food Safety Authority (EFSA) as stated in Council Regulation (EC) 178/2002 [14].

Network analyses are useful ways of visualising the countries that are importing animals from a great number of other countries (high level of indegree) and countries that are exporting to a high number of countries (outdegree), these are values that can change temporally. They have been used to find out movement between farms of different species, for example, fish movement between farms in Scotland [15] and a study of pig and cattle movement between farms in Sweden [16]. Countries with a high indegree, which for the purposes of this study has a maximum number of 27 (the number of countries, i.e. (nodes, within this study and the EU as of 2011) that could be used to rank countries, can be more vulnerable to introducing disease due to importing animals from a greater number of countries than those with a low indegree whilst countries with a high outdegree may have a great ability to be able to transmit a disease to many countries; this highlights the importance of understanding levels of disease within trading countries. Information about the indegree and outdegree of farms was used by Frössling et al. (2012) [17] to investigate whether it could be used to target the surveillance of two cattle diseases in Sweden, based on a threshold of in- and out-degrees. They found a positive association between a positive test result and the purchase of animals and proposed approaches to design risk-based surveillance based on cattle movement data. Networks can also be used to quantify the proportion of international partners trading with each other (dyadic contacts) compared with the maximum number of national trading partners available for trade within an area allowing a comparison to be made between species and production systems [16]. The higher the density the more connected countries are with respect to the animal being traded and the more countries that may be at risk from contracting a disease from buying in infected livestock. A measure of mixing within a network is to look at its transitivity which indicates whether countries that a country is trading animals to are also trading animals with each other (a triad) [18]. The greater the level of transitivity the faster a disease can spread between countries and potentially infect many countries within the European area [19]. Transitivity and density for different communities of wild and domestic ungulates were investigated for the propensity to transmit *E. coli* by VanderWaal et al. (2014) [20]. However, the network may only consider the point of origin and destination and not necessarily consider the route itself that may involve briefly stopping in other countries where a disease transmission event may occur, for example FMD in France [9].

We hypothesise that the description of trade networks can inform the design of more efficient animal health surveillance systems that may enable a more rapid investigation or response to be implemented. Different species being transported for different purposes will have networks of different densities and different countries with the greatest indegree or outdegree. The aim of this project was to map live animal trade networks in EU countries and assess potential differences between species and purposes of transport. This was done by illustrating the number of live animal imports and exports between 27 EU countries including the number of country contacts and numbers of livestock units (LSU, a unit that takes into account the age, sex, purpose of animals with dairy cows having a reference number of 1) moved determining the density of networks and similarities of networks between species.

Results

Table 1 illustrates the median livestock intra-community movements (expressed in livestock units) and the densities of the transport networks. By far the most heavily moved animal species within Europe in 2011 were poultry for slaughter and breeding, followed by poultry for 'other' purposes, pigs for fattening, pigs for slaughter and cattle for fattening; goats were the least traded species. Generally more LSUs were transported for fattening than for slaughter.

The density of movement (Table 1) shows that there was greater connectivity for cattle than for the heavily traded poultry. Breeding networks were found to be denser than those for other purposes. This may be due to the number of consignments needed to move the relative units of animals. The geographical trade flows are shown in Figures 1, 2, 3, 4, 5 and 6. The transitivity indicates that disease would spread more slowly for 'other' purposes of animal movement than for breeding,

Table 1 The median and interquartile range of livestock units (LSU) being transported within the Europe Union for different purposes, the density and transitivity of each transport network

Trade purpose	LSU median (IQR)	Density	Transitivity
Cattle breeding	207 (34–947.5)	0.35	0.64
Cattle fattening	1267 (203–8283)	0.23	0.56
Cattle slaughter	647 (138.8-5381)	0.13	0.56
Cattle other	15 (3–115.5)	0.08	0.28
Pig breeding	86.5 (10–964)	0.24	0.62
Pig fattening	1762 (227.1-8923)	0.13	0.58
Pig slaughter	1433 (175.5-12260)	0.17	0.62
Pig other	7.8 (0.6-41.4)	0.06	0.36
Sheep breeding	6.1 (1.25-26.05)	0.16	0.47
Sheep fattening	130.7 (30–589.4)	0.11	0.44
Sheep slaughter	113.2 (32.33-564.2)	0.11	0.44
Sheep other	5.3 (0.35-46.75)	0.05	0.22
Goat breeding	1.8 (0.4-8.2)	0.09	0.34
Goat fattening	20.7 (3.25-53)	0.03	0.18
Goat slaughter	31.2 (5.1-255.2)	0.03	0.30
Goat other	0.4 (0.22-2.875)	0.03	0.25
Poultry breeding	2152 (376.6-13760)	0.24	0.55
Poultry slaughter	2645 (549.9-26530)	0.1	0.43
Poultry other	1570 (303.3-7353)	0.2	0.50
Equine breeding	4.4 (1.6-21)	0.17	0.49
Equine registered	9.6 (2.8-39.6)	0.45	0.67
Equine slaughter	145.6 (8.4-458)	0.05	0.31
Equine other	7.2 (1.6-37.2)	0.21	0.58

fattening or slaughter with the exception of poultry and equines.

Figures 1, 2, 3, 4, 5 and 6 show the in- and outdegrees of livestock unit movements in the EU on the left and the geographical trade flows in the right, which are separated by species and by purpose of trade. The axes of the graphs of the in- and outdegrees reflect the numbers of trading partners. The countries in the top right received and exported animals with the greatest number of countries, whilst the bottom left indicates those that have little or no export or import trade with other countries. Some countries are found in the top right corner with regards to many different animal movements e.g. Germany, whilst others rarely buy or sell to the other 26 countries considered in this study e.g. Cyprus, Finland and Sweden, whilst other countries import from many countries and export to few e.g. Italy.

Very few shipments of weaned cattle, sheep and goats require a rest period of 24 hours (Additional file 1), whereas many unweaned animals would require a 24 hour break in their journey from their point of origin to their

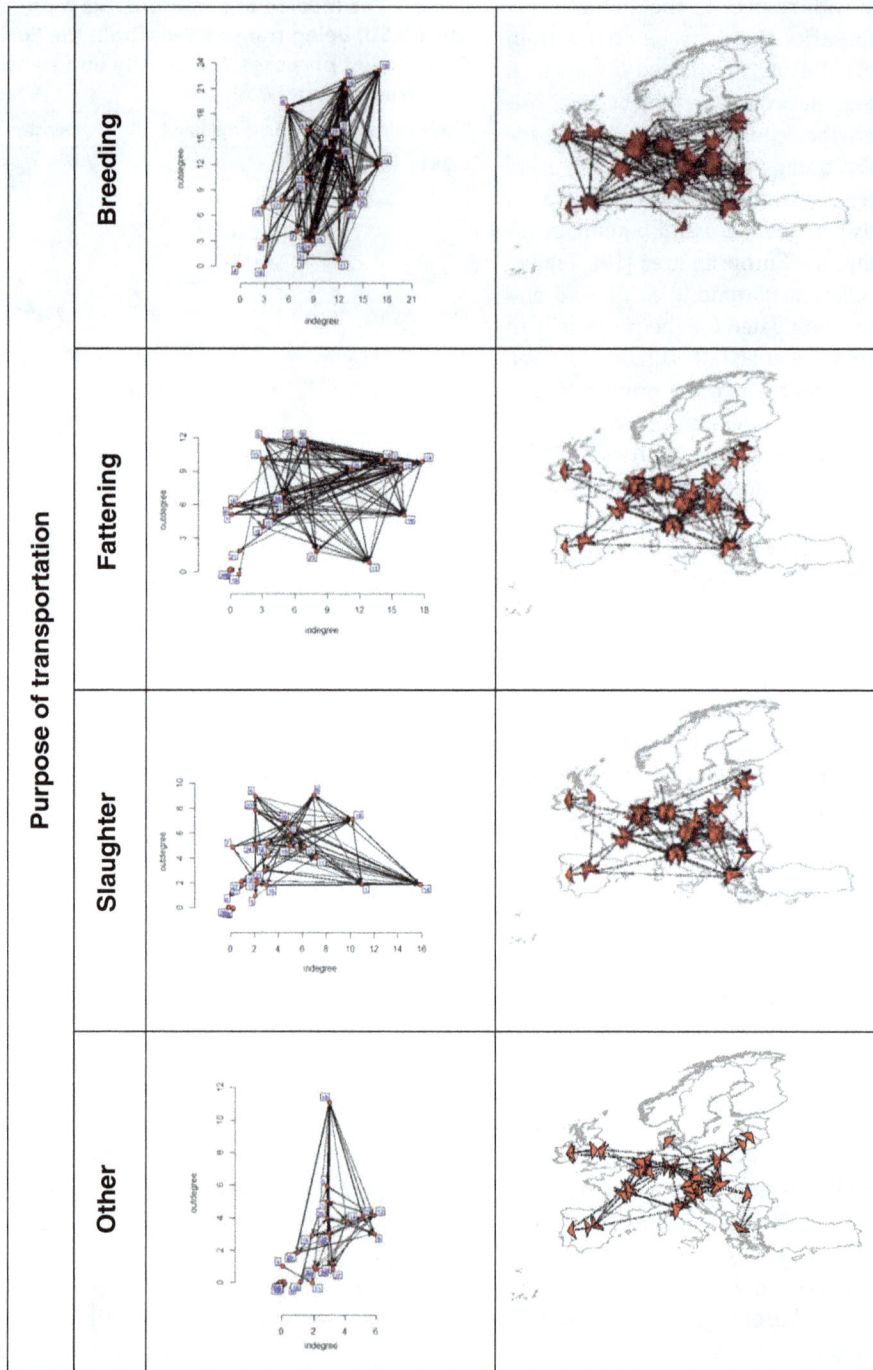

Figure 1 The outdegree is shown against the indegree for the trade of cattle for different purposes on the left column of the table and the geographical movement across Europe is shown on the right column of the table. The arrows between the countries indicate trade between the countries. The numbers in the figures refer to the corresponding countries: [1] Austria, [2] Belgium, [3] Bulgaria, [4] Cyprus, [5] Czech Republic, [6] Denmark, [7] Estonia, [8] Finland, [9] France, [10] Germany, [11] Greece, [12] Hungary, [13] Ireland, [14] Italy, [15] Lithuania, [16] Latvia, [17] Luxembourg, [18] Malta, [19] Netherlands, [20] Poland, [21] Portugal, [22] Romania, [23] Slovakia, [24] Slovenia, [25] Spain, [26] Sweden and [27] UK.

final destination (Additional file 2) as would most journeys of poultry 72 hours after hatching (Additional file 3).

The proportion of national populations imported and exported could be calculated for all species except equines for which there was no data for the year 2011 (Additional file 4). Goats were the species where imports and exports were a low proportion of the national population in comparison with pigs where many countries were importing

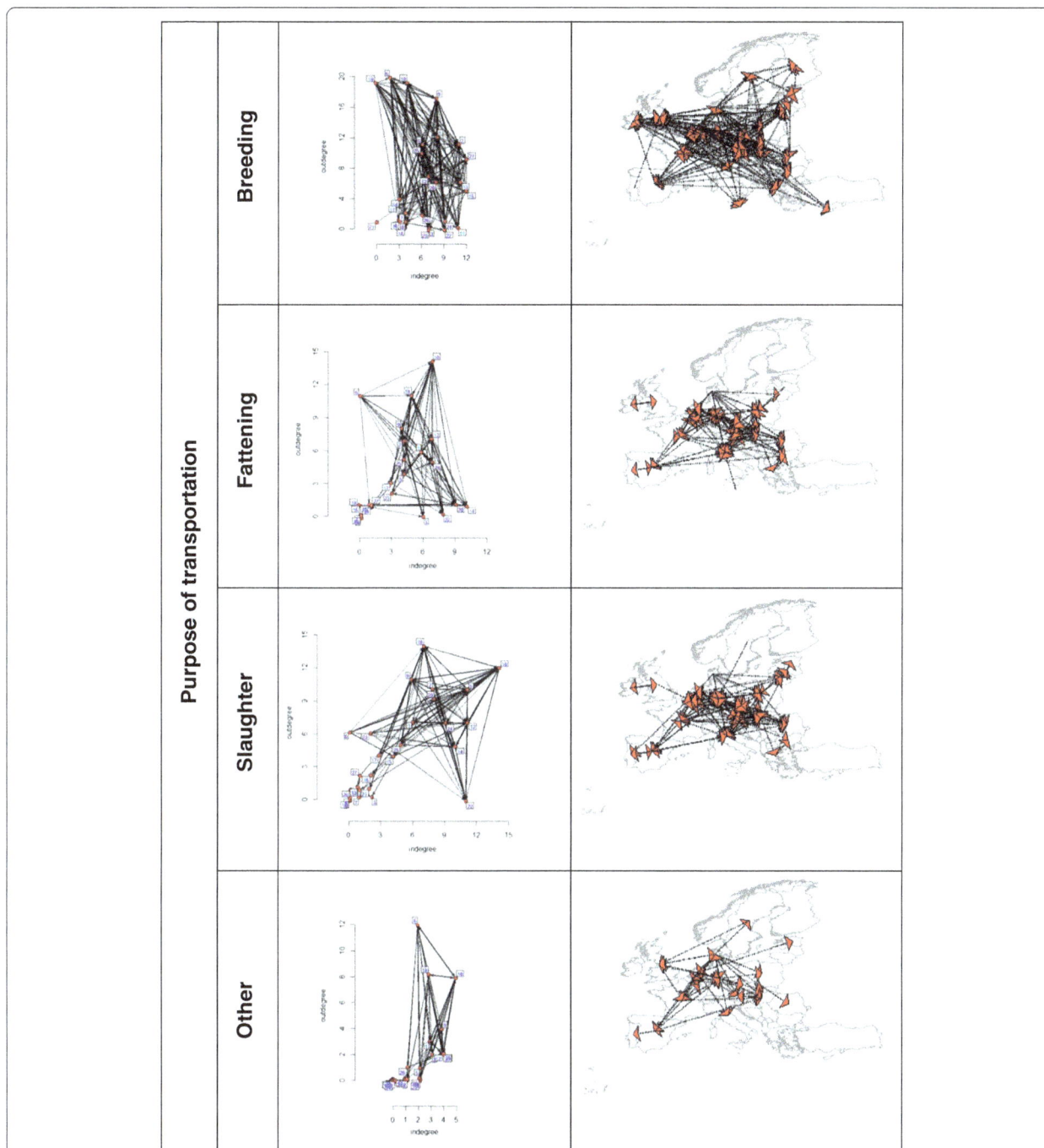

Figure 2 The outdegree is shown against the indegree for the trade of pigs for different purposes on the left column of the table and the geographical movement across Europe is shown on the right column of the table. The arrows between the countries indicate trade between the countries. The numbers in the figures refer to the corresponding countries: [1] Austria, [2] Belgium, [3] Bulgaria, [4] Cyprus, [5] Czech Republic, [6] Denmark, [7] Estonia, [8] Finland, [9] France, [10] Germany, [11] Greece, [12] Hungary, [13] Ireland, [14] Italy, [15] Lithuania, [16] Latvia, [17] Luxembourg, [18] Malta, [19] Netherlands, [20] Poland, [21] Portugal, [22] Romania, [23] Slovakia, [24] Slovenia, [25] Spain, [26] Sweden and [27] UK.

and exporting high proportions of their national population, the officially recorded number of animals of that species in the particular country.

Discussion

The poultry and pig sectors had the greatest number of LSU movements, which are being used to indicate

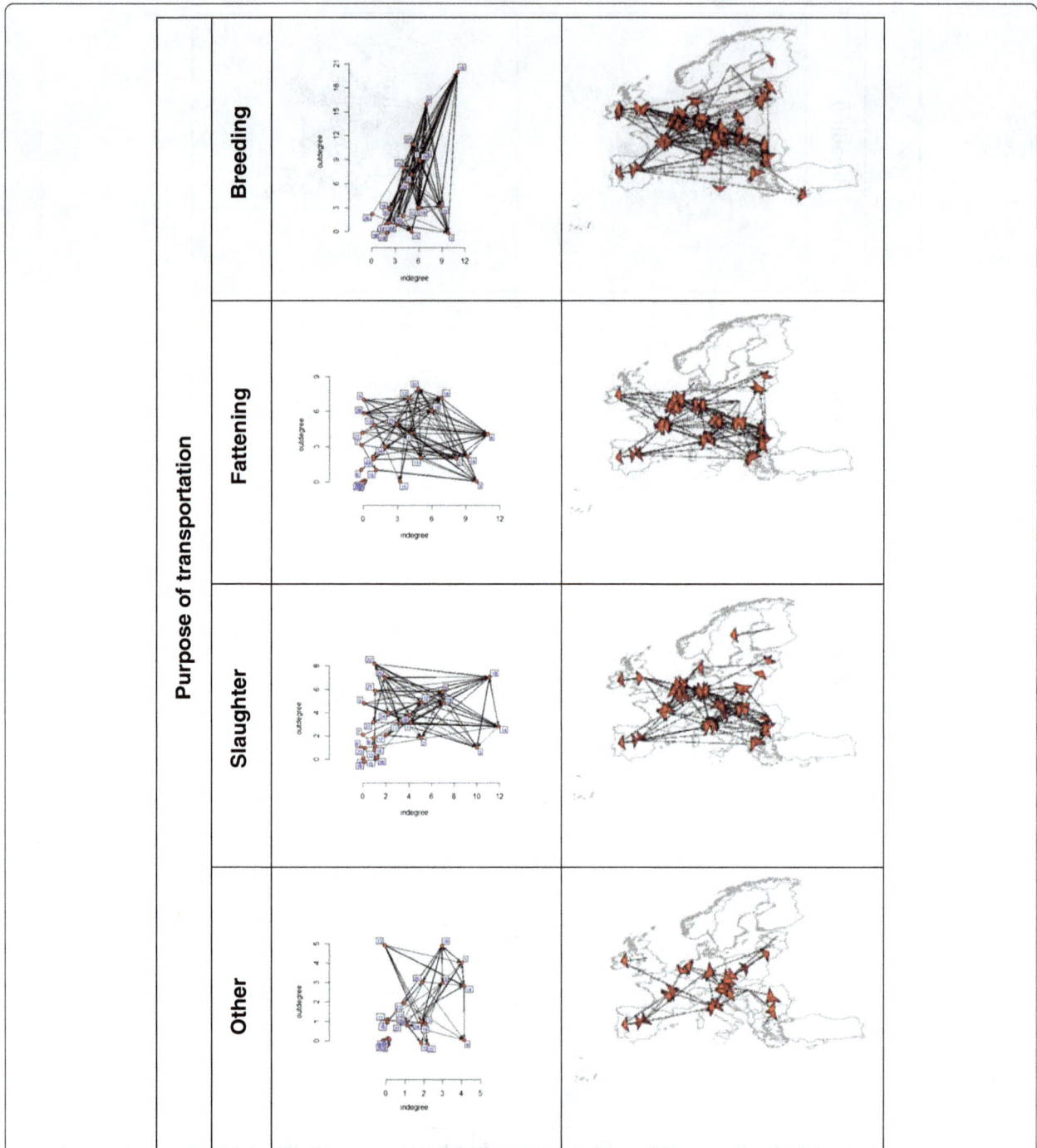

Figure 3 The outdegree is shown against the indegree for the trade of sheep for different purposes on the left column of the table and the geographical movement across Europe is shown on the right column of the table. The arrows between the countries indicate trade between the countries. The numbers in the figures refer to the corresponding countries: [1] Austria, [2] Belgium, [3] Bulgaria, [4] Cyprus, [5] Czech Republic, [6] Denmark, [7] Estonia, [8] Finland, [9] France, [10] Germany, [11] Greece, [12] Hungary, [13] Ireland, [14] Italy, [15] Lithuania, [16] Latvia, [17] Luxembourg, [18] Malta, [19] Netherlands, [20] Poland, [21] Portugal, [22] Romania, [23] Slovakia, [24] Slovenia, [25] Spain, [26] Sweden and [27] UK.

the potential opportunities of pathogen introduction and spread, implying that they require more attention in terms of disease prevention and management, while the equine and goat sectors had the greatest and lowest densities of movements respectively. In addition to LSU movements larger proportions of national pig populations are imported

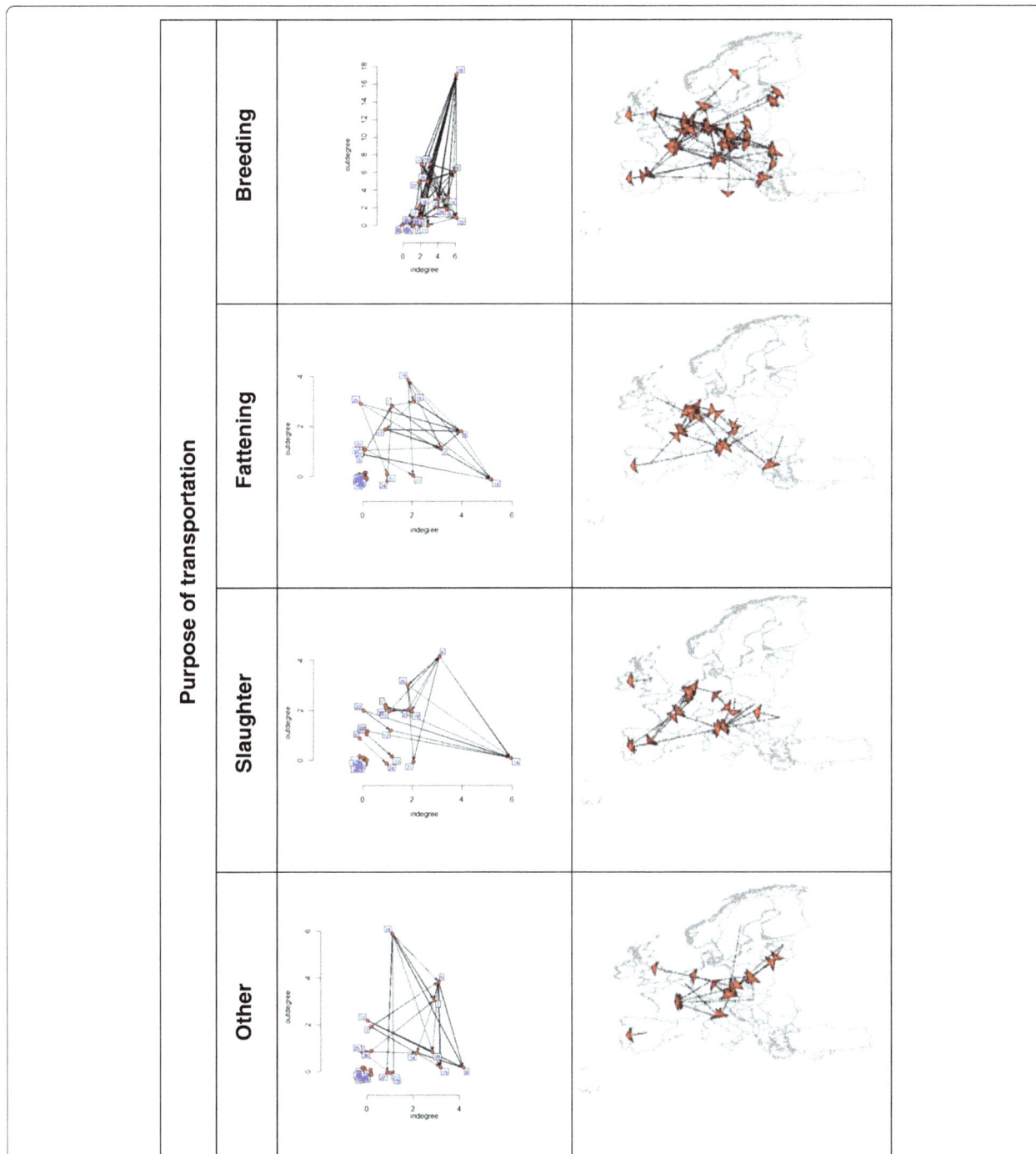

Figure 4 The outdegree is shown against the indegree for the trade of goats for different purposes on the left column of the table and the geographical movement across Europe is shown on the right column of the table. The arrows between the countries indicate trade between the countries. The numbers in the figures refer to the corresponding countries: [1] Austria, [2] Belgium, [3] Bulgaria, [4] Cyprus, [5] Czech Republic, [6] Denmark, [7] Estonia, [8] Finland, [9] France, [10] Germany, [11] Greece, [12] Hungary, [13] Ireland, [14] Italy, [15] Lithuania, [16] Latvia, [17] Luxembourg, [18] Malta, [19] Netherlands, [20] Poland, [21] Portugal, [22] Romania, [23] Slovakia, [24] Slovenia, [25] Spain, [26] Sweden and [27] UK.

compared with species such as goats increasing the possibility for the introduction of infected animals to an existing population. For poultry, the highest numbers of LSUs moved were for slaughter, which may present less of a risk

of introducing disease to an existing population, as the animals are likely to be transported from the production site directly to the slaughter point. However, many poultry journeys would require a break in transit emphasising the

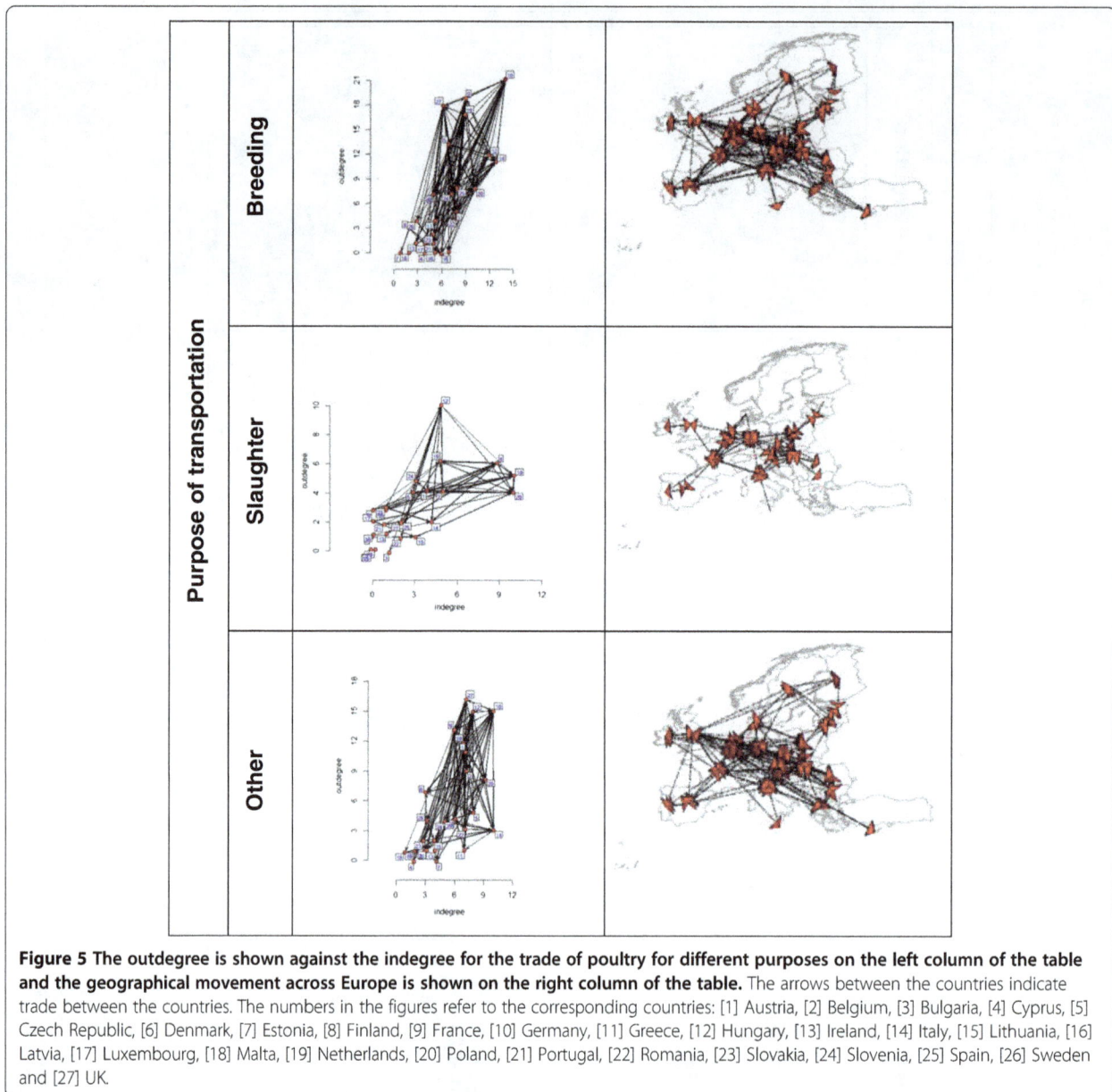

Figure 5 The outdegree is shown against the indegree for the trade of poultry for different purposes on the left column of the table and the geographical movement across Europe is shown on the right column of the table. The arrows between the countries indicate trade between the countries. The numbers in the figures refer to the corresponding countries: [1] Austria, [2] Belgium, [3] Bulgaria, [4] Cyprus, [5] Czech Republic, [6] Denmark, [7] Estonia, [8] Finland, [9] France, [10] Germany, [11] Greece, [12] Hungary, [13] Ireland, [14] Italy, [15] Lithuania, [16] Latvia, [17] Luxembourg, [18] Malta, [19] Netherlands, [20] Poland, [21] Portugal, [22] Romania, [23] Slovakia, [24] Slovenia, [25] Spain, [26] Sweden and [27] UK.

vulnerability of the chain and need for adequate surveillance. Poultry for breeding had the second highest LSU movements overall, which likely reflects the current structure of commercial poultry production. Pure line grandparent and parent stock for breeding are produced by only a limited number of breeding organisations worldwide. For example, the two companies Aviagen and Cobb, have a market share of more than 85% of the commercial broilers produced in the EU and use their global network of distributors to serve almost all European countries [21]. The breeder farms supplied with young breeding stock have links to hatcheries that produce day old chicks, broiler or layer farms, and slaughterhouses. This system leads to transport of

young breeders, hatching eggs and day old chicks. In pigs, heavy movements were recorded for fattening, which reflects ongoing changes in production centres in the EU. In fact, more than two thirds of breeding pigs are produced in Denmark, Germany, Spain, France, the Netherlands and Poland with half of the breeding pigs at regional level being concentrated in eleven regions in these six countries [22]. Germany is the main importer of fattening pigs, with an indegree of 7 and Denmark is the main exporter with an outdegree of 11. Moreover, pigs for breeding and fattening as well as poultry for breeding were shown to have among the highest transitivities, indicating that disease spread in these networks would be fast if uncontained. Hence, solely taking into

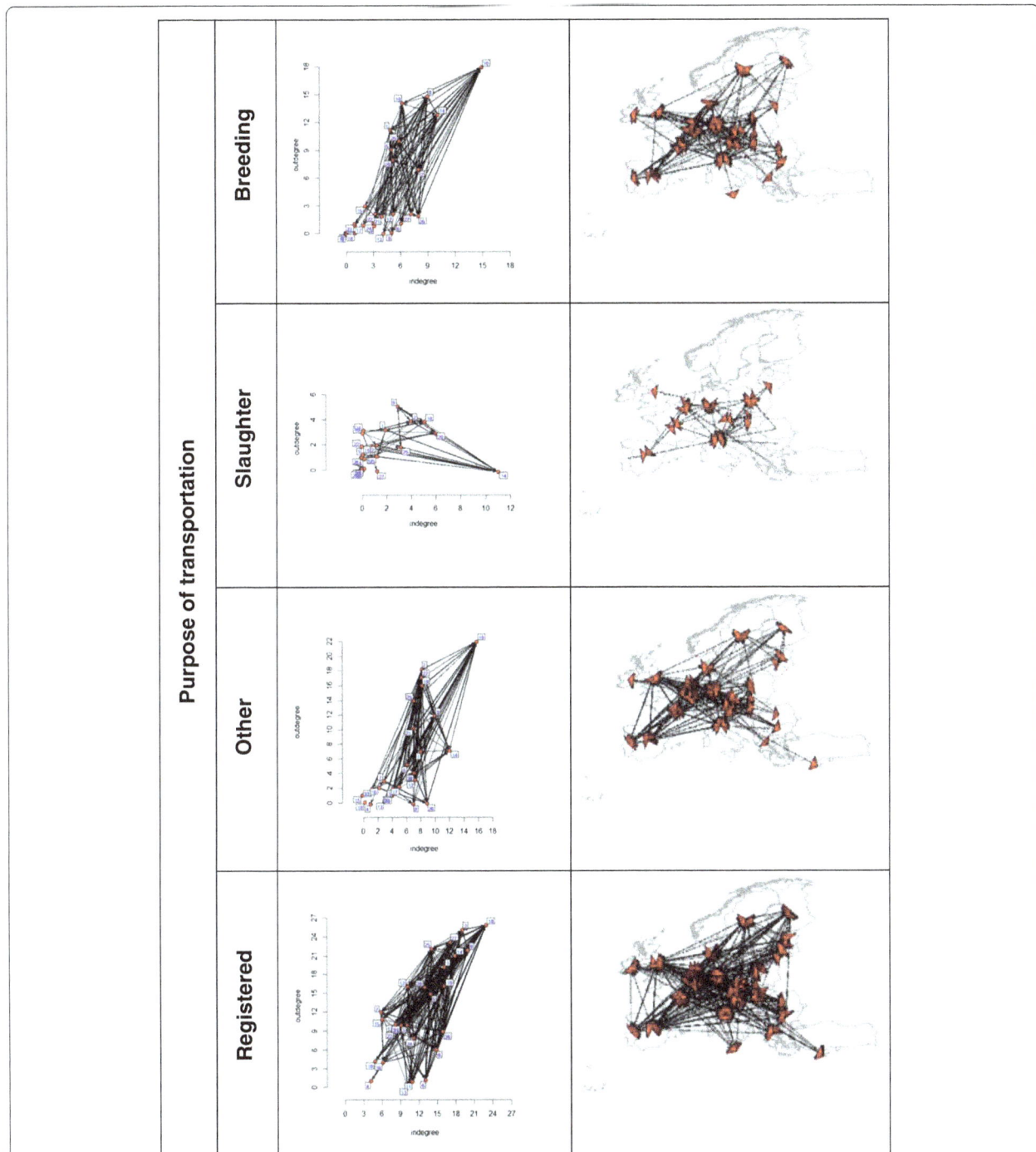

Figure 6 The outdegree is shown against the indegree for the trade of equines for different purposes on the left column of the table and the geographical movement across Europe is shown on the right column of the table. The arrows between the countries indicate trade between the countries. The numbers in the figures refer to the corresponding countries: [1] Austria, [2] Belgium, [3] Bulgaria, [4] Cyprus, [5] Czech Republic, [6] Denmark, [7] Estonia, [8] Finland, [9] France, [10] Germany, [11] Greece, [12] Hungary, [13] Ireland, [14] Italy, [15] Lithuania, [16] Latvia, [17] Luxembourg, [18] Malta, [19] Netherlands, [20] Poland, [21] Portugal, [22] Romania, [23] Slovakia, [24] Slovenia, [25] Spain, [26] Sweden and [27] UK.

account trade data, surveillance efforts would need to focus on poultry for breeding and pigs for breeding and fattening. However, a mapping of surveillance in seven European countries showed that the highest proportion of surveillance components in place were for cattle [23]. Similarly, a recent literature review on animal health issues (including zoonoses) researched in the EU showed that cattle and buffalo were the species most frequently studied in the EU [24]; this may reflect differ-ences in resource allocation for surveillance and disease mitigation. The reasons for this may be that cattle harbour or are perceived to harbour more pathogens than other species, that outbreaks in cattle systems have higher impact, that cattle receives more attention than other species for cultural or historical reasons, or that disease prevention and management in cattle systems are of lower quality. Currently, there are no multi-pathogen, multi-species systematic risk assessments available at EU level that would allow a comparison of these factors. Breeding networks were found to be more highly connected with more trade between countries indicating disease may spread more easily through them. This is of concern as these animals are not intended to be slaugh-tered on arrival and will produce new animals, therefore stringent precautions are needed to protect these popula-tions, particularly if they are diseases not covered by EU legislation, for example the diseases listed in Council Regulation (EC) 722/2013 [25]. The density of inter-national agri-trade calculated by Ercsey-Ravasz et al. (2012) [26] was 0.33 which was comparable with density of many networks in this study. However, in national networks the densities and transitivities are smaller, which are due to the greater number of farms involved in national animal production compared with the number of countries involved in this study. The cattle trade network in France had a very low annual level of transitivity indicat-ing that disease spread would be slower than that between European countries [27]. The pig and cattle networks in Sweden had lower transitivities than international net-works of these species [16] as did the transitivity of pig movements in Denmark [28] and the UK [29].

The location of countries in Figures 1, 2, 3, 4, 5 and 6 gave an indication of where surveillance could be targeted with countries in the upper right quadrant both importing and exporting high numbers of LSU, which means that they need to monitor both production to export healthy animals and import processes to avoid introduction of disease. Countries in the lower right quadrant may need to consider strengthening surveillance related to import processes. Many national studies have found that the majority of animal movements are between premises with lower indegrees and outdegrees as shown in a study by Smith et al. 2013 [29], this reduces the likelihood of disease transmission to many different areas, reducing the level of surveillance needed. Many countries trading cattle were found to have an in or out degree equal or greater than five. This was the threshold that was calculated to require enhanced surveillance for bovine coronavirus in a study on trade and cattle in Sweden by Frössling et al. 2012 [17]. Consequently, there seems to be ample opportunity to take advantage of trade network data to enhance surveillance. The evolution of trade networks over time at the EU level

could be monitored using indegrees, outdegrees, and transi-tivity. Such monitoring would provide information at the systems level and allow observations of changes in net-works over time and where consequent surveillance efforts should be focused. Higher-level surveillance capturing trends or changes in trade patterns could complement existing surveillance systems that are commonly disease centered. The differences across countries in terms of inde-grees and outdegrees also bring up the question of who has the responsibility for disease control, including surveillance – the buyer, the seller or relevant food business operator depending on the stage of livestock production [30]. While the draft new EU Animal Health Law [31] refers to listed diseases and pre-dominantly supports disease centered surveillance, it also creates a framework for the better use of the synergies between surveillance undertaken by the different actors in the field to ensure the most effective and cost efficient use of surveillance resources as well as pro-motion of data availability and facilitation of data exchange.

Transportation itself is stressful for animals as indicated in many studies in many species for example cortisol in pigs [32]; heart rate and cortisol in cattle [33]; cortisol in lambs [34]; cortisol in horses [35]; increasing susceptibility to disease and may enhance the likelihood of shedding pathogenic agents in transit or in the receiving country, which may lead to infection in other animals. It is common to refer to malaise post-transportation as shipping illness [36]. However, pathogens may be introduced or spread from transporters and not just from the animals that they transport. Studies have demonstrated that transporters need to be thoroughly cleaned to prevent them from acting as a source of pathogens to subsequently carried animals, for example to prevent transmission of porcine reproduct-ive and respiratory syndrome virus, that can survive in transporters, being transferred to pigs [37]. Rest stops are infrequent for some species, however, if animals from more than one origin are rested in the same place it may allow for disease spread. This is most likely to impact animals traded for breeding and fattening purposes that have more LSUs and are more highly connected than animals already at slaughter weight. These are animals that will live in the receiving country for a period of time that may enable pathogen transfer. Many of the highly connected countries (with high in and out degrees in the top right of Figures 1, 2, 3, 4, 5 and 6) for example Germany are geographically located in an area (Central Europe) that minimises the distances and therefore time that animals have to travel reducing the need for rest breaks and the consequent potential for pathogen transfer. Many of the long distances are from countries that rarely trade with mainland Europe for example Cyprus. Many animals undergo long journeys between countries. The time in transit is a concern with regards of the potential for disease to spread along trade routes [9].

This has implications for policy around the planning of livestock production and slaughter. Ideally, large production facilities would not be placed adjacent to well-known and used trade routes and or resting points. However, such information is only of use to policy makers if it is captured in a systematic and continuous way allowing to monitor trends, change and modify policies accordingly if deemed necessary.

Limitations

The analyses have only considered the spatial aspect of trade and not taken into account temporal variations that may occur altering the relationships between the countries (nodes) and the respective network, and affect the likelihood of an animal being infectious with a disease. Animal populations fluctuate within a year and the population recorded in December was used to calculate the proportion of animals being imported or exported into a country, therefore it may have under or overestimated the actual population at the time of movement. For example the majority of lambs are born between January and April increasing the sheep population until they reach slaughter weight and are culled, which occurs before December. Networks are highly dynamic and these changes in movements between countries will need to be considered by surveillance programs using this approach. One method that may address this is to use exponential random graph models that can incorporate a range of different distributions of connectivity between the nodes to create many different networks, which can be compared with the data to find a model that best fits the current trade pattern [38].

The distances that animals are transported between countries may be shorter or longer than the distances between centroids. In addition, there are many different routes across Europe that may be used and this may be worth investigating in future analyses with regards to distance, time and mixing between countries. This means that our calculations for whether particular species need a rest break for movement between particular countries are generalised so that there may be fewer or greater numbers of animals being rested en-route to their destination country altering the potential for pathogen exposure.

The analyses did not take into account the numbers of convoys or animals and the mixing of animals: from different farms per convoy, at resting places, at borders, when received by individuals and at markets in the country of destination. These factors will have an impact on contact between potentially naïve and infectious animals, pathogen exposure and susceptibility.

The analyses could not take into animals being bought and sold on to more than one country i.e. the chain of infection [16] and assumed that an animal moved once between countries in its lifetime.

Conclusions

Creating networks has enabled us to visualise the countries that have a higher level of involvement in animal trade. Using network analysis we were able to determine the extent to which a disease may spread, the production systems where disease spread may be more rapid, for example registered horses and breeding cattle, pigs and poultry, and facilitates comparisons with networks in other areas. Similarities between countries, species and production purposes has the potential to inform international surveillance policies that take into account trade patterns. The study has highlighted the vulnerability of the pig network to disease, which is of increasing concern due to the proximity of African Swine Fever to the EU and the potential for wildlife to introduce the disease [11]. This information could complement the national movement recording systems that are mandatory for cattle throughout the EU [39] that will soon be implemented in sheep and goats now that their form of identification tags have been decided upon [40], and being planned for porcines [41] to produce a more robust surveillance plan.

Methods

Data on numbers of live cattle, goats, horses, pigs, poultry and sheep movements in 27 EU countries were obtained from Directorate General Sanco Animal Health DG Sanco unit G2 activity report for the year 2011 obtained from http://ec.europa.eu/food/animal/resources/publications_en.htm. The data obtained related to the production purpose of the animals, which fell into five categories: breeding, fattening, slaughter, registered and other (e.g. pets, show animals). These categories were analysed separately and combined for each species.

The numbers of animals were converted into livestock units to enable comparison between species using the following conversion factors derived from the Eurostat glossary on statistics (2013) [42]: pigs 0.5 (breeding), pigs 0.3 (other), goats 0.1, sheep 0.1, horses 0.8 and poultry 0.014. All data were obtained at a national level from publically accessible databases and no animal experimentation occurred nor consultation with animal owners therefore ethical approval was not needed.

All the analyses and associated network figures were created and carried out using R 3.0.1. [43]. Networks were created from adjacency matrices and their densities were calculated using network function found in R package Network [44]. The in and out degrees were calculated and respective graphs were produced using the degree and network.layout.degree functions in R package Network [44]. The transitivity of each network was calculated using the gtrans function in the SNA package [45]. Trade maps in the Figures 1, 2, 3, 4, 5 and 6 were produced by merging shapefiles of all the countries of Europe downloaded from maplibrary.org (www.gadm.org/, 2010, gadm version 9) into one polygon (Europe) using ArcGIS 10.1 [46]. The map of Europe was then read into R using the function readShapePoly found in the Maptools package [47]. Centroids (the co-ordinates for the centre of a country) were calculated for each country and linked with respective importing and exporting countries were calculated using the calcCentroid function in R package PBSmapping [48]. Curved lines and arrows were drawn between the centroids for each movement using the gcIntermediate function found in the geosphere package [49].

To be able to relate the numbers of animals being traded with the animal populations of the countries, the numbers of animals of each species were obtained for 2011 from the Eurostat database. The data used was for December as this was the only calendar month available for all species. A movement:standing population ratio was calculated for both animal imports and exports through adding the total number of breeding, fattening, slaughter, registered and other animals being moved and dividing by the total population of animals of that species in the exporting or importing country.

To illustrate the number of animal journeys that require 24 hour rest periods during transit, distances that animals would have to travel were approximated by estimating arc distances from one capital city to the other using www.timeanddate.com. The time in transit before animals are required to have a 24 hour rest period were obtained from Council Regulation EC 1/2005 [4]. The Regulation states that unweaned cattle, goats, sheep, pigs and horses require a 24 hour rest period after 18 hours of travel. Weaned cattle, goats and sheep can be in transit for 28 hours without a rest, whereas weaned pigs and domestic horses need to be rested after 24 hours of transportation. Any animal being transported by boat should be rested for 12 hours at the port after being unloaded. The law for poultry and rabbits states that they can travel for up to 12 hours without food or water and whereas chicks within 72 hours of hatching can travel for up to 24 hours without food or water. To gauge whether a journey between two rest points would need a break the following equation was used given the assumption that a vehicle would be travelling at an average 80 kilometres an hour.

$$24 \text{ hour rest period} = \frac{Distance\ between\ cities}{Duration\ of\ travel\ before\ 24\ hours\ rest\ period * 80\ km/h}$$

Additional files

Additional file 1: Journeys that would require rest breaks due to being over 28 hours long or over 24 hours long. These data are displayed in tables.

Additional file 2: Journeys that would require rest breaks for unweaned animals. The data are displayed in a table.

Additional file 3: Journeys that would require rest breaks for poultry other than chicks <72 hours old. The data are displayed in a table.

Additional file 4: The proportions of national animal imports and exports compared with the national population. These data are displayed in separate tables for each species.

Abbreviations
AI: Avian influenza; BSE: Bovine spongiform encephalopathy; BTV: Bluetongue virus; EU: European Union; FAO: Food and Agricultural Organisation of the United Nations; FMD: Foot and mouth disease; IQR: Interquartile range; LSU: Livestock units; SBV: Schmallenberg virus; TRACES: Trade Control and Expert System.

Competing interests
The authors declare that they have no competing interests.

Authors' contributions
JH obtained the data and undertook the analyses. JH, BH and JR interpreted the results and had an equal contribution to the manuscript. All authors have read and approved the final manuscript.

Acknowledgements
BH acknowledges financial support from the Leverhulme Centre for Integrative Research on Agriculture and Health (LCIRAH).

Author details
[1]University of Liverpool- Institute of Infection and Global Health, The Farr Institute@HeRC, 2nd Floor - Block F, Waterhouse building, Liverpool L69 3GL, UK. [2]Leverhulme Centre for Integrative Research on Agriculture and Health, Royal Veterinary College, Hawkshead Lane, North Mymms, Hatfield, Hertfordshire AL9 7TA, UK. [3]Department of Production and Population Health, Royal Veterinary College, Hawkshead Lane, North Mymms, Hatfield, Hertfordshire AL9 7TA, UK.

References
1. Di Nardo A, Knowles NJ, Paton DJ. Combining livestock trade patterns with phylogenetics to help understand the spread of foot and mouth disease in sub-Saharan Africa, the Middle East and Southeast Asia. Rev Sci Tech. 2011;30:63–85.
2. Carolan DJ, Wells GA, Wilesmith JW. BSE in Oman. Vet Rec. 1990;126:92.
3. Chen SS, Charlton KM, Balachandran AV, O'Connor BP, Jenson CC. Bovine spongiform encephalopathy identified in a cow imported to Canada from the United Kingdom–a case report. Can Vet J. 1996;37:38–40.
4. European Union Council Regulation (EC) 1/2005. The protection of animals during transport and related operations and amending Directives 64/432/EEC and 93/119/EC and Regulation (EC) No 1255/97. Off J Eur Union. 2005; L3/1:1–44.
5. European Union Council Regulation (EC) 623/2003. Commision decision of 19 August 2003 concerning the development of an integrated computerised veterinary system known as Traces. Off J Eur Union. 2003; L216:58–9.
6. Hoinville LJ, Alban L, Drewe JA, Gibbens JC, Gustafson L, Häsler B, et al. Proposed terms and concepts for describing and evaluating animal-health surveillance systems. Prev Vet Med. 2013;112:1–12.
7. Braks M, van der Giessen J, Kretzschmar M, van Pelt W, Scholte E-J, Reusken C, et al. Towards an integrated approach in surveillance of vector-borne diseases in Europe. Parasit Vectors. 2011;4:192.
8. Ashworth SW, Mainland DD. The economic impact of BSE on the UK beef industry. Outlook Agric. 1995;24:151–4.
9. Bouma A, Elbers ARW, Dekker A, de Koeijer A, Bartels C, Vellema P, et al. The foot-and-mouth disease epidemic in The Netherlands in 2001. Prev Vet Med. 2003;57:155–66.

10. Fegan N, Higgs G, Duffy LL, Barlow RS. The effects of transport and lairage on counts of Escherichia coli O157 in the feces and on the hides of individual cattle. Foodborne Pathog Dis. 2009;6:1113–20.

11. Roberts H, Lopez M, Hartley M. International disease monitoring, April to June 2011. Vet Rec. 2011;169:118–21.

12. Howe KS, Häsler B, Stärk KDC. Economic principles for resource allocation decisions at national level to mitigate the effects of disease in farm animal populations. Epidemiol Infect. 2013;141:91–101.

13. European Union Council Regulation (EC) 854/2004. The laying down specific rules for the organisation of official controls on products of animal origin intended for human consumption. Off J Eur Union. 2004;L226:83–127.

14. European Union. Council regulation (EC) 178/2002. Laying down the general principles and requirements of food law, establishing the European Food Safety Authority and laying down procedures in matters of food safety. Off J Eur Union. 2002;L31:1–24.

15. Green DM, Gregory A, Munro LA. Small- and large-scale network structure of live fish movements in Scotland. Prev Vet Med. 2009;91:261–9.

16. Nöremark M, Håkansson N, Lewerin SS, Lindberg A, Jonsson A. Network analysis of cattle and pig movements in Sweden: measures relevant for disease control and risk based surveillance. Prev Vet Med. 2011;99:78–90.

17. Frössling J, Ohlson A, Björkman C, Håkansson N, Nöremark M. Application of network analysis parameters in risk-based surveillance - examples based on cattle trade data and bovine infections in Sweden. Prev Vet Med. 2012;105:202–8.

18. Watts DJ, Strogatz SH. Collective dynamics of "small-world" networks. Nature. 1998;393:440–2.

19. Read JM, Keeling MJ. Disease evolution on networks: the role of contact structure. Proc Biol Sci. 2003;270:699–708.

20. VanderWaal KL, Atwill ER, Isbell LA, McCowan B. Quantifying microbe transmission networks for wild and domestic ungulates in Kenya. Biol Conserv. 2014;169:136–46.

21. Van Horne PLM. Chapter 3 Production and consumption of poultry meat and eggs in the European Union. 2008. p. 1–21.

22. Gewest V. Pig farming in the EU, a changing sector. Eurostat Stat Focus 2010 (Agriculture and fisheries). 2010;8:1–12.

23. Häsler B, Bisdorff B, Brouwer A, Comin A, Dórea FC, Drewe J, et al. Mapping of surveillance and livestock systems, infrastructure, trade flows and decision-making processes to explore the potential of surveillance at a systems level. Cuba: In ICAHS Conf May; 2014.

24. LinkTAD. Review of the Emerging Animal Health and Food Security Issues. 2014.

25. European Union. Council Regulation (EC) 722/2013 Approving annumal and multiannual programmes and the financial contribution from the Union for the eradication, control and monitoring of certain animal diseases and zoonoses presented by the member states for 2014 and the following years (2013/722/EU). Off J Eur Union. 2013;328:101:101–17.

26. Ercsey-Ravasz M, Toroczkai Z, Lakner Z, Baranyi J. Complexity of the international agro-food trade network and its impact on food safety. PLoS One. 2012;7:e37810.

27. Rautureau S, Dufour B, Durand B. Vulnerability of Animal Trade Networks to The Spread of Infectious Diseases: A Methodological Approach Applied to Evaluation and Emergency Control Strategies in Cattle, France, 2005. Transbound Emerg Dis. 2010;58:110–20.

28. Bigras-Poulin M, Barfod K, Mortensen S, Greiner M. Relationship of trade patterns of the Danish swine industry animal movements network to potential disease spread. Prev Vet Med. 2007;80:143–65.

29. Smith RP, Cook AJC, Christley RM. Descriptive and social network analysis of pig transport data recorded by quality assured pig farms in the UK. Prev Vet Med. 2013;108:167–77.

30. European Union Council Regulation (EC) 853/2004. Laying down of specific hygiene rules on the hygiene of foodstuffs. Off J Eur Union. 2004;L139:55–206.

31. European Union. Council Regulation (EC) 722/2013. Approving annual and multiannual programmes and the financial contribution from the Union for the eradication, control and monitoring of certain animal diseases and zoonoses presented by the member states for 2014 and the following years. Off J Eur Union. 2013;L328:101–17.

32. McGlone JJ, Salak JL, Lumpkin EA, Nicholson RI, Gibson M, Norman RL. Shipping stress and social status effects on pig performance, plasma cortisol, natural killer cell activity, and leukocyte numbers. J Anim Sci. 1993;71:888–96.

33. Grigor PN, Cockram MS, Steele WB, McIntyre J, Williams CL, Leushuis IE, et al. A comparison of the welfare and meat quality of veal calves slaughtered on the farm with those subjected to transportation and lairage. Livest Prod Sci. 2004;91:219–28.

34. Tadich N, Gallo C, Brito ML, Broom DM. Effects of weaning and 48 h transport by road and ferry on some blood indicators of welfare in lambs. Livest Sci. 2009;121:132–6.

35. Werner M, Gallo C. Effects of transport, lairage and stunning on the concentrations of some blood constituents in horses destined for slaughter. Livest Sci. 2008;115:94–8.

36. Storz J, Purdy CW, Lin X, Burrell M, Truax RE, Briggs RE, et al. Isolation of respiratory bovine coronavirus, other cytocidal viruses, and Pasteurella spp of shipping fever. J Am Vet Medicial Assoc. 2000;216:1599–604.

37. Dee S, Deen J, Burns D, Douthit G, Pijoan C. An evaluation of disinfectants for the sanitation of porcine reproductive and respiratory syndrome virus-contaminated transport vehicles at cold temperatures. Can J Vet Res. 2005;69:64–70.

38. Robins G, Pattison P, Kalish Y, Lusher D. An introduction to exponential random graph (p*) models for social networks. Soc Networks. 2007;29:173–91.

39. European Union. Council Regulation (EC) 1760/2000: Implementing Regulation (EC) No 1760/2000 of the European Parliament and of the Council as regards eartags, passports and holding registers. Off J Eur Union. 2004;L163:65–70.

40. European Commission. CELEX 52007DC0711: Report from the Commission to the Council on the implementation of electronic identification in sheep and goats, vol. 0711. 2007. p. 1–13.

41. European Union. Council Regulation (EC) 71/2008: The identification and registration of pigs. Off J Eur Union. 2008;L213:31–6.

42. Eurostat Glossary. Eurostat Glossary: livestock unit (LSU) – statistics explained. URL http://ec.europa.eu/eurostat/statistics-explained/index.php/Glossary:Livestock_unit_(LSU), accessed 02/08/2013.

43. R Core Team: R. A language environment for statistical programming. 2013. URL http://www.r-project.org.

44. Carter A, Butts T, Hunter D, Handcock M, Bender-demoll S, Butts MCT. Package network. 2014. URL http://CRAN.R-project.org/package=network.

45. Carter A, Butts T, Butts MCT. Package sna. 2014. URL http://CRAN.R-project.org/package=sna.

46. ESRI. ArcGIS Desktop: Release 10. Environmental Systems Research Institute: Redlands, CA; 2011.

47. Bivand R, Lewin-Koh N. Maptools: Tools for reading and handling spatial objects. 2014. URL http://CRAN.R-project.org/package=maptools.

48. Schnute JT, Boers N, Haigh R, Grandin C, Johnson A, WP and AF. PBSmapping: mapping fisheries data and spatial analysis tools. 2014. URL: http://CRAN.R-project.org/package=PBSmapping.

49. Hijmans RJ, Williams E and Vennes C. Geosphere: spherical trigonometry. R package version 1.2-28. 2012. URL http://CRAN.R-project.org/package=geosphere.

8

Investigating the introduction of porcine epidemic diarrhea virus into an Ohio swine operation

Andrew S Bowman[1*], Roger A Krogwold[2], Todd Price[3], Matt Davis[4] and Steven J Moeller[5]

Abstract

Background: Porcine Epidemic Diarrhea virus (PEDV) is a highly transmissible coronavirus that causes a severe enteric disease that is particularly deadly for neonatal piglets. Since its introduction to the United States in 2013, PEDV has spread quickly across the country and has caused significant financial losses to pork producers. With no fully licensed vaccines currently available in the United States, prevention and control of PEDV disease is heavily reliant on biosecurity measures. Despite proven, effective biosecurity practices, multiple sites and production stages, within and across designated production flows in an Ohio swine operation broke with confirmed PEDV in January 2014, leading the producer and attending veterinarian to investigate the route of introduction.

Case presentation: On January 12, 2014, several sows within a production flow were noted with signs of enteric illness. Within a few days, illness had spread to most of the sows in the facility and was confirmed by RT-PCR to be PEDV. Within a short time period, confirmed disease was present on multiple sites within and across breeding and post weaning production flows of the operation and mortality approached 100% in neonatal piglets. After an epidemiologic investigation, an outsourced, pelleted piglet diet was identified for assessment, and a bioassay, where naïve piglets were fed the suspected feed pellets, was initiated to test the pellets for infectious PEDV.

Conclusions: The epidemiological investigation provided strong evidence for contaminated feed as the source of the outbreak. In addition, feed pellets collected from unopened bags at the affected sites tested positive for PEDV using RT-PCR. However, the bioassay study was not able to show infectivity when feeding the suspected feed pellets to a small number of naïve piglets. The results highlight the critical need for surveillance of feed and feed components to further define transmission avenues in an effort to limit the spread of PEDV throughout the U.S. swine industry.

Keywords: Feed, PEDV, Swine

Background

Porcine epidemic diarrhea virus (PEDV) is a coronavirus of the genus *Alphacoronavirus*. Disease from PEDV is characterized by vomiting, anorexia, and watery diarrhea in swine. The virus is particularly deadly for neonatal pigs for which malabsorption and dehydration [1-3] can result in mortality rates approaching 80%-100% [2,4]. Disease caused by PEDV is clinically indistinguishable from transmissible gastroenteritis virus and cannot be diagnosed on presentation alone [4]. Because attempts at virus isolation have only resulted in limited or temporary success, with virus isolation rates as low as 4% [5], diagnosticians heavily rely upon RT-PCR tests to directly detect viral nucleic acid and diagnose PEDV.

PEDV was first identified in Belgium in 1978 and in the 1980s and 1990s, PEDV was found throughout Belgium, England, Germany, France, the Netherlands, and Switzerland [6]. Since the European emergence, PEDV has affected the pork industries in Philippines, South Korea, and China [7]. In May 2013, the United States confirmed the first cases of PEDV on farms in Iowa and Indiana [2], after which the virus spread quickly throughout the country. While the mode of PEDV introduction to the U.S. remains unknown, comparison of available sequence data indicates the PEDV

* Correspondence: bowman.214@osu.edu
[1]The Ohio State University College of Veterinary Medicine, 1920 Coffey Road, Columbus, OH 43210, USA
Full list of author information is available at the end of the article

strains detected in the Unites States have an ancestry linked to PEDV strains detected in China. At the end of 2013, sequenced U.S. strains had greater than 99.0% sequence identity and several strains shared unique nucleotides with a Chinese PEDV strain isolated in the Anhui Province (AH2012) [2,3]. Unexpected genetic similarity of U.S. PEDV strains to a bat coronavirus isolated in southeastern China may provide evidence for the role of cross-species transmission in the development of emergent strains that spread to the United States [3].

Transmission of PEDV occurs via the fecal-oral route [7] and fecal contamination of fomites may play a role in the introduction of the virus to swine. An investigation of 575 livestock trailers at 6 harvest facilities in the United States showed that all truck drivers stepped into the harvest facility at least once, and the proportion of PEDV contaminated trailers increased from 6.6% before unloading to 9.2% after unloading [8]. These data indicate that contaminated transport vehicles and personnel could be associated with the rapid spread of the virus throughout the US. At present, PEDV prevention and control in the U.S. are heavily dependent on biosecurity procedures.

While transportation equipment might play a role in the spread of PEDV, on-farm investigations into several PEDV outbreaks in the United States have indicated that contaminated feed could be a pathway of viral introduction; however, scientific support of this route is regularly debated. Dee *et al.* showed that material collected from the inside of feed bins during a PEDV outbreak was infectious when concentrated and inoculated into pigs [9]. One Canadian report showed spray-dried porcine plasma, a component used in some swine feed, was infectious to pigs, but the complete feed containing spray-dried porcine plasma was not infectious in an experimental setting [10]. On the other hand, a study team has provided contrary evidence with an unsuccessful attempt to infect pigs with spray-dried porcine plasma and data that indicates PEDV is inactivated during spray-dried porcine plasma production process [11,12].

In January 2014, an outbreak of PEDV was confirmed in a multi-site, multiple flow swine operation in Ohio. After a thorough epidemiologic investigation, contaminated feed was identified as the likely source of pathogen introduction, a finding supported by a positive RT-PCR result from testing the feed source. Of note, RT-PCR detects viral RNA, and thus can only confirm the presence of viral nucleic acid in a sample, not necessarily presence of viable and infectious virus. Since PEDV isolation is very difficult in numerous testing and research laboratories, virus isolation attempts from feed pellets could not be relied on to detect viable, infectious virus. Consequently, a bioassay was initiated where samples of feed cryopreserved by the attending veterinarian during the

outbreak were later fed to naïve piglets in an attempt to demonstrate feed infectivity. This report will discuss the aforementioned epidemiologic investigation and subsequent bioassay findings.

Case presentation

The Ohio swine operation (Figure 1), consisting of 3 multi-site, farrow-to-finish production flows (referred to as flows A-C, each having two breed-wean sites) and a multiplier herd (referred to as D, with a single breed-wean site) had no prior cases of PEDV and was determined to have effective biosecurity measures in place evidenced by the absence of Porcine Reproductive and Respiratory Syndrome Virus (PRRSV) during more than the prior seven years. Routine oral fluid testing of pigs in flow B on January 8, 2014 and surveillance testing in flow C in November and December 2013 were all negative for PEDV. At time of weaning, pigs move from breed-wean premises to wean-to-finish barns for flow A and to nursery facilities and then finisher sites for flows B and C. Weaned pigs from flow D, the multiplier herd, are raised in gilt developer units or wean-to-finish barns.

Disease outbreak

On the morning of January 12, 2014, four lactating sows from the one of the breed-wean units in flow A (unit A1) were noted with vomiting and diarrhea. The illness spread rapidly and by 4:00 pm, 80 litters showed signs of diarrhea, vomiting, and dehydration. Within a few days, 80% of sows on the site showed similar clinical signs. Fecal samples taken January 15, 2014 were positive for PEDV using RT-PCR. Forty-two percent mortality was observed in piglets in the A1 farrowing unit. Beyond the sow unit, a wean-to-finish barn in flow A that received pigs on January 10th from both flow A breed-wean units (A1 and A2) reported loose stools on January 12th and had confirmation of PEDV with RT-PCR positive fecal samples collected the same day. Also within flow A, one wean-to-finish barn that was filled with piglets from both flow A breed-wean units (A1 and A2) on January 10th and 12th had fecal samples test PEDV RT-PCR positive on January 15, 2014. In addition, on January 15th, a third wean to finish barn that received pigs from both flow A sow farms on January 9th had fecal samples test PEDV positive. A schematic of flow A is shown in Figure 1A.

While no PEDV-like disease was observed in either breed-wean units in flow C, pigs in 3 nurseries within flow C did test PEDV RT-PCR positive between January 14th and January 20th, 2014 (Figure 1C). On January 22, 2014 one breed-wean unit within flow B (B1) began experiencing PEDV-like disease. On that same day, an oral fluid sample from one of the nurseries in flow B that received pigs from both flow B breed-wean units (B1 and

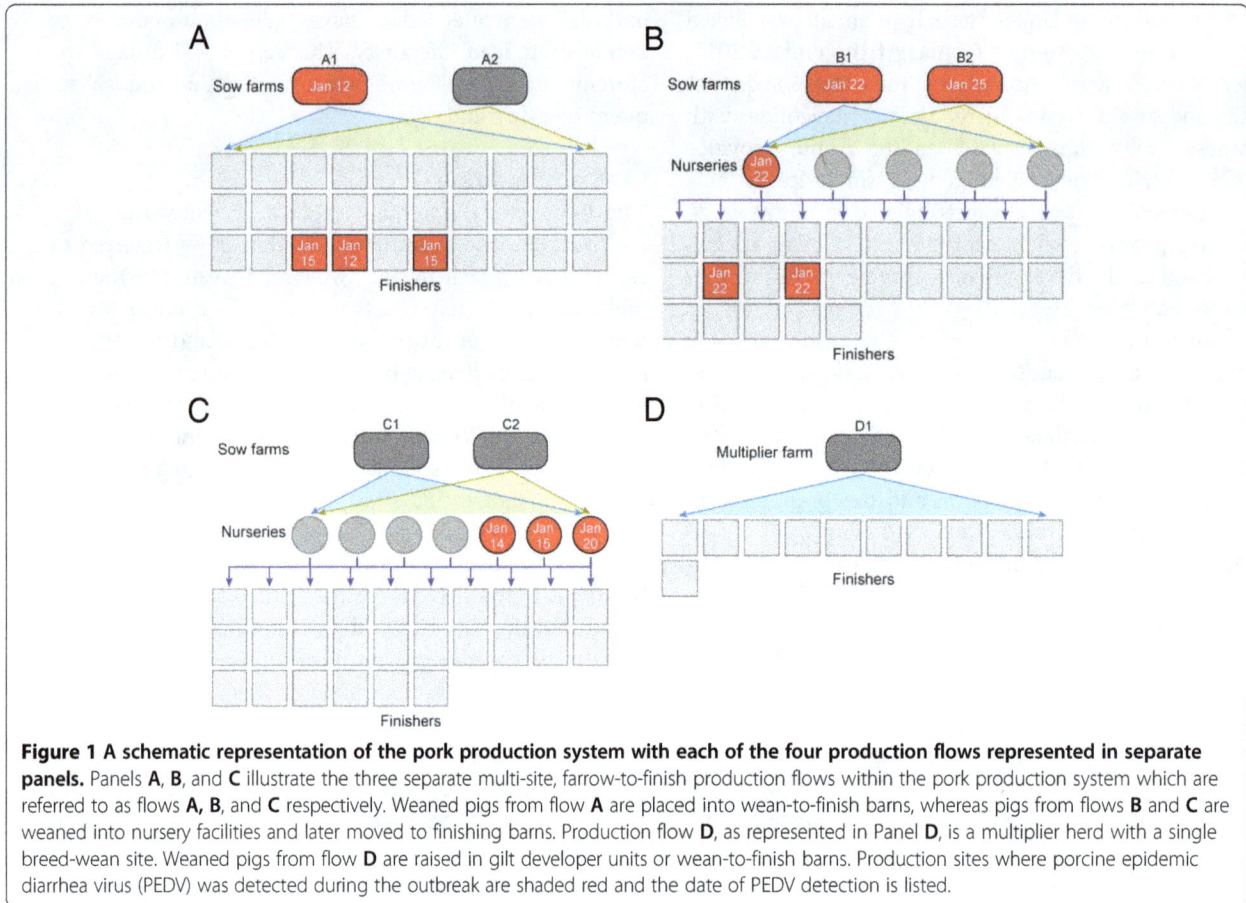

Figure 1 A schematic representation of the pork production system with each of the four production flows represented in separate panels. Panels **A**, **B**, and **C** illustrate the three separate multi-site, farrow-to-finish production flows within the pork production system which are referred to as flows **A**, **B**, and **C** respectively. Weaned pigs from flow **A** are placed into wean-to-finish barns, whereas pigs from flows **B** and **C** are weaned into nursery facilities and later moved to finishing barns. Production flow **D**, as represented in Panel **D**, is a multiplier herd with a single breed-wean site. Weaned pigs from flow **D** are raised in gilt developer units or wean-to-finish barns. Production sites where porcine epidemic diarrhea virus (PEDV) was detected during the outbreak are shaded red and the date of PEDV detection is listed.

B2) on January 15th, 17th, and 20th, 2014 tested PEDV PCR positive (Figure 1B). Also on January 22nd, two finishing barns in flow B had a PEDV PCR positive oral fluid test. By January 25th, the second breed-wean unit in flow B (B2) was also experiencing the disease. Overall, mortality among neonatal piglets was close to 100% in flow B.

Epidemiological investigation

Five American Association of Swine Veterinarians (AASV) PEDV questionnaires were completed by a USDA epidemiologist and an Ohio Department of Agriculture Veterinary Medical Officer in conjunction with swine operation representatives and the operation's local veterinarian. Several potential pathways of pathogen introduction to the swine operation, including human introduction, delivery of contaminated supplies, aerosol spread, contaminated pig transport vehicles, and contaminated feed or feed ingredients were considered and evaluated.

It is unlikely PEDV was introduced to the operation by visitors or workers. There were no foreign visitors, and no employees had visited foreign countries within 10 days of the outbreak. Nor did any employee have swine at their place of residence or associated farm enterprises. All swine

operation employees and non-employee contractors follow meticulous biosecurity procedures to enter a facility, and movement of people from one facility to another within the same day is limited to production managers only, which typically occur only within the same flow. Effectiveness of the biosecurity measures in place was evidenced by the absence of PRRS cases for over seven years.

Veterinary, vaccine, and semen supplies delivered by supply vendors were also considered as a potential source of PEDV introduction to the swine operation, but were subsequently ruled out as likely sources for several reasons. First, supplies are delivered to buildings separate from the swine housing areas and they are not shared among different flows. Disease, however, broke out separately in geographically and personnel isolated units from 3 different flows. In addition, supplies were disinfected in a fume chamber within the enclosed room whereby the incoming materials were placed on an elevated metal grate and a mister system applied a quaternary ammonium/glutaraldehyde combination disinfectant (Synergize, Preserve International, Reno, NV) and allowed to stand for 15 minutes before entry into site. This practice was considered to greatly reduce the likelihood of contaminated supplies as the potential route of PEDV introduction.

Airborne spread could be considered with PEDV [13], as coronaviruses classified within the same group as PEDV (group 1 coronaviruses) include those that cause enteric or respiratory infection. Porcine respiratory coronavirus is a mutant of transmissible gastroenteritis virus and is an example of a group 1 coronavirus that is spread through droplets and aerosols [14]. Aerosols or droplets are unlikely to be responsible for the spread of disease on this swine operation because most units are not located geographically close to each other, and disease broke on multiple separate units from 3 separate flows across a period of 13 days. Additional factors that could be involved in virus transmission such as water supply and shavings used during transport of young pigs are not probable because pigs on all sites have equal exposure to these factors but not all sites were involved in the outbreak.

Lowe *et al.* have shown that contaminated transport vehicles are likely to be involved in rapid spread of PEDV because it is common to transport pigs to harvest facilities on vehicles that have not been disinfected between loads [8]. In relation to the swine operation involved in this outbreak, it is improbable that contaminated vehicles were involved. First, the operation is closed, meaning no swine are brought on site unless they are owned by the entity and managed under the stringent biosecurity procedures displayed by the operation. Second, the operation maintains 3 truck wash facilities where written protocols are followed to thoroughly clean, wash and disinfect all company trucks. The production company regularly audits the truck wash facilities and was actively testing trucks, trailers, drying equipment, and wash bays for PEDV; all samples taken prior to the outbreak and during the first week of the outbreak were negative for PEDV. Cull animals are hauled on cull-only trailers controlled by the production system and are washed, disinfected, dried and inspected prior to use. Cull animals are transferred to a neutral location where the animals are transferred onto a third party hauler's washed and disinfected trailer for market delivery. Finisher trucks are not disinfected at company truck washes but rather at truck washes external to the production system. Given lack of production system control over these external truck washes, finishing trucks are perceived as a higher biosecurity risk to the operation; however, trucks transporting finisher swine go only to harvest facilities and do not come in contact with pigs or sows from breed-wean units within the operation.

This operation primarily uses feed produced by the operation's on-site feed mill, with exception of an outsourced starter pellet fed to piglets at the time of weaning and a commercial meal mix used to start nursery pigs on pellets. It was determined that neither feed supplied by the operation's own mill, nor the commercial meal mix were likely to be involved in the transmission of PEDV to pigs on the operation. Prior to the outbreak, the same internal feed ingredients and commercial meal mix had been used with no ill effects. Also, internal feed ingredients were used across all swine units within the operation, but not all swine units were involved in the outbreak.

Because the timing of the outbreak seemed to coincide with the switch to a new source of starter pellet feed, the attending veterinarian and farm officials suspected the new supplier's starter pelleted diet was the source of pathogen introduction. Results of the epidemiologic investigation indicated PEDV genetic material presence in the starter feed, validating this suspicion.

Starter feed pellets as a source of pathogen introduction

Starter feed pellets from the new supplier were offered to piglets in the A1 farrowing facility during the week of January 6, 2014. By January 12, 2014, clinical signs of PEDV were present among sows and piglets in the A1 facility. Starter feed pellets were subjected to standard biosecurity procedures to enter into the facility. In short, feed bags are placed into clean bins from the facility, and bins loaded with feed are disinfected in a fume chamber as they are transferred into the facility. Following this protocol eliminates contamination from the outer surface of the bag as the source and indicates feed ingredients are likely the source of contamination. Supporting the introduced pellets as a likely source, the A2 breed-wean site within the same flow, which never received the new supply of feed pellets, remained PEDV negative. Pigs in one nursery in flow B (BN1), 3 nurseries in flow C (CN5, CN6 and CN7 west barn), and one wean-to-finish unit in the multiplier herd (D) were also started on the new supplier's feed pellets. All of these sites were subsequently found to be PCR positive for PEDV except the flow D wean-to-finish unit. It is thought that differences in pellet storage conditions may account for this inconsistency from the flow D unit. Flows B and C store their feed pellets in a room separate from the barn. During winter, these rooms are estimated to be at 40°F (approximately 4°C). The units in flow D store their pellets within the barn where temperatures are around 80°F (approximately 27°C). Storage in higher temperatures may have inactivated the virus. This hypothesis is supported in a study by Jung and Chae where storage of fecal samples at temperatures 21°C and greater resulted in a decline in PEDV nucleic acid detection by RT-PCR when compared to those stored at 4°C [15].

Another inconsistency was that two contract finisher facilities in flow B and both B flow breed-wean units also broke with disease or tested positive for PEDV, even though these facilities did not receive the new supplier's pellets. Because PEDV is highly transmissible, spread of disease from the units where it broke to the breed-wean units by human error cannot be ruled out. Of note, the same person does chores at the B1 farrowing unit and the BN1 nursery where pigs were fed the implicated pellets. Also, the two flow B finisher facilities had just received pigs and do share a person who does chores between them, but that person did not have direct contact with any of the sow units.

Along with the timing of the outbreak that coincided with the switch to new supplier's feed pellets, strong evidence for these feed pellets as the source of the outbreak comes from PCR testing of the new supplier's pellets. Pellets from the BN1 nursery tested PEDV positive by RT-PCR on January 17, 2014 (C_t value = 32.95). Additionally, three lots of feed pellets from BN2 nursery, which had been cleaned and disinfected and was empty of pigs at the time, tested positive for PEDV by RT-PCR (mean C_t value = 32.58). Pigs that had left this nursery and were now in a finisher facility tested negative for PEDV, showing this nursery had been negative for PEDV while it was housing pigs. Similar findings result from testing of units within flow C. Feeder pigs that left the facility at the end of December and beginning of January were tested and found to be PEDV negative, confirming that no disease was present prior to January 12. One of the afflicted flow C nursery sites (CN7) consists of 2 barns labeled east and west. CN7 west barn received new pigs, pellets from the new supplier, and subsequently broke with PEDV. At the same time, the CN7 east barn housed PEDV negative pigs weighing approximately 50 lbs. from the previous placement. These pigs stayed PEDV negative after moving offsite all the way through marketing. Interestingly, CN7 west barn had pellets from both the old and new suppliers in the barn at the time of the outbreak. The test results showed swabs taken on the outside of both old and new suppliers' pellet feedbags were PEDV RT-PCR positive (mean C_t value = 31.93). Therefore, pellet samples were collected with care to avoid contamination from the exterior of the bags. Briefly, the top 25 cm of the feedbags were wiped with a 0.52% solution of sodium hypochlorite. Bags were then opened by cutting the top of the bag off with a scalpel to ensure a minimum risk for potential dust contamination. Feed samples were retrieved from the center of each bag by the attending veterinarian who was wearing a sterile obstetrical sleeve. The samples were placed into a sterile plastic bag, sealed, and submitted for testing. PEDV RT-PCR was positive (mean C_t value = 33.34) for the new supplier's pellets and PEDV RT-PCR negative for the old supplier's pellets. These results were interpreted to mean that the exterior of the feedbags had become contaminated with PEDV in the barn during the outbreak; however, since PEDV was detected in the interior of the unopened bags of the new supplier's pellets, PEDV contamination of this feed had to occur prior to delivery at the barn.

Building on the RT-PCR results from new supplier's feed pellets on the swine operation, back-up pellets of the same lots at the new supplier's manufacturing facility also tested RT-PCR positive (mean C_t value = 32.97). Testing of individual ingredients at the new supplier's facility yielded several positive results. Strong evidence implicating pellets from the new supplier as the contamination source based on the PEDV RT-PCR positive results is firmly supported by findings of the epidemiologic investigation. The epidemiologic investigation also concluded that virus isolation from pellets would be critical evidence that the pellets caused the outbreak.

Bioassay design

Since PEDV is very difficult to isolate, a bioassay was initiated to determine if the pellets in question could infect naïve piglets. During the outbreak at the swine operation, the attending herd veterinarian aseptically collected aliquots (as described above) of the RT-PCR positive pelleted feed from the farm and mixed them with sterile phosphate buffered saline to make a mash. These moistened, mash aliquots were stored at −20°C until the bioassay could be performed.

Ten, 10-day-old pigs, were obtained from a commercial sow herd. Sows from the source herd, the facility where the bioassay was performed, and the piglets were all confirmed to be negative for PEDV by RT-PCR at the start of the bioassay. Serum, collected from the pigs prior to leaving the source farm, tested negative for PEDV antibodies using an indirect immunofluorescence assay. During a 108 hour acclimation period, pigs were fed a commercial swine starter feed and rectal swabs from the pigs, feed samples, and environmental swabs were all collected on a daily basis. Following the acclimation period, the pigs were provided ad libitum access to the RT-PCR positive mash along with dry pellets from the same lot for 7 days, and observed for clinical signs of PEDV. Feed samples, environmental swabs, and rectal swabs were collected each day of the study. After 7 days, the pigs were euthanized and intestinal tissues were submitted for diagnostic testing.

Bioassay results

The environment, starter feed, and pigs were PEDV negative using RT-PCR prior to the study and during the 108 hour acclimation period. Mash aliquots and pelleted feed obtained from the swine operation site tested weakly PEDV positive with RT-PCR during the 7 day study (mean Ct = 36.5). Pigs were observed to be very healthy during the bioassay and no clinical signs of disease were observed in the pigs during the bioassay.

Environmental and rectal swabs collected daily during the study were negative for PEDV using RT-PCR. Microscopic examination of intestinal tissues collected from the piglets at the end of the study revealed no significant morphologic lesions.

Although the bioassay results did not confirm the feed pellets in question were infectious, feed cannot be ruled out as the cause of this outbreak. In the present study, the sensitivity of the bioassay was limited by the amount of feed the individual pigs and the small number of pigs collectively could consume during the trial period. Even if infectious virus was present in the feed used for the bioassay, the mean C_t value of 36.5 indicates it would be present at very low concentration. In addition, the pigs evaluated appeared healthy, with what was likely limited disease challenge resulting in little immune or digestive system compromise. In a field setting where there are thousands of pigs consuming tons of feed, and known, observable presence of unthrifty pigs with potentially compromised digestive or immune systems, it is conceivable that a very small amount of infectious PEDV in a food source would be capable of initiating an outbreak that would rapidly spread through the population of susceptible animals. In addition, the present bioassay portion of the study may have been hindered by the 28 day lag from the time the feed was manufactured and the initiation of the bioassay. The time lag likely decreased the viability of any infectious PEDV that was present in the feed at the time of delivery to the farm.

Conclusions

Because the timing of this outbreak coincided with a switch to new out-sourced feed pellets and due to the strong evidence provided by PEDV positive RT-PCR results of these feed pellets at both the swine operation and the supplier, it is believed that contaminated feed pellets were the source of this outbreak. A study reported subsequent to completion of the present study proved that contaminated feed can serve as a vehicle to transmit PEDV to naïve pigs [9]. The results of the epidemiologic investigation, proof of concept by other investigators and the presence of PEDV RNA from unopened bags of feed all support feed as the source of the outbreak. The inability of a bioassay to prove the feed pellets were infectious after the outbreak occurred must be considered, but the low sensitivity of this assay does not rule out feed as possible source. The results of the present and other studies demonstrate the need for strict biosecurity practices and thorough testing for feed and feed ingredients used in the pork industry for which, PEDV outbreaks can cause devastating financial losses and PEDV surveillance and prevention efforts are of the utmost importance.

Competing interests
The authors declare that they have no competing interests.

Authors' contributions
ASB performed the bioassay and drafted the manuscript. RAK led the epidemiological investigation and assisted with preparation of the manuscript. TP and MD performed field activities. SJM performed the bioassay and assisted with manuscript preparation. All authors read and approved the final manuscript.

Acknowledgements
We thank Jody Edwards for her expertise in scientific writing and editing and Tim Vojt for his medical illustration services. Funding was provided by the National Pork Checkoff, PIC North America and the U.S. Department of Agriculture. Partial funding for Open Access was provided by The Ohio State University Open Access Fund. Any mention of trade names or commercial products is solely for the purpose of providing specific information and does not imply recommendation or endorsement by the US Department of Agriculture. The contents herein are solely the responsibility of the authors and do not necessarily represent the official views of the National Pork Board, PIC North America or the U.S. Department of Agriculture.

Author details
[1]The Ohio State University College of Veterinary Medicine, 1920 Coffey Road, Columbus, OH 43210, USA. [2]USDA, APHIS, Veterinary Services, Pickerington, OH 43147, USA. [3]North Central Veterinary Service, Sycamore, OH 44882, USA. [4]Hord Livestock Company, Bucyrus, OH 44820, USA. [5]The Ohio State University College of Agriculture, Columbus, OH 43210, USA.

References
1. Jung K, Wang Q, Scheuer KA, Lu Z, Zhang Y, Saif LJ. Pathology of US porcine epidemic diarrhea virus strain PC21A in gnotobiotic pigs. Emerg Infect Dis. 2014;20(4):662–5.
2. Stevenson GW, Hoang H, Schwartz KJ, Burrough ER, Sun D, Madson D, et al. Emergence of Porcine epidemic diarrhea virus in the United States: clinical signs, lesions, and viral genomic sequences. J Vet Diagn Invest. 2013;25(5):649–54.
3. Huang YW, Dickerman AW, Pineyro P, Li L, Fang L, Kiehne R, et al. Origin, evolution, and genotyping of emergent porcine epidemic diarrhea virus strains in the United States. mBio. 2013;4(5):e00737–00713.
4. Cima G. Fighting a deadly pig disease. Industry, veterinarians trying to contain PED virus, new to the US. J Am Vet Med Assoc. 2013;243(4):469–70.
5. Chen Q, Li G, Stasko J, Thomas JT, Stensland WR, Pillatzki AE, et al. Isolation and characterization of porcine epidemic diarrhea viruses associated with the 2013 disease outbreak among swine in the United States. J Clin Microbiol. 2014;52(1):234–43.
6. Pensaert MB, de Bouck P. A new coronavirus-like particle associated with diarrhea in swine. Arch Virol. 1978;58(3):243–7.
7. Song D, Park B. Porcine epidemic diarrhoea virus: a comprehensive review of molecular epidemiology, diagnosis, and vaccines. Virus Genes. 2012;44(2):167–75.
8. Lowe J, Gauger P, Harmon K, Zhang J, Connor J, Yeske P, et al. Role of transportation in spread of porcine epidemic diarrhea virus infection, United States. Emerg Infect Dis. 2014;20(5):872–4.
9. Dee S, Clement T, Schelkopf A, Nerem J, Knudsen D, Christopher-Hennings J, et al. An evaluation of contaminated complete feed as a vehicle for porcine epidemic diarrhea virus infection of naive pigs following consumption via natural feeding behavior: proof of concept. BMC Vet Res. 2014;10(1):176.
10. Pasick J, Berhane Y, Ojkic D, Maxie G, Embury-Hyatt C, Swekla K, et al. Investigation into the Role of Potentially Contaminated Feed as a Source of the First-Detected Outbreaks of Porcine Epidemic Diarrhea in Canada. Transbound Emerg Dis. 2014;61(5):397–410.
11. Gerber PF, Xiao CT, Chen Q, Zhang J, Halbur PG, Opriessnig T. The spray-drying process is sufficient to inactivate infectious porcine epidemic diarrhea virus in plasma. Vet Microbiol. 2014;174(1-2):86–92.
12. Opriessnig T, Xiao CT, Gerber PF, Zhang J, Halbur PG. Porcine epidemic diarrhea virus RNA present in commercial spray-dried porcine plasma is not infectious to naive pigs. PLoS ONE. 2014;9(8):e104766.
13. Alonso C, Goede DP, Morrison RB, Davies PR, Rovira A, Marthaler DG, et al. Evidence of infectivity of airborne porcine epidemic diarrhea virus and detection of airborne viral RNA at long distances from infected herds. Vet Res. 2014;45(1):73.

14. Saif LJ. Animal coronaviruses: what can they teach us about the severe acute respiratory syndrome? Rev Sci Tech. 2004;23(2):643–60.
15. Jung K, Chae C. Effect of temperature on the detection of porcine epidemic diarrhea virus and transmissible gastroenteritis virus in fecal samples by reverse transcription-polymerase chain reaction. J Vet Diagn Invest. 2004;16(3):237–9.

9

Synovial fluid pharmacokinetics of tulathromycin, gamithromycin and florfenicol after a single subcutaneous dose in cattle

Meredyth L Jones[1]*, Kevin E Washburn[1], Virginia R Fajt[2], Somchai Rice[3] and Johann F Coetzee[3,4]

Abstract

Background: Deep digital septic conditions represent some of the most refractory causes of severe lameness in cattle. The objective of this study was to determine the distribution of tulathromycin, gamithromycin and florfenicol into the synovial fluid of the metatarsophalangeal (MTP) joint of cattle after single subcutaneous administration of drug to evaluate the potential usefulness of these single-dose, long-acting antimicrobials for treating bacterial infections of the joints in cattle.

Results: Twelve cross-bred beef cows were randomly assigned to one of the drugs. Following subcutaneous administration, arthrocentesis of the left metatarsophalangeal joint was performed at various time points up to 240 hours post-injection, and samples were analyzed for drug concentration. In synovial fluid, florfenicol pharmacokinetic parameters estimates were: mean T_{max} 7 +/− 2 hours, mean $t_{1/2}$ 64.9 +/− 20.1 hours and mean AUC_{0-inf} 154.0 +/− 26.2 ug*h/mL. Gamithromycin synovial fluid pharmacokinetic parameters estimates were: mean T_{max} 8 hours, mean $t_{1/2}$ 77.9 +/− 30.0 hours, and AUC_{0-inf} 6.5 +/− 2.9 ug*h/mL. Tulathromycin pharmacokinetic parameters estimates in synovial fluid were: T_{max} 19 +/− 10 hours, $t_{1/2}$ 109 +/− 53.9 hours, and AUC_{0-inf} 57.6 +/− 28.2 ug h/mL.

Conclusions: In conclusion, synovial fluid concentrations of all three antimicrobials were higher for a longer duration than that of previously reported plasma values. Although clinical data are needed to confirm microbiological efficacy, florfenicol achieved a synovial fluid concentration greater than the MIC_{90} for *F. necrophorum* for at least 6 days.

Keywords: Synovial fluid, Tulathromycin, Gamithromycin, Florfenicol, Pharmacokinetics, Bovine

Background

Lameness is an important cause of production loss and culling in all classes of cattle, making it a significant economic and welfare concern. In a survey of beef cattle operations in the US, 31.6% of herds with greater than 200 cows reported selling cattle due to lameness [1], while 8.4% of death losses of breeding cattle were due to lameness or injury [2], making it the second most common single identifiable cause of death. Deep digital septic conditions represent some of the most refractory conditions causing severe lameness. In a recent report, septic arthritis, tenosynovitis and pedal osteitis represented 15.2% of all beef cattle lameness cases presented to a veterinary teaching hospital [3].

Medical therapy alone is rarely associated with successful resolution of deep septic conditions of the digit, and medical therapy is more often used in combination with surgical approaches, including digit amputation or joint resection. Even when medical therapy is contemplated, there are currently no antimicrobials approved for the treatment of deep limb sepsis in cattle in the United States. When used for deep digital sepsis, antimicrobial drugs are administered by various routes, including systemic, regional intravenous (IV), and intra-articular. Perceived concerns over the ability to achieve sufficient concentrations of drug in the synovial structures by systemic administration has resulted in increased use of local techniques, designed to provide high concentration of drug at the site of infection to increase efficacy. Antimicrobials that exhibit concentration-dependent bacterial killing are most suited for this type of therapy, as these techniques allow for injection of

* Correspondence: mjones@cvm.tamu.edu
[1]Large Animal Clinical Sciences, Texas A&M University College of Veterinary Medicine & Biomedical Sciences, College Station, TX 77843, USA
Full list of author information is available at the end of the article

high concentrations of the agent at the site of infection. However, prohibitions against extralabel use in the U.S. or voluntary industry bans preclude the use of the concentration-dependent aminoglycosides, fluoroquinolones and metronidazole in cattle. Regional IV perfusion of ceftiofur [4], tetracycline [5], cefazolin [6] and florfenicol [7] has been evaluated in cattle, but these drugs are considered to depend on time > Minimum Inhibitory Concentration (MIC) to maximize efficacy, which means frequent treatment. However, regional IV perfusion in cattle requires chute restraint, placement of a tourniquet, and daily administration of an antimicrobial drug intravenously in the distal limb. In addition, the cephalosporins may not be administered via an extralabel route in cattle in the U.S, precluding regional IV perfusion.

We propose that drugs with a high volume of distribution should achieve sufficient intra-synovial concentrations by a more easily accomplished route of administration and may produce therapeutic concentrations within joints. Additionally, use of long-acting antimicrobial formulations (that is, longer than 24 hours) would limit the frequency of animal handling and potential disturbance of a surgical site. Tulathromycin, gamithromycin and florfenicol have high volumes of distribution in cattle [8-10] and are available as long-acting formulations. They are expected to demonstrate a time-dependent mode of action, for which the time > MIC for a given pathogen correlates with efficacy, although the pharmacodynamic parameter for any long-acting formulation has not been established. Their spectrum of activity includes Gram-negative anaerobes common in digital disease [11], namely *Fusobacterium necrophorum*, as well as mycoplasmas that have been implicated in arthritis, making these reasonable choices for an investigation to determine whether systemic antimicrobials for deep limb sepsis and septic arthritis of the distal limb might be possible. Finally, synovial fluid concentrations have not been previously assessed with these drugs.

The objective of this study was to determine the distribution of tulathromycin, gamithromycin and florfenicol into the synovial fluid of the metatarsophalangeal (MTP) joint of cattle after a single subcutaneous dose of drug to evaluate the potential usefulness of these drugs for bacterial infections of the joint in cattle. We hypothesized that tulathromycin, gamithromycin and florfenicol would reach detectable, therapeutic and sustained concentrations in synovial fluid following a single parenteral dose.

Methods
Animals
Twelve cross-bred beef cows with ages ranging from 2 to 12 years (mean: 6.4 years) were selected for inclusion in this study based on apparent health upon evaluation and no evidence of lameness. Cows were 13–83 days postpartum

(mean: 47.2 days), were lactating, and weighed between 480.5 kg and 823.6 kg (mean: 622 kg). Body condition scores of cows ranged from 3.5-7/9 (mean: 4.8/9) [12].

Experimental design
Four days prior to the start of each of 4 treatment periods, three of the 12 cows were selected if they had already calved (non-random selection). At the study site, they were housed in a paddock and fed *ad libitum* coastal Bermuda grass hay and 2 kg of 20% protein range cubes per cow twice daily. The 3 cows in each treatment period were randomly assigned to a treatment group (tulathromycin, gamithromycin or florfenicol), with the result that four cows were administered each of the three drugs over the course of the study.

On the first day for each treatment period (3 cows/period), cows were weighed on a platform floor scale. Each cow was then restrained in a hydraulic chute with overturning capability. Cows were then overturned and foot restraints applied. The region of the lateral aspect of the metatarsophalangeal (MTP) joint of the left limb was clipped and surgically prepared. Arthrocentesis was performed using a 20ga, 3.8 cm needle and 1.0 mL synovial fluid removed (Time 0). A portion of this sample was evaluated on a refractometer for total protein concentration, and the remainder was placed in a storage tube (Falcon, Tewksbury, MA, USA). A light bandage was placed over the MTP joint, and the cows were returned to standing. Synovial fluid samples were stored at –80°C. Each cow was then administered the assigned antimicrobial subcutaneously (SC) in the neck (tulathromycin 2.5 mg/kg (Draxxin, Pfizer, New York, NY, USA), gamithromycin 6 mg/kg (Zactran, Merial, Duluth, GA, USA), or florfenicol 40 mg/kg (Nuflor Gold, Intervet, Summit, NJ, USA)). If the total dose exceeded 10 mL, multiple injection sites were used. Additional 0.5 mL synovial fluid samples were collected from the MTP joint at 4, 8, 24, 48, 72, 168 and 240 hours post injection, had total protein concentration determined, and were stored at –80°C until completion of the study for determination of drug concentration. Cattle were monitored twice daily for demeanor, appetite, lameness score (1-5/5; 1 – normal, 5 – severely lame) [13], and swelling or drainage from the arthrocentesis site. Each three-cow treatment cycle was repeated four times, resulting in 4 cows receiving each treatment drug. Individual records were maintained for each cow to ensure post-treatment meat withdrawal times were followed.

Procedures used in this study were approved by the Texas A&M University Institutional Animal Care and Use Committee.

Laboratory analysis
Stored synovial fluid samples were analyzed at the Iowa State University Pharmacology Analytical Support Team

(PhAST). Synovial fluid concentrations of florfenicol, gamithromycin and tulathromycin were measured with high-pressure liquid chromatography–tandem mass spectrometry utilizing a LTQ ion trap mass spectrometer (Thermo Scientific, San Jose, CA, USA) coupled to an Agilent 1100 series pump and Autosampler (Agilent Technologies, Santa Clara, CA, USA). Synovial fluid samples or synovial fluid standards were prepared as follows: Briefly, frozen samples or standards were thawed at room temperature. A 200 μL synovial fluid sample was diluted with 0.5 mL of ultrapure water and 0.5 mL of ammonium acetate buffer, pH 4.5. 100 ng and 50 ng of thiamphenicol and roxithromycin, respectively, were added to each tube as internal standards and vigorously mixed by vortex. The samples were centrifuged at 2000 rpm for 20 minutes to pellet solids. The entire diluted supernatant was applied to a solid phase extraction (SPE) cartridge, Strata X-C 33 Polymeric Strong Cation (100 mg/3 mL, Phenomenex, Torrance, CA, USA) which was preconditioned prior with methanol (1 mL), equilibrated with water (1 mL), followed by ammonium acetate buffer, pH 4.5 (1 mL) utilizing gravity for filtration. The sample was subsequently washed with ultrapure water (1 mL), followed by 5% methanol in water (v/v) (1 mL). The SPE cartridges were dried under flow of nitrogen for 5 minutes. Florfenicol (and thiamphenicol) was eluted with 2 fractions of 1 mL portions of 70:30 acetonitrile: methanol into a glass test tube. The SPE cartridges were dried a second time under flow of nitrogen for 5 minutes. Macrolides were eluted from the same column with 2 fractions of a 1 mL 5% ammonium hydroxide in 70:30 acetonitrile: methanol and collected in the same tube as previously described. Samples were evaporated to dryness at 48°C under a stream of nitrogen, reconstituted with 100 μL 25% (v/v) acetonitrile in water. An additional 50 μL of ultrapure water was added, and the entire 150 μL sample was transferred into an injection vial for LC-MS/MS analysis with the injection volume set to 20 μL. The mobile phases consisted of A: 0.1% formic acid in water and B: 0.1% formic acid in acetonitrile at a flow rate of 0.27 mL/min. The mobile phase began at 10% B with a linear gradient to 95% B at 7 minutes, which was maintained for 2 minutes, followed by re-equilibration to 10% B. Separation was achieved with an ACE3 C18 column (150 mm × 2.1 mm, 3 μm particles, Advanced Chromatography Technologies, LTD (MacMod, Chadds Ford, PA, USA) maintained at 40°C.

Florfenicol eluted at 6.03 minutes, gamithromycin eluted at 5.64 minutes, tulathromycin eluted at 4.79 minutes, roxithromycin eluted at 6.75 minutes, and thiamphenicol eluted at 5.10 minutes. Three SRM transitions were monitored for all target analytes. The quantifying ions for florfenicol were 218.89, 335.94, and 357.25 m/z. The quantifying ions for gamithromycin were 462.44, 601.50, and 619.47 m/z. The quantifying ions for tulathromycin

were 230.96, 251.14, and 289.36 m/z. The quantifying ions for internal standards roxithromycin and thiamphenicol were 522.34, 558.22, and 679.35 m/z and 227.10, 290.05, and 282.00 m/z, respectively. Synovial fluid concentration of target analytes in unknown samples were calculated by the Xcalibur software based on the calibration curve. Results were then viewed in the Quan Browser portion of the Xcalibur software. The standard curve determined using bovine synovial fluid ranged 1 to 1000 ng/mL for florfenicol and 1 to 5000 ng/mL for the macrolides and was accepted when the correlation coefficient exceeded 0.99 and measured values were within 15% of the actual values. Sample concentrations not bracketed by range of the standard curve were repeated using a lesser volume of synovial fluid and final concentrations were back-calculated using the appropriate dilution factor dependent on the volume of synovial fluid analyzed. The inter-assay CV for mid and high range controls (100 ng/mL and 500 ng/mL from the calibration curve) were 3.1 for florfenicol, 5.7 for gamithromycin, and 4.3 for tulathromycin. There was insufficient volume of unknown samples for duplicate runs, and intra-assay CV was not determined.

Noncompartmental analysis was performed using industry standard software (WinNonLin 6.3, Pharsight) to estimate the pharmacokinetic parameters in synovial fluid for each individual animal. The following parameters were estimated for each animal: time of peak serum drug concentration (T_{max}), peak drug concentration (C_{max}), apparent elimination half-life ($t_{1/2}$, calculated as $\ln(2)/\lambda_z$, λ_z being the first order rate constant associated with the terminal portion of the time-concentration curve as estimated by linear regression of time vs. log concentration), area under the time-concentration curve from time zero to the last observed concentration (AUC_{0-obs}, calculated by the linear trapezoidal rule), area under the time-concentration curve from time zero extrapolated to infinity (AUC_{0-inf}, calculated by adding the last observed concentration divided by λ_z to the AUC_{0-obs}), area under the moment curve from time zero to last observed concentration ($AUMC_{0-obs}$), area under the moment curve from time zero extrapolated to infinity ($AUMC_{0-inf}$), mean resident time estimated using time zero to last observed concentrations (MRT_{0-obs}, calculated as $AUMC_{0-obs}/AUC_{0-obs}$), and mean residence time estimated using time zero to infinity (MRT_{0-inf}, calculated as $AUMC_{0-inf}/AUC_{0-inf}$). Mean parameters for each drug were then calculated from individual animal estimates.

Results

All synovial fluid samples were successfully collected as scheduled (see Figures 1, 2 and 3 for synovial fluid concentrations). Cows remained apparently healthy throughout

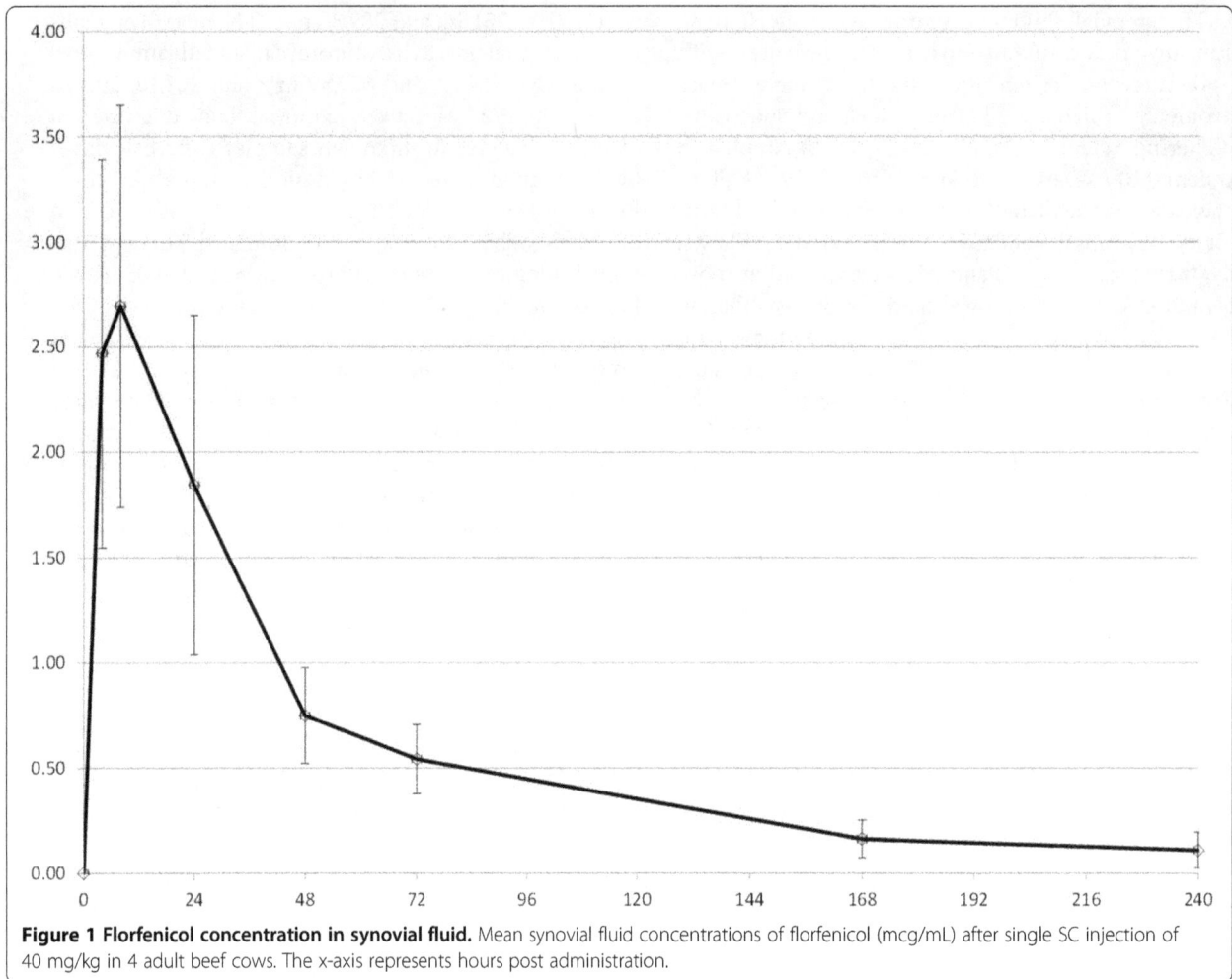

Figure 1 Florfenicol concentration in synovial fluid. Mean synovial fluid concentrations of florfenicol (mcg/mL) after single SC injection of 40 mg/kg in 4 adult beef cows. The x-axis represents hours post administration.

the study as indicated by normal attitude and appetite. No cow was scored with a lameness score greater than 1 (normal) at any point in the study. Mild swelling was noted in some cows at the site of arthrocentesis; this swelling never interfered with sampling nor was painful to pressure or produced drainage. Total protein levels were measured on all synovial fluid samples and ranged from 0.1-1.6 g/dL (mean: 0.52 g/dL).

Mean synovial fluid pharmacokinetic parameters for florfenicol, gamithromycin and tulathromycin were calculated (Table 1).

Discussion

The objective of our study was to demonstrate that potentially effective concentrations of 3 antimicrobial drugs are achieved in synovial fluid after subcutaneous administration of a single dose of long-acting time-dependent drugs, so that logistically challenging methods of drug administration such as regional IV infusion can be avoided. Our sampling strategy focused on determining concentrations in the elimination phase of drug disposition,

because we were mainly interested in demonstrating overall drug exposure and elimination rate to compare with previously described plasma disposition of the drugs [9,14-16]. Characterizing the rate of distribution of drugs into the joint space was a low priority, so we purposely did not collect many samples in the early hours after drug administration but did sample up to 240 hours. We chose not to evaluate comparative plasma concentrations in the present study due to financial constraints, and because published data are available. This sampling strategy therefore might have resulted in inaccurate estimates of C_{max}. Published mean plasma C_{max} estimate for florfenicol was 5.9 mcg/mL [17], approximately twice our estimate of 2.7 mcg/ml. For gamithromycin, C_{max} has been estimated to be 0.75 mcg/mL [9], significantly higher than our estimate of 0.14 mcg/mL. And the C_{max} estimate for tulathromycin was 0.28 mcg/mL [16] in one study, which is lower than our estimate of 0.79 mcg/ml. However, because we had a limited number of samples in the time range of the reported plasma T_{max} of all 3 drugs (5 hrs for florfenicol [17], 8 hrs for gamithromycin [9], 3 hrs for tulathromycin [16]), and

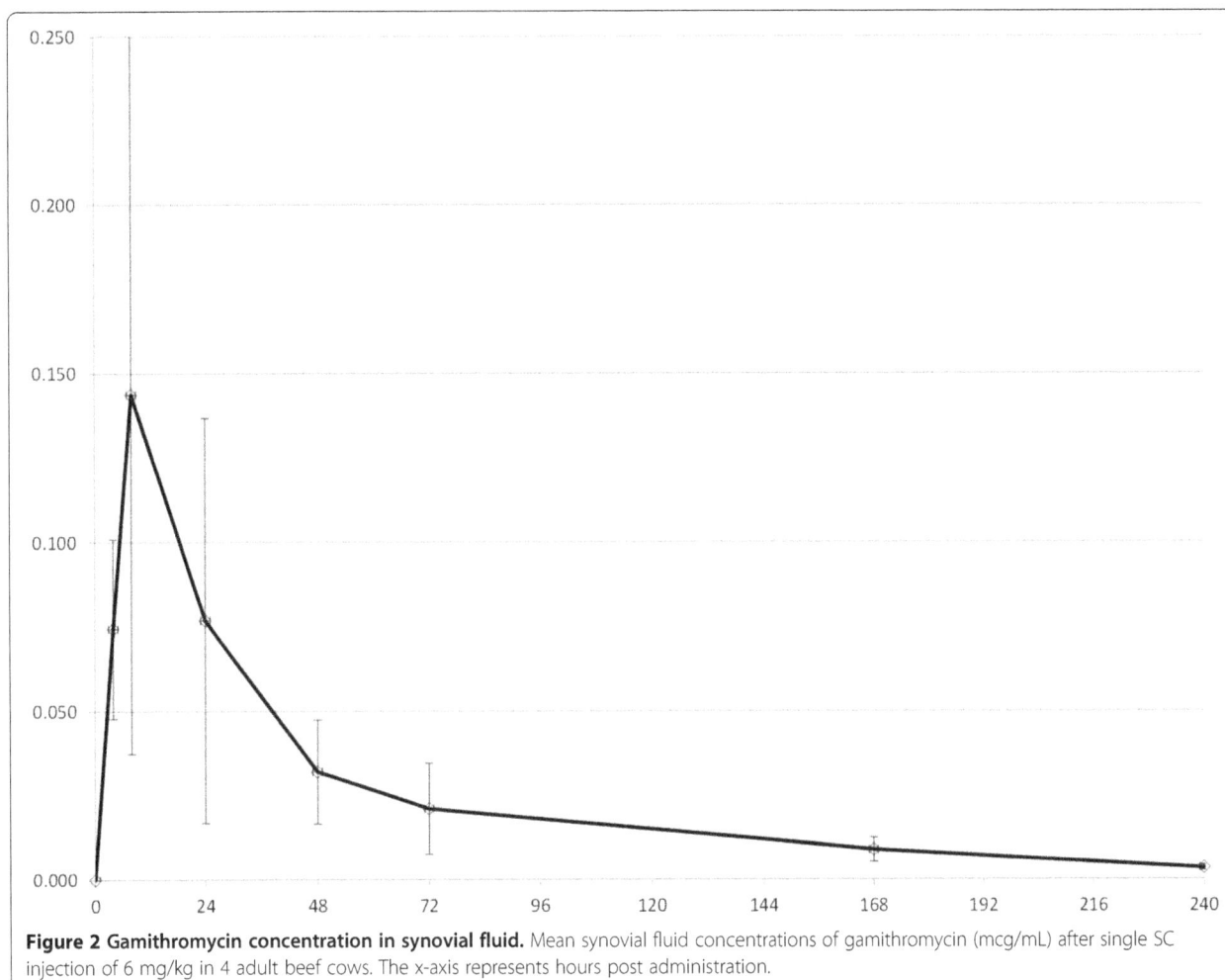

Figure 2 Gamithromycin concentration in synovial fluid. Mean synovial fluid concentrations of gamithromycin (mcg/mL) after single SC injection of 6 mg/kg in 4 adult beef cows. The x-axis represents hours post administration.

because we expect drug distribution into the joint space to not be immediate, these differences are probably of little significance clinically.

More important are the comparisons between plasma $t_{1/2}$ and synovial $t_{1/2}$ as well as between the time synovial concentrations remain above MIC of target organisms as compared to plasma concentrations. We assumed that the appropriate pharmacodynamic parameter was time > MIC, but pharmacodynamic parameters for long-acting formulations or for macrolides have not been well characterized in the literature. $T_{1/2}$ of florfenicol in synovial fluid was estimated to be approximately 65 hrs, compared to reported plasma $t_{1/2}$ of 38 hrs [17]. $T_{1/2}$ of gamithromycin in synovial fluid was estimated to be 78 hrs vs. 51 hrs in plasma as previously reported [9]. Finally, $t_{1/2}$ of tulathromycin in synovial fluid was estimated in the present study to be 109 hrs, as compared to the published plasma $t_{1/2}$ of 64 hrs [16]. Therefore, it appears that drug elimination from synovial fluid is slower than from plasma due to delayed presentation to the organs of elimination, a potential advantage for medical therapy.

Equally important to compare is the amount of time that synovial fluid concentrations remained above a particular concentration, since this is likely to be predictive of efficacy. Recognizing that a direct comparison between pathogen MIC and synovial fluid concentration is not defensible in the absence of supportive clinical data, a qualitative comparison is helpful in suggesting the potential for efficacy. Synovial concentrations of florfenicol in the present study remained above 0.5 mcg/mL for approximately 72 hours, which is similar to the previously reported plasma concentrations. Synovial concentrations of gamithromycin in the present study compared favorably with previously reported plasma concentrations: synovial concentrations were 0.02 mcg/mL at 72 hrs, as compared to 0.026 mcg/mL previously reported. Finally, synovial concentration of tulathromycin in the present study averaged 0.078 mcg/mL at 168 hrs, whereas previously reported estimates (from visual examination of graphical data) were between 0.01 and 0.02 mcg/mL.

MICs for several target pathogens for these 3 drugs have been reported: Synovial fluid concentrations of florfenicol

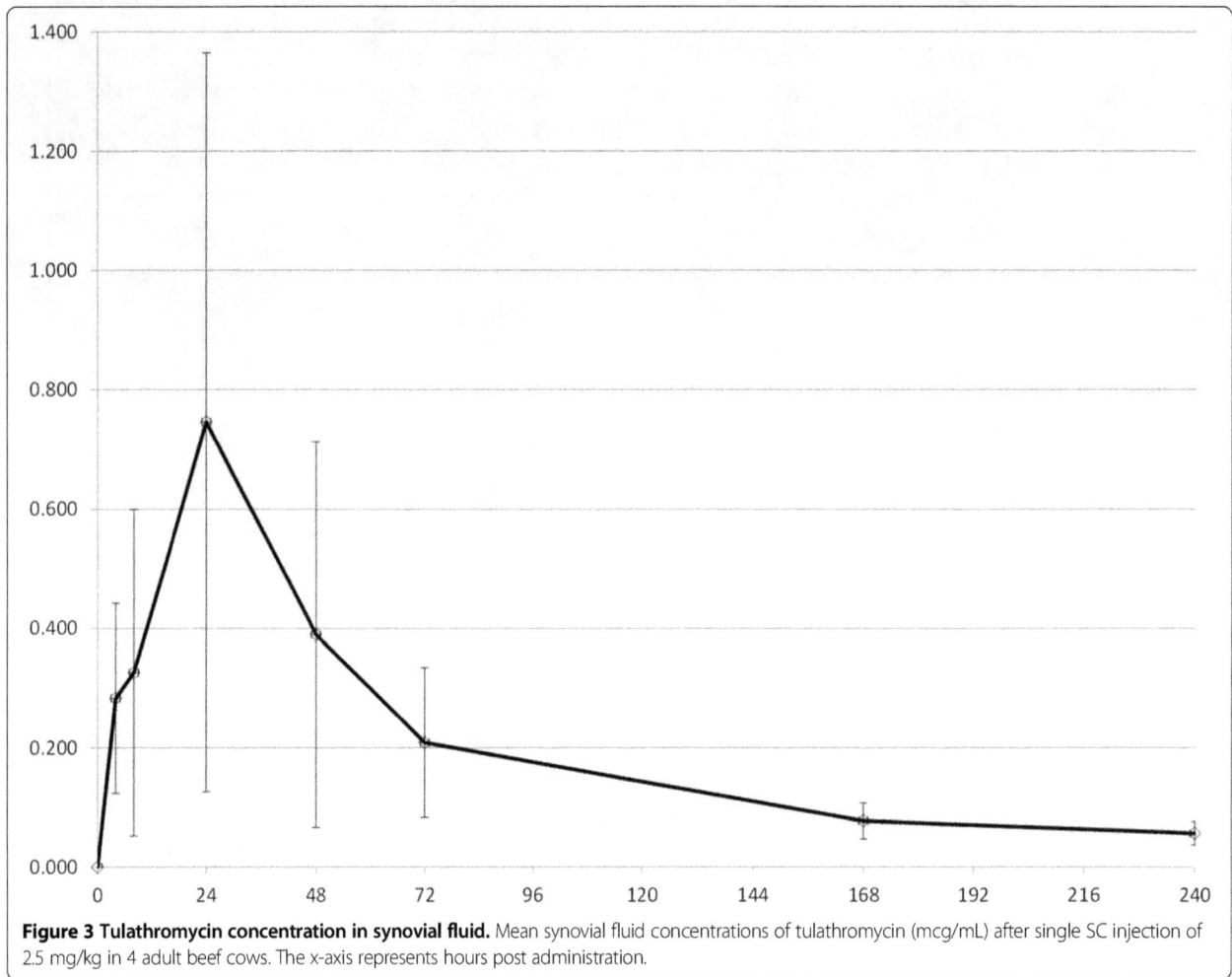

Figure 3 Tulathromycin concentration in synovial fluid. Mean synovial fluid concentrations of tulathromycin (mcg/mL) after single SC injection of 2.5 mg/kg in 4 adult beef cows. The x-axis represents hours post administration.

Table 1 Synovial fluid pharmacokinetic parameters

		Florfenicol		Gamithromycin		Tulathromycin	
		Mean	SD	Mean	SD	Mean	SD
C_{max}	mcg/mL	2.71	0.93	0.14	0.11	0.79	0.57
T_{max}	hr	7	2	8	0	19	10
λz	/hr	0.0115	0.0035	0.0099	0.0038	0.0077	0.0038
$t_{\frac{1}{2}\lambda z}$	hr	64.9	20.1	77.9	30.0	109.0	53.9
AUC_{last}	mcg*hr/mL	142.0	17.5	6.2	2.8	49.7	29.1
AUC_{0-inf}	mcg*hr/mL	154.0	26.2	6.5	2.9	57.6	28.2
AUC % Extrap		7.1	6.3	6.2	2.8	18.1	12.1
$AUMC_{0-obs}$	mcg*hr^2/mL	7623	2577	331	122	3323	1577
$AUMC_{0-inf}$	mcg*hr^2/mL	11860	7054	469	124	6490	1311
MRT_{0-obs}	hr	53.5	15.4	55.9	14.2	71.7	14.4
MRT_{0-inf}	hr	74.1	32.9	75.2	12.3	136.5	65.0

T_{max}: time of peak serum drug concentration; C_{max}: peak drug concentration; $t_{1/2}$: apparent elimination half-life calculated as $\ln(2)/\lambda_z$, λ_z being the first order rate constant associated with the terminal portion of the time-concentration curve; AUC_{0-obs}: area under the time-concentration curve from time zero to the last observed concentration; AUC_{0-inf}: area under the time-concentration curve from time zero extrapolated to infinity; $AUMC_{0-obs}$: area under the moment curve from time zero to the last observed concentration; $AUMC_{0-inf}$: area under the moment curve from time zero extrapolated to infinity; MRT_{0-obs}: Mean Resident Time calculated as $AUMC_{0-obs}/AUC_{0-obs}$; MRT_{0-inf}: Mean Residence Time calculated as $AUMC_{0-inf}/AUC_{0-inf}$.

Mean pharmacokinetic parameters in synovial fluid estimated via noncompartmental analysis after SC administration of florfenicol (40 mg/kg), gamithromycin (6 mg/kg), and tulathromycin (2.5 mg/kg) (n = 4/group).

in the present study would be expected to be above *Fusobacterium necrophorum* and *Bacteroides melaninogenicus* MIC (MIC$_{90}$: 0.25 mcg/mL) for at least 6 days, but not above reported MICs for *Trueperella pyogenes* (MIC$_{90}$: 16 mcg/mL [18]), although these were uterine isolates. Susceptibility data related to gamithromycin and Gram-negative anaerobic isolates likely to be responsible for digital sepsis are not available, so predictions cannot be made for this drug. Synovial fluid concentrations of tulathromycin do not appear to remain above the reported MIC$_{50}$ of *Fusobacterium necrophorum* (2 mcg/mL); however, tulathromycin is approved for use in the treatment of footrot, and the plasma concentrations also do not reach these concentrations, so the PK/PD relationship is likely more complicated than a simple comparison of concentration to MIC. One important caveat to these comparisons of pharmacokinetic values to published data on florfenicol and tulathromycin is that there have been two commercially available florfenicol preparations (Nuflor, Schering Plough, Summit, NJ, USA; Nuflor Gold, Intervet, Roseland, NJ, USA), and one study of tulathromycin was performed using prototype formulations [15].

A question might arise about the impact of sample collection on inflammation in the joint and its effects on drug concentrations. A previous study [7] used indwelling catheters to facilitate sample collection to evaluate synovial fluid pharmacokinetics after regional perfusion in the metatarsophalangeal joint. Synovial fluid samples for this project, however, were readily obtained with needle arthrocentesis at each time point. This technique potentially minimized inflammation in the joint by eliminating the use of an indwelling foreign body for 240 hours. While total protein concentration of synovial fluid as measured on a refractometer is an imperfect indicator of inflammation, the values obtained at each time point fell well below medial total protein levels seen in cattle with various forms of noninfectious joint disease [19]. This, combined with no clinical evidence of inflammation (swelling, drainage, lameness) in any study joint, provides an indication that this procedure is both effective at obtaining sufficient sample for drug analysis and minimizing inflammatory response. Systemic administration of antimicrobial drugs may also help prevent septicemia of the digital vasculature, which has been reported after regional IV perfusion of lidocaine when digital sepsis was present [20].

No products used in this study are approved for use in lactating dairy cattle and their use may only be advocated in beef cattle and non-lactating dairy cattle. Products including ampicillin, ceftiofur and oxytetracycline make more appropriate choices for dairy cattle, but need to be evaluated for their synovial fluid pharmacokinetics in adult cattle. Oxytetracycline concentrations in synovial fluid have been evaluated after IM injection in

healthy calves [21,22], and IV administration in calves with experimentally-induced synovitis [23], but these drugs were not included in the present study.

Conclusions

In conclusion, synovial fluid concentrations of all three drugs were higher for a longer duration than that of previously reported plasma values. Although florfenicol achieved a synovial fluid concentration greater than the MIC$_{90}$ for *F. necrophorum* for at least 6 days, clinical data are needed to confirm microbiological efficacy.

Abbreviations
AUC: Area under the curve; AUMC: Area under the moment curve; Cmax: Peak drug concentration; MIC: Minimum inhibitory concentration; MRT: Mean residence time; MTP: Metatarsophalangeal; t1/2: Elimination half-life; Tmax: Time of peak drug concentration.

Competing interests
The authors declare that they have no competing interests.

Authors' contributions
MLJ conceived of the study and participated in its design, participated in treatments, sample collection and data analysis and was the primary author of the manuscript. KEW conceived of the study and participated in its design, participated in treatments, sample collection and data analysis and revised the manuscript. VRF significantly contributed to the conception and design of the study, pharmacokinetic data analysis and revised the manuscript. SR contributed sample analysis and generation of data, co-authored the section of the manuscript on Laboratory Analysis and revised the manuscript. JFC contributed sample analysis and generation of data, co-authored the section of the manuscript on Laboratory Analysis and revised the manuscript. All authors read and approved the final manuscript.

Acknowledgements
This project was funded by a grant from the Texas A&M University Department of Large Animal Clinical Sciences. This funding body provided funds for animal care, research supplies, and sample analysis.
The open access publishing fees for this article have been covered by the Texas A&M University Online Access to Knowledge (OAK) Fund, supported by the University Libraries and the Office of the Vice President for Research. Corresponding products used in this project were provided by Merck Animal Health and Zoetis.

Author details
[1]Large Animal Clinical Sciences, Texas A&M University College of Veterinary Medicine & Biomedical Sciences, College Station, TX 77843, USA. [2]Veterinary Physiology and Pharmacology, Texas A&M University College of Veterinary Medicine & Biomedical Sciences, College Station, TX 77843, USA. [3]Pharmacology Analytical Support Team (PhAST), Veterinary Diagnostic Laboratory, Iowa State University College of Veterinary Medicine, Ames, IA 50011, USA. [4]Veterinary Diagnostic and Production Animal Medicine, Iowa State University College of Veterinary Medicine, Ames, IA 50011, USA.

References
1. USDA National Animal Heath Monitoring Service. Beef 2007–2008 part IV: reference of beef Cow-calf management practices in the United States. 2010.
2. USDA National Animal Heath Monitoring Service. Beef 2007–2008 part V: reference of beef Cow-calf management practices in the United States. 2010.
3. Fraser B, Miesner M, Anderson D, Laflin S, Jones M. Lameness in beef cattle: retrospective study of foot disorders (2007–2010) [abstract]. J Vet Intern Med. 2011;25:686–7.
4. Navarre CB, Zhang L, Sunkara G, Duran SH, Kompella UB. Ceftiofur distribution in plasma and joint fluid following regional limb injection in cattle. J Vet Pharm Therap. 1999;22:13–9.

5. Rodrigues CA, Hussni CA, Nascimento ES, Esteban C, Perri SH. Pharmacokinetics of tetracycline in plasma, synovial fluid and milk using single intravenous and single intravenous regional doses in dairy cattle with papillomatous digital dermatitis. J Vet PharmTherap. 2010;33:363–70.

6. Gagnon H, Ferguson IG, Papich MG, Bailey IV. Single-dose pharmacokinetics of cefazolin in bovine synovial fluid after intravenous regional injection. J Vet Pharm Therap. 1994;17:31–7.

7. Gilliam JN, Streeter RN, Papich MG, Washburn KE, Payton ME. Pharmacokinetics of florfenicol in serum and synovial fluid after regional intravenous perfusion in the distal portion of the hind limb of adult cows. Am J Vet Res. 2008;69:997–1004.

8. Evans NA. Tulathromycin: an overview of a new triamilide antibiotic for livestock respiratory disease. Vet Therap. 2005;6:83–95.

9. Huang RA, Letendre LT, Banav N, Fischer J, Somerville B. Pharmacokinetics of gamithromycin in cattle with comparison of plasma and lung tissue concentrations and plasma antibacterial activity. J Vet PharmTherap. 2010;33:227–37.

10. Lobell RD, Varma KJ, Johnson JC, Sams RA, Gerken DF, Ashcraft SM. Pharmacokinetics of florfenicol following intravenous and intramuscular doses to cattle. J Vet Pharm Therap. 1994;17:253–8.

11. Bergsten C. Infectious diseases of the digits. In: Greenough PR, Weaver AD, editors. Lameness in cattle. 3rd ed. Philadelphia: Saunders; 1997. p. 89–100.

12. Texas A&M AgriLife Research and Extension Center at Vernon: Guide to Body Condition Scoring Cattle. [http://vernon.tamu.edu/center-programs/range-animal-nutrition-program/decision-aids-for-cattle-producers/body-condition-scoring-photo-guide/overview-of-body-condition-scoring-system/#guide]

13. Sprecher DJ, Hostetler DE, Kaneene JB. A lameness scoring system that uses posture and gait to predict dairy cattle reproductive performance. Therio. 1997;47:1179–87.

14. Sidhu P, Rassouli A, Illambas J, Potter T, Pelligand L, Rycroft A, et al. Pharmacokinetic-pharmacodynamic integration and modelling of florfenicol in calves. J Vet Pharm Therap. 2014;37:231–42.

15. Nowakowski MA, Inskeep PB, Risk JE, Skogerboe TL, Benchaoui HA, Meinert TR, et al. Pharmacokinetics and lung tissue concentrations of tulathromycin, a new triamilide antibiotic, in cattle. Vet Therap. 2004;5:60–74.

16. Cox SR, McLaughlin C, Fielder AE, Yancey MF, Bowersock TL, Garcia-Tapia D, et al. Rapid and prolonged distribution of tulathromycin into lung homogenate and pulmonary epithelial lining fluid of Holstein calves following single subcutaneous administration of 2.5 mg/kg body weight. Int J Appl Res Vet Med. 2010;8:129–37.

17. Nuflor Gold [package insert]. Roseland, NJ: Intervet Inc.; 2009.

18. Santos TM, Caixeta LS, Machado VS, Rauf AK, Gilbert RO, Bicalho RC. Antimicrobial resistance and presence of virulence factor genes in *Arcanobacterium pyogenes* isolated from the uterus of postpartum dairy cows. Vet Micro. 2010;145:84–9.

19. Rohde C, Anderson DE, Desrochers A, St-Jean G, Hull BL, Rings DM. Synovial fluid analysis in cattle: a review of 130 cases. Vet Surg. 2000;29:341–6.

20. Simpson KM, Streeter RN, Taylor JD, Gull TB, Step DL. Bacteremia in the pedal circulation following regional intravenous perfusion of a 2% lidocaine solution in cattle with deep digital sepsis. J Am Vet Med Assoc. 2014;245:565–70.

21. Landoni MF, Errecalde JO. Tissue concentrations of a long-acting oxytetracycline formulation after intramuscular administration in cattle. Rev Sci Tech. 1992;11:909–15.

22. Bengtsson B, Franklin A, Luthman J, Jacobsson SO. Concentrations of sulphadimidine, oxytetracycline and penicillin G in serum, synovial fluid and tissue cage fluid after parenteral administration to calves. J Vet Pharm Therap. 1989;12:37–45.

23. Guard CL, Byman KW, Schwark WS. Effect of experimental synovitis on disposition of penicillin and oxytetracycline in neonatal calves. Cornell Vet. 1989;79:161–71.

10

The effect of Zhangfei/CREBZF on cell growth, differentiation, apoptosis, migration, and the unfolded protein response in several canine osteosarcoma cell lines

Rui Zhang[1,3], Douglas H Thamm[2] and Vikram Misra[1*]

Abstract

Background: We had previously shown that the bLZip domain-containing transcription factor, Zhangfei/CREBZF inhibits the growth and the unfolded protein response (UPR) in cells of the D–17 canine osteosarcoma (OS) line and that the effects of Zhangfei are mediated by it stabilizing the tumour suppressor protein p53. To determine if our observations with D-17 cells applied more universally to canine OS, we examined three other independently isolated canine OS cell lines—Abrams, McKinley and Gracie.

Results: Like D–17, the three cell lines expressed p53 proteins that were capable of activating promoters with p53 response elements on their own, and synergistically with Zhangfei. Furthermore, as with D–17 cells, Zhangfei suppressed the growth and UPR-related transcripts in the OS cell lines. Zhangfei also induced the activation of osteocalcin expression, a marker of osteoblast differentiation and triggered programmed cell death.

Conclusions: Osteosarcomas are common malignancies in large breeds of dogs. Although there has been dramatic progress in their treatment, these therapies often fail, leading to recurrence of the tumour and metastatic spread. Our results indicate that induction of the expression of Zhangfei in OS, where p53 is functional, may be an effective modality for the treatment of OS.

Keywords: Canine osteosarcoma, Zhangfei/CREBZF, p53, Apoptosis, Osteocalcin

Background

Osteosarcoma (OS) is the most common primary malignant bone tumour in children and adolescents, although its incidence in dogs is ten times greater than in humans [1]. Spontaneously occurring osteosarcomas in dogs are an ideal model for cancer research due to their anatomical and physiological similarities with human counterparts (reviewed by [2-4]).

We had previously shown that the basic leucine zipper (bLZip) domain-containing transcription factor, Zhangfei/CREBZF/SMILE inhibits the growth and the unfolded protein response (UPR) in the D–17 canine osteosarcoma (OS) cell line [5] and that the effects of Zhangfei are mediated by stabilizing the tumour suppressor protein p53 [6]. To determine if our observations with D–17 cells applied more universally to canine OS, we examined three other independently isolated canine OS cell lines—Abrams, McKinley [7-10] and Gracie [11]. The purpose of this study was to determine the inhibitory role of Zhangfei in these OS cell lines by exploring its potential involvement in growth, differentiation, apoptosis, and metastasis.

Zhangfei was initially identified through its interaction with the host cell factor (HCF1) a protein required for the initiation of herpes simplex virus gene expression [12]. Unlike other bLZip transcription factors, Zhangfei appears to be incapable of binding to consensus bLZip response elements as a homodimer [13]. Instead, it fulfills its role in transcriptional regulation by hetero-dimerizing with and modulating other transcription factors or signaling molecules, such as

* Correspondence: vikram.misra@usask.ca
[1]Department of Microbiology, Western College of Veterinary Medicine, University of Saskatchewan, Saskatoon, SK, Canada
Full list of author information is available at the end of the article

Luman/CREB3 [14], Xbp1 [15], ATF4 [16], SMAD 1,5,8 [17], herpes simplex virus VP16 [18], and p53 [19].

Results and discussion
All four canine OS cells lines express functional p53
To confirm the effects of Zhangfei we had observed in D–17 OS cells we examined three other canine OS cell lines. We have shown that Zhangfei exerts its effect on cell growth and the UPR by stabilizing p53 [6] and it therefore has no effect on cancer cells that do not possess functional p53. To assess the status of p53 in the canine cell lines we amplified p53 transcripts from the cells using PCR and determined the nucleotide sequences of the products. Figure 1B shows the derived amino acid sequences of p53 from the cell lines and the reference sequence from the canine genome database. All four cell lines contained transcripts for p53 that, with the exception of a few amino acid variations, were identical to the reference sequence. None of the amino acid polymorphisms in the sequences were at positions identified as important for p53 function [20] (Figure 1A,B).

To determine if the p53 proteins in the cell lines were functionally active, we transfected the cells with a plasmid that expressed the reporter protein chloramphenicol acetyl transferase (CAT) regulated by a promoter with two copies of a p53 response element (pCATp53RE). As a negative control, cells were transfected with a plasmid (pCAT3B) without the response elements. Parallel cultures were transfected with a plasmid expressing Zhangfei. Figure 1C shows that expression of CAT was activated in all four cell lines in a p53 response element–dependent manner and that the presence of Zhangfei enhanced expression.

Cellular outcome following ectopic expression of Zhangfei: growth arrest, apoptosis and differentiation
We next compared the effect of Zhangfei on the growth characteristics of Abrams, McKinley, and Gracie cells with its effect on D–17 cells. The cells were infected with adenovirus expressing either Zhangfei (Adeno-ZF) or the control protein β-galactosidase (Adeno-LacZ). Cell growth was monitored by the WST-1 Cell Proliferation Assay. In agreement with previous results, all four Adeno-ZF-infected cells failed to divide as early as day 1 after infection as determined by their ability to convert WST-1 Cell Proliferation reagent and absorb light at 405 nm. Mock infected cells continued to grow for three days and the growth of Adeno-LacZ-infected cells was indistinguishable from mock-infected cells (Figure 2). Apoptosis was induced in all four cell lines as a result of Zhangfei expression (Figure 3). D–17 and Abrams appeared to be more sensitive as cultures had substantial numbers of apoptotic cells at 24 hr. The response in McKinley and Gracie, was slower with cultures showing

20 to 34% apoptotic cells by 48 hr. Since the level of p53 in response to Zhangfei was similar in all the cell lines the quantitative differences in the induction of apoptosis suggests that Zhangfei may have effects that are, at least partially, independent of p53.

Since the effect of Zhangfei was most dramatic on D–17 and Abrams cells we selected them for further analysis. Zhangfei may stop cell growth by inducing differentiation and/or causing apoptosis, we therefore performed a transcript level analysis of the OS differentiation marker—osteocalcin [21] in D–17 and Abrams cells infected with either Adeno-ZF or Adeno-LacZ. Compared with LacZ-expressing and even vitamin D3-treated cells (negative and positive controls, respectively), Zhangfei significantly increased the expression of osteocalcin transcripts in a time-dependent manner (Figure 4).

Expression of Zhangfei inhibits the ability of canine osteosarcoma cells to close a scratch wound
Migratory behaviour in cancer cells is a typical hallmark of malignancy. To investigate whether ectopic expression of Zhangfei correlated with altered migratory behaviour, we performed cell motility assays on the canine OS cultures. Following scratch wounding, wound closure was significantly slower in cultures (D–17 and Abrams canine cells) infected with Adeno-ZF compared to cultures infected with Adeno-LacZ or mock-infected cells (Figure 5), showing that the ectopic expression of Zhangfei indeed causes decreased cell motility in canine osteosarcoma cells. However, it is also possible that the decrease in ability of Zhangfei-expressing cells to grow heal the scratch wound may be because of a decrease in growth rates rather than a decrease in the ability to migrate.

Zhangfei negatively regulates the UPR in canine osteosarcomas
The unfolded protein response (UPR) is an adaptive cellular stress response that alleviates ER stress or, failing, induces apoptosis. In previous studies, we found Zhangfei was a negative regulator of the UPR in D–17 canine OS cells [5]. To investigate if Zhangfei could consistently suppress the UPR in other canine OS cells, the four canine OS cell lines infected with either Adeno-ZF or Adeno-LacZ were treated with the UPR pharmacological inducer thapsigargin, or were deprived of glucose. The latter treatment is a known physiological inducer of the UPR. Both treatments increased the level of transcripts for UPR transcripts Xbp1s, HERP, CHOP and GRP78 (Figure 6A) and Zhangfei suppressed the transcripts in thapsigargin treated (Figure 6B) and glucose deprived (Figure 6C) cells. In contrast, LacZ had no obvious effect. In addition, this decrease in mRNA was reflected in a decrease in UPR proteins (Xbp1s, HERP, and GRP78) in thapsigargin-treated D–17

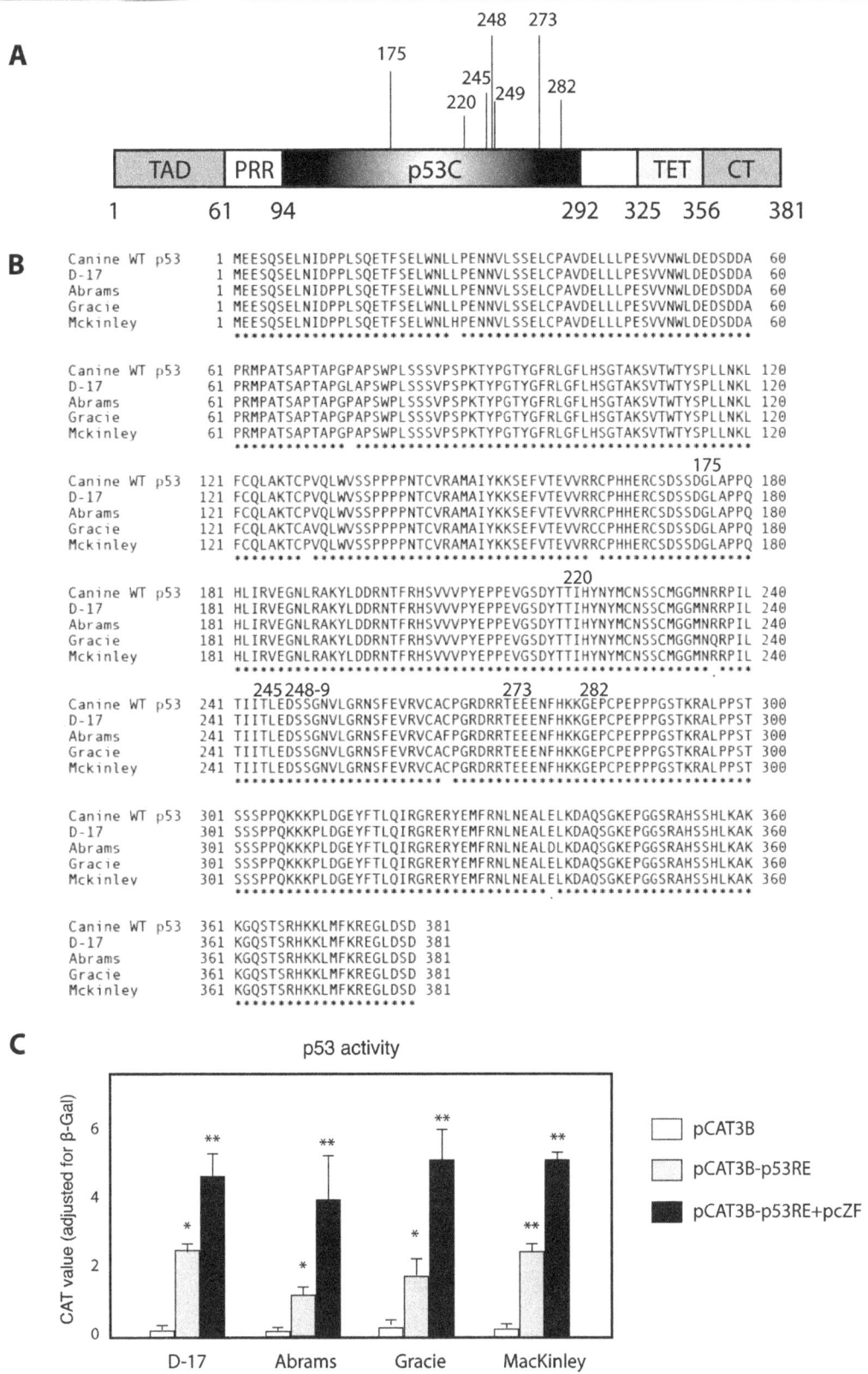

Figure 1 (See legend on next page.)

(See figure on previous page.)

Figure 1 p53 in dog osteosarcoma cell lines. (A) Schematic structure of full-length p53. TAD: N-terminal transactivation domain; PRR: proline-rich region; p53C: central DNA-binding domain; TET: tetramerization domain; CT: extreme carboxyl terminus. p53C is the domain where most cancer-associated p53 mutations are located. The numbers below the diagram indicate amino acid residues delineating the domains and numbers above the diagram represent the residues with highest frequency of oncogenic missense mutations [20]. **(B)** Derived amino acid sequence alignment of p53s from 4 dog OS cell lines and dog wild-type p53. The residues that have high mutant frequency were marked above the diagram. Accession numbers: KP279761, KP279762, KP279763, KP279764 **(C)** p53 proteins of dog OS cell lines have transcriptional activity, and Zhangfei enhances p53-dependent transactivation. D–17, Abrams, McKinley, and Gracie cells were transfected with 0.5 μg of pCAT3B or pCAT3B-p53RE, in the presence or absence of 1 μg of pcZF. 24 h after transfection, the CAT activity was determined. Values represented the relative CAT activity (adjusted by β-galactosidase) of different treatments. Standard deviations from means of three individual experiments are shown. Significance of differences of the means (*$P < 0.05$, **$P < 0.01$) were determined using ANOVA.

[5] and Abrams (Figure 6D) cells. Figure 6E, which showed intracellular proteins detected by immunofluorescence, also supported these data—the Xbp1s protein was undetectable in D–17 and Abrams cells expressing Zhangfei.

Conclusions

Canine OS is an aggressive tumour that accounts for approximately 85% of primary bone tumours in the dog [22]. OS causes local skeletal destruction resulting in osteoproductive and osteolytic lesions, and it is highly metastatic to the lungs. Although there has been dramatic progress in the standard treatments of OS, including amputation, chemotherapy, and palliative radiation therapy, these therapies often fail, leading to recurrence of the tumour and metastatic spread [23-26]. Over the years, combined therapies, such as chemotherapy combined with immune modulators, have been practiced on dog OS [27,28], although with poor overall survival times.

The dog is a well-established model for spontaneous OS in humans, owing to striking similarity in biology and gene expression. The large size of dogs, relative outbreeding, and immunocompetence increase their model potential. Furthermore, dogs with spontaneous tumors

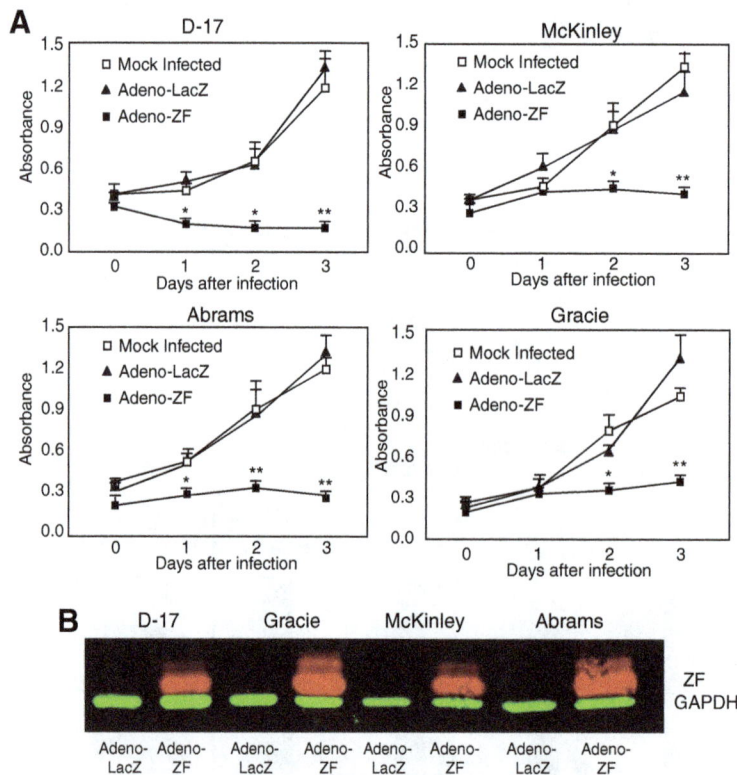

Figure 2 Ectopic expression of Zhangfei suppresses cell growth in canine osteosarcomas. D–17, Abrams, McKinley, and Gracie canine OS cells were mock-infected or infected with adenovirus vectors expressing either Zhangfei (Adeno-ZF) or β-galactosidase (Adeno-LacZ) and growth rates were measured **(A)** by absorbance at 405 nm with WST-1 at different time points after infection. Error bars indicate standard deviations from means of three individual experiments. Standard deviations from means of three individual experiments are shown and significance (*$P < 0.05$, **$P < 0.01$) was determined using ANOVA. **(B).** Zhangfei was detected by immunoblotting using antiserum against Zhangfei.

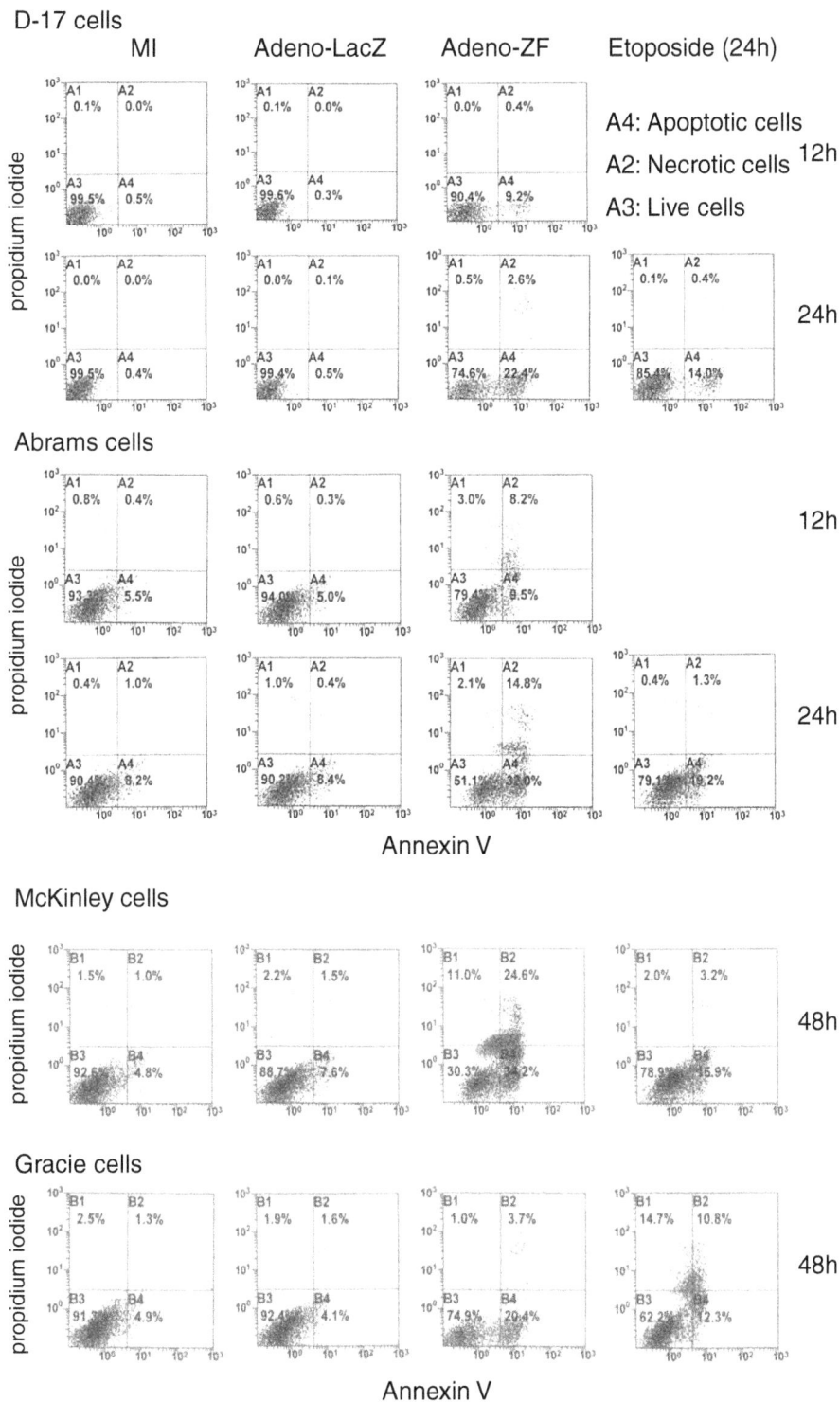

Figure 3 Zhangfei causes canine osteosarcoma cells to commit apoptosis. D–17, Abrams, McKinley and Gracie cells, mock-infected or infected with Adeno-ZF or Adeno-LacZ or treated with 50 μM etoposide (positive control) were stained with fluorescent Annexin V and propidium iodide. Unstained cells or cells staining with either or both dyes were enumerated by FACS. A4 represents the percentage of total cells undergoing apoptosis. For McKinley and Gracie only reading for 48 hr are shown. Differences between LacZ and ZF-expressing cells were more pronounced at that time-point.

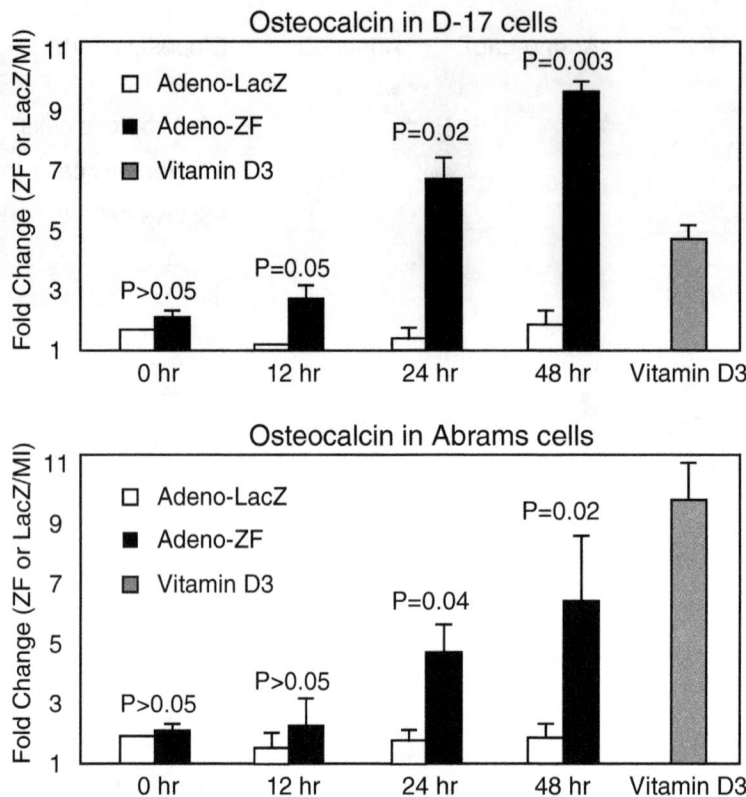

Figure 4 Zhangfei induces differentiation of canine osteosarcoma cells. D–17 and Abrams cells were either mock-infected or infected with Adeno-ZF or Adeno-LacZ. The positive control cells were treated with 10^{-5} mM vitamin D3. The mRNA levels of osteoblast differentiation marker (osteocalcin) were estimated by qRT-PCR. Standard deviations from means and P values as calculated using a Student T-test are shown.

naturally develop therapy resistance and metastasis. In addition, tumor burdens in spontaneously arising cancers of dogs are more similar to humans than the experimentally induced tumors found in murine models, which may be important with regard to biologic factors such as hypoxia and clonal variation. The size of canine tumors also allows for serial imaging and tissue collection over time [29].

In previous studies, we found that the transcription factor CREBZF/Zhangfei suppressed the growth of D–17 dog OS cells [5]. Herein, we further discovered that the growth suppressive effects of Zhangfei were applicable to three other independently isolated canine OS cell lines as well.

The unfolded protein response (UPR) is an adaptive response induced by endoplasmic reticulum (ER) stress, which alleviates ER stress by up-regulating the expression of ER-resident chaperons [30], inducing ER-associated protein degradation (ERAD), and down-regulating the synthesis of new proteins [31,32]. If these mechanisms are not sufficient to alleviate ER stress, then an apoptosis program is initiated to induce cell death. Our previous results [15] suggest that Zhangfei is a potential regulator of the UPR, and it might accelerate UPR feedback mechanisms

by interacting with the UPR mediator-Xbp1 and targeting it for proteasomal degradation. In the present study, the strong inhibitory effects of Zhangfei on both pharmacological (thapsigargin) and physiological (glucose deprivation) –induced UPR was also observed in the four canine OS cell lines we examined.

Zhangfei suppresses the UPR and cell growth by stabilizing the tumour suppressor protein p53 [6]. All four canine OS cell lines we examined express functional p53 (Figure 1). These results suggest that the induction of Zhangfei expression in canine OS may be an effective strategy for suppressing cell growth and metastasis. However, the strategy would likely only be successful with OS that have functional p53. A large proportion of human cancers have deleted or otherwise non-functional p53. At present we do not know the proportion of canine OS that have inactive p53. Some studies [33] suggest that most canine OS do not have deletions or major rearrangements in the gene for p53. Although 30–50% of p53 coding sequences in canine OS have polymorphisms [33-35] the effect of these changes on p53 functionality is unknown. It is therefore difficult to determine how universally applicable Zhangfei would be as a modality for treating canine OS. The role of p53 in canine OS is also

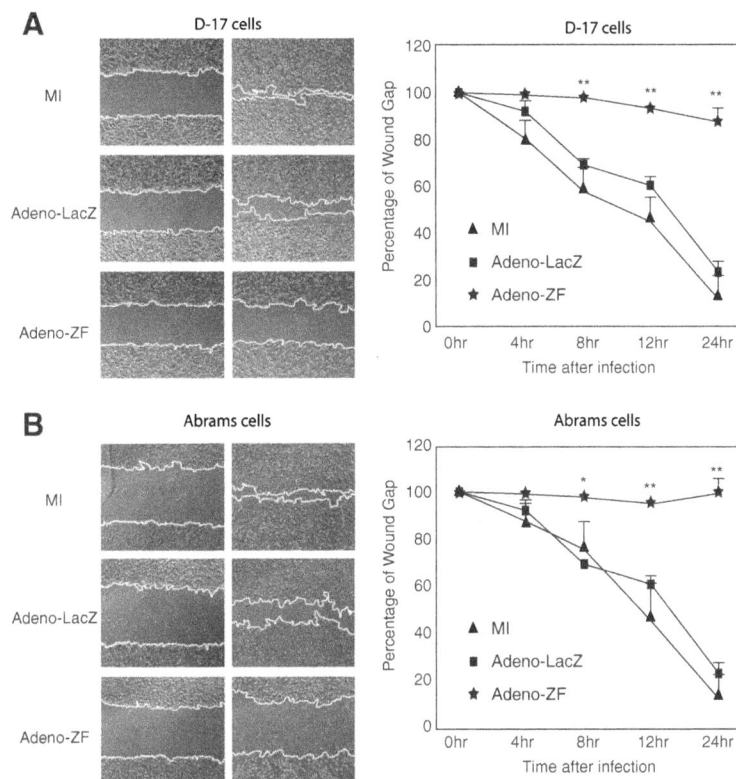

Figure 5 Ectopic expression of Zhangfei causes decreased ability of canine osteosarcoma cells to repair a scratch wound. (A) Scratch wounds were made in 100% confluent cultures of D–17 or Abrams cells mock-infected or infected with Adeno-ZF or Adeno-LacZ. Phase contrast images were taken at 0, 4, 8, 12, and 24 hours after infection from identical regions. **(B)** The wound size relative to the starting wound size was measured at each time point after infection in three independent experiments and expressed as a percentage reduction in wound size + standard deviation. Significance of differences of means (*$P < 0.05$, **$P < 0.01$) were determined using ANOVA.

controversial. The expression of ectopic p53 in canine OS cells, both *in vitro* and *in vivo* models leads to reduced tumour growth and an increase in apoptotic cells [5,36,37]. In contrast, other studies in both humans [38] and dogs [39,40] suggest that increased p53 expression in OS correlates with more aggressive tumours and decreases survival time.

Methods

Cells and tissue culture

Canine osteosarcoma D–17 cells, obtained from the American Type Tissue Culture Collection, were grown in MEM-Alpha containing 10% fetal bovine serum (FBS). Canine Abrams, McKinley and Gracie cell lines were grown in Dulbecco's minimal essential medium containing penicillin, streptomycin and 10% newborn calf serum. All media, serum and antibiotics were purchased from Invitrogen (Carlsbad, California). Abrams cells were derived from metastatic OS nodules whereas McKinley and Gracie cells were from primary tumours. All cell lines were confirmed to be of canine origin by multispecies multiplex PCR and identified by short tandem repeat analysis as described [41].

Adenovirus Vectors Expressing Zhangfei and ß-galactosidase (LacZ)

These vectors were constructed, grown, and purified using the Adeno-X Expression System (Clontech). They were created in our laboratory as described earlier [14]. Cells were infected with Adeno-Zhangfei, Adeno-LacZ (expressing *E. coli* ß-galactosidase, LacZ) or mock-infected. A multiplicity of infection (MOI) of 100 plaque-forming units (pfu) per cell was used.

WST-1 cell proliferation and viability assay

To determine the growth rate of cells, 10^4 cells/well were seeded into 96-well plates. 24 h later cells were either mock infected or infected with adenovirus vectors expressing Zhangfei (Adeno-ZF) or ß-galactosidase (Adeno-LacZ). Cell proliferation was assessed using Cell Proliferation Reagent WST-1 (Roche, Mannheim, Germany) according to the manufacturer's specifications.

Annexin V-apoptosis assay

Cells were collected after trypsinization and stained with Annexin V and propidium iodide (PI) using an Annexin V kit (Calbiochem) following manufacturer's instructions. As

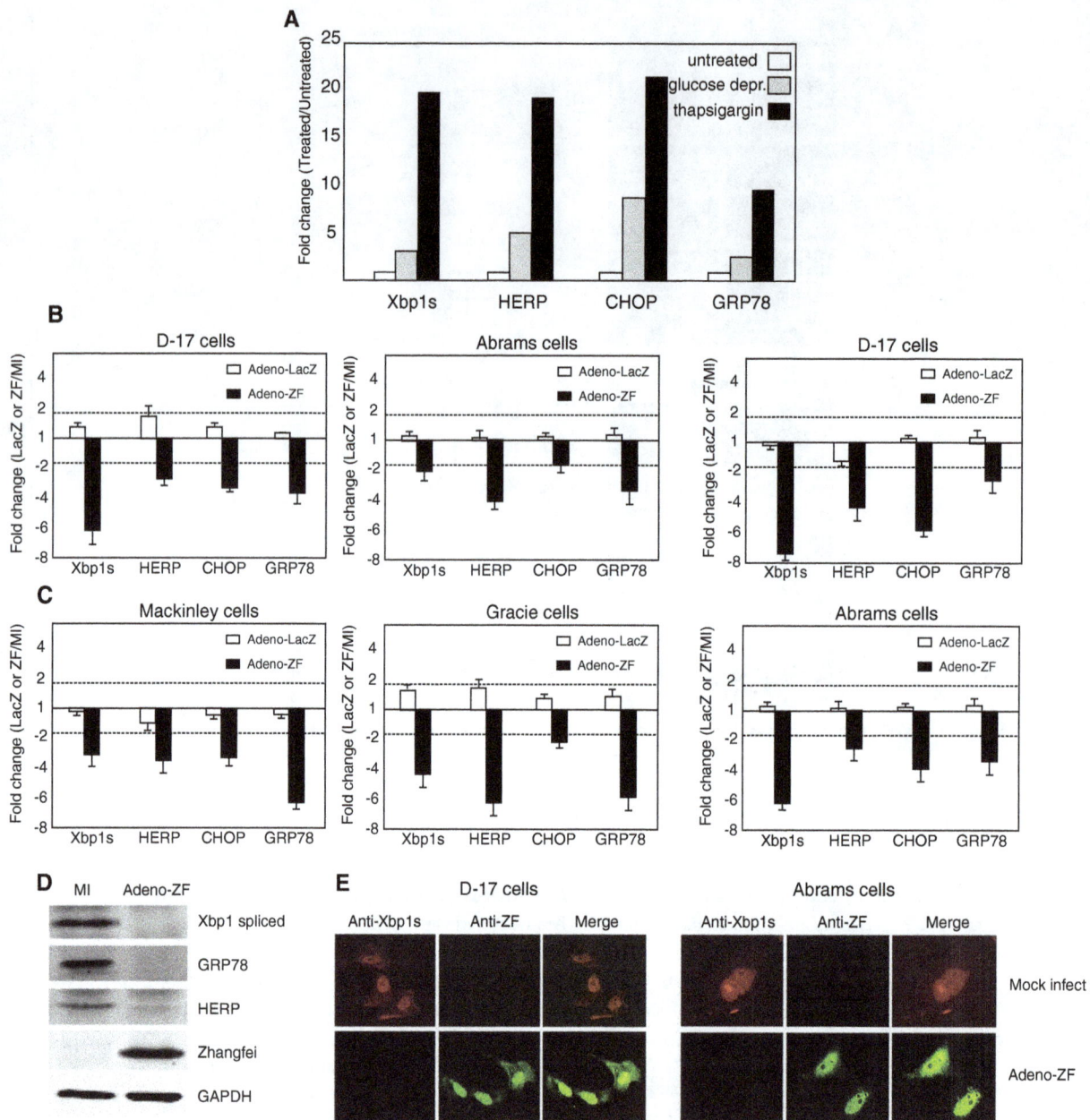

Figure 6 Zhangfei negatively regulates the Unfolded Protein Responses (UPR) in canine osteosarcomas. (A) D–17 cells were left untreated, treated with thapsigargin or grown in glucose free medium. Twelve hours later cells were harvested and transcripts for the UPR- linked genes Xbp1s, HERP, CHOP and GRP78 estimated by qRT-PCR. Cells were mock-infected or infected with either Adeno-ZF or Adeno-LacZ and then treated with thapsigargin **(B)** or deprived of glucose **(C)**. 24 hr later cells were harvested and transcripts for UPR genes estimated. Proteins in thapsigargin-treated mock-infected and Adeno-ZF-infected cells were detected by immunoblots **(D)** and immunofluorescence **(E)**. Dotted lines in A and B indicate a 2-fold difference. Values greater than 2 fold were considered significant.

a positive control cells were treated with 50 μM etopocide (Calbiochem) for 24 hr. Cells were analyzed in a Coulter EPICS XL flow cytometer. In this assay, early apoptotic cells stained with Annexin V but not with PI while late apoptotic or necrotic cells stained with both Annexin V and PI.

Scratch wound healing assay

Scratch wounds more than 5 mm in length and of equal thickness were made in 100% confluent cultures of D–17 or Abrams cells mock-infected or infected with Adeno-ZF or Adeno-LacZ with a 10 μL disposable micropipette tip. Phase contrast images were obtained at 0, 4, 8, 12, and

24 hours after infection from identical regions. The wound size at each time point after infection relative to the starting wound size was measured using Photoshop software in three independent experiments.

Quantitative real-time PCR (qPCR)
Total RNA was extracted using RNeasy Plus Mini Kit from Qiagen (Mississauga, ON, Canada). Gene expression was analyzed by RT-PCR using Brilliant II SYBR Green QPCR Master Mix Kit (Agilent Technologies). Levels of GAPDH were used to normalize the samples. All reactions were analyzed in duplicate and each experiment was repeated at least twice. Relative fold changes of transcript levels were calculated as $2^{\Delta\Delta\ Ct}$. Nucleotide sequences of the primers used are in Table 1. The identity of all products was confirmed by electrophoretic mobility on mobility on agarose gels and by determining nucleotide sequence. Only results with homogeneous thermal disassociation profiles were considered.

PCR and sequencing of p53 genes
The sequences of PCR primers used for canine p53 amplification were: canine p53-forward: GGTGACTG CAATGGAGGAGTCGCA, canine p53-reverse: TCAGT CTGAGTCAAGCCCTTCTCT. RNA was purified from cells using the RNEasy Plus mini kit with a genomic DNA elimination step (Qiagen) and RNA converted to cDNA with the Quantitect Reverse Transcription kit (Qiagen) using instructions supplied by the manufacturer. Two-step RT-PCR reactions used TopTaq emzyme (Qiagen) and were performed in a PCR machine. Sequences were aligned using the software, MacVector. Nucleotide sequences for coding sequences for p53 transcripts recovered from D17, Abrams, McKinley and Gracie cell lines were submitted to GenBank/NCBI and were assigned the following accession numbers: KP279761, KP279762, KP279763, KP279764.

Table 1 Sequence of primers used for qRT-PCR

Xbp1	spliced-forward	TCTGCTGAGTCCGCAGCAGG
	spliced-reverse	TAAGGAACTGGGTCCTTCT
HERP	forward	CCGAGCCTGAGCCCGTCACG
	reverse	CTTTGGAAGCAAGTCCTTGA
CHOP	forward	TGGAAGCCTGGTATGAGGAC
	reverse	TGCCACTTTCCTCTCGTTCT
GRP78	forward	GGCTTGGATAAGAGGGAAGG
	reverse	GGTAGAACGGAACAGGTCCA
osteocalcin	forward	AAGCRGGAGGGCAGCAGGT
	reverse	CYGRTARGCYTCCTGRAAGC
GAPDH	forward	TGCCTCCTGCACCACCAACTGC
	reverse	GGGCCATCCACAGTCTTCTGGG

All sequences are in the 5′–3′ direction.

Plasmids and chloramphenicol acetyl transferase (CAT) assay
The construction of pcZF [12], a plasmid that expresses Zhangfei in mammalian cells, has been described. The CAT reporter plasmid pCAT3B-p53RE was constructed by transferring oligonucleotides containing two copies of p53 responsive element, GGTCAAGTTGGGACACGTC CaaGAGCTAAGTCCTGACATGTCT (IDT, Coralville, Iowa), to pCAT3Basic (Promega), which contains the coding sequence for CAT linked to a basal promoter. Oligonucleotides representing the p53 responsive elements with overhanging 5′ terminal KpnI and 3′ terminal BglII sites were annealed and ligated to pCAT3Basic cut with the same enzymes.

In CAT assay, D–17, Abrams, Gracie and McKinley cells were transfected with 0.5 μg of pCAT3B-p53RE, in the presence or absence of a plasmid expressing Zhangfei (pcZF, 1 μg), using Lipofectamine 2000 (Invitrogen) as described in the manufacturer's instructions. The promoterless parental reporter plasmid, pCAT3B was included as a control to show basal CAT activity. 250 ng of pCMVBGal, a plasmid specifying β-galactosidase, were added to each transfection as an internal control. 24 h after transfection, the CAT activity was determined by ELISA. CAT values were normalized to β-galactosidase.

Antibodies, immunoblotting and immunofluorescence
The antibodies used were mouse anti-FLAG (Sigma), rabbit anti-Zhangfei serum [12], rabbit anti-Xbp1 (Abcam, Cambridge, MA), rabbit anti-HERP (Abcam, Cambridge, MA), rabbit anti-GRP78 (Abcam, Cambridge, MA), and mouse anti-GAPDH (Chemicon, Billerica, MA). Suppliers of antibodies against Xbp1, HERP, GRP78 and GAPDH indicated that they recognized canine proteins. Secondary antibodies were goat anti-mouse Alexa488, goat anti-rabbit Alexa546 and goat anti-rabbit Cy5 (Invitrogen). Cells were processed for immunoblotting and immunofluorescence as described previously [5,12].

Statistical analysis
Statistical analysis of data was performed by Student T-test or ANOVA using IBM SPSS statistics version 21.0.0 software. ANOVA tests with LSDpost hoc comparison was used to analyze the differences between multi-group means and their associated procedures by adding individuals as a treatment variable, and a paired T-test was used to evaluate the effects of one treatment compared with no treatment/control. A P value of less than 0.05 was considered to be statistically significant for both tests.

Availability of supporting data
Accession numbers sequences supporting the results of this article are available in the GenBank repository, [GenBank: KP279761, GenBank:KP279762, GenBank:KP279763, GenBank:KP279764]."

Ethics and biosafety statement

All experiments were done following biosafety procedures and precautions approved by the University of Saskatchewan Biosafety committee and under Biosafety Permit VMB-03. All experiment were done on established cell lines and no animals were used.

Abbreviations

bLZip: Basic leucine zipper; CERBZF: Cyclic AMP response element binding protein Zhangfei; UPR: Unfolded protein response; OS: Osteosarcoma; p53: 53,000 molecular weight protein; Xbp1: X-box binding protein one; ATF4: Activation transcription factor four; SMAD: Homologue of *small body size* (*C. elegans*) and *mothers against decapentaplegic* (*Drosophila*); VP16: Herpes simplex virus virion protein sixteen; LacZ: Beta galactosidase; GRP78: Glucose responsive protein 78,000 molecular weight; HERP: Homocysteine-responsive endoplasmic reticulum resident protein; CHOP: C/EBP homologous protein; ERAD: Endoplasmic reticulum resident protein degradation; FBS: Foetal bovine serum; MOI: Multiplicity of infection; PI: Propidium iodide; GAPDH: Glyceraldehyde 3-phosphate dehydrogenase; qPCR: Quantitative polymerase chain reaction; CAT: Chloramphenicol acetyl transferase.

Competing interests

The authors declare that they have no competing interests.

Authors' contributions

RZ, VM and DHT conceived of the experiments and DHT provided the cell lines. RZ performed all the experiments and prepared the initial manuscript and figures. VM, DHT and RZ edited, approved and prepared the final manuscript.

Acknowledgements

This work was supported by a Discovery grant to VM from the Natural Sciences and Engineering Research Council (NSERC) of Canada and a grant from the Western College of Veterinary Medicine (WCVM) Companion Animal Research Fund and the Kaye Canine Foundation. RZ was supported by scholarships from the Government of China (China Scholarship Council, RZ-2010635007) and the University of Saskatchewan College of Graduate Studies and Research.

Author details

[1]Department of Microbiology, Western College of Veterinary Medicine, University of Saskatchewan, Saskatoon, SK, Canada. [2]Flint Animal Cancer Center, Colorado State University, Fort Collins, CO, USA. [3]Present address: Department of Basic Veterinary Medicine, College of Veterinary Medicine, China Agricultural University, Beijing, China.

References

1. Withrow SJ, Wilkins RM. Cross talk from pets to people: translational osteosarcoma treatments. ILAR J. 2010;51(3):208–213.
2. Mueller F, Fuchs B, Kaser-Hotz B. Comparative biology of human and canine osteosarcoma. Anticancer Res. 2007;27(1A):155–164.
3. Khanna C, London C, Vail D, Mazcko C, Hirschfeld S. Guiding the optimal translation of new cancer treatments from canine to human cancer patients. Clin Cancer Res. 2009;15(18):5671–5677.
4. Paoloni M, Khanna C. Translation of new cancer treatments from pet dogs to humans. Nat Rev Cancer. 2008;8(2):147–156.
5. Bergeron T, Zhang R, Elliot K, Rapin N, MacDonald V, Linn K. The effect of Zhangfei on the unfolded protein response and growth of cells derived from canine and human osteosarcomas. Vet Comp Oncol. 2013;11(2):140–50.
6. Zhang R, Misra V. Effects of cyclic AMP response element binding protein-Zhangfei (CREBZF) on the unfolded protein response and cell growth are exerted through the tumor suppressor p53. Cell Cycle. 2014;13(2):279–92.
7. Legare ME, Bush J, Ashley AK, Kato T, Hanneman WH. Cellular and phenotypic characterization of canine osteosarcoma cell lines. J Cancer. 2011;2:262–270.
8. MacEwen EG, Kutzke J, Carew J, Pastor J, Schmidt JA, Tsan R, et al. c-Met tyrosine kinase receptor expression and function in human and canine osteosarcoma cells. Clin Exp Metastasis. 2003;20(5):421–430.
9. MacEwen EG, Pastor J, Kutzke J, Tsan R, Kurzman ID, Thamm DH, et al. IGF-1 receptor contributes to the malignant phenotype in human and canine osteosarcoma. J Cell Biochem. 2004;92(1):77–91.
10. Schwartz AL, Custis JT, Harmon JF, Powers BE, Chubb LS, LaRue SM, et al. Orthotopic model of canine osteosarcoma in athymic rats for evaluation of stereotactic radiotherapy. Am J Vet Res. 2013;74(3):452–458.
11. Maeda J, Yurkon CR, Fujisawa H, Kaneko M, Genet SC, Roybal EJ, et al. Genomic instability and telomere fusion of canine osteosarcoma cells. PLoS One. 2012;7(8):e43355.
12. Lu R, Misra V: Z. Second cellular protein interacts with herpes simplex virus accessory factor HCF in a manner similar to Luman and VP16. Nucleic Acids Res. 2000;28(12):2446–2454.
13. Cockram GP, Hogan MR, Burnett HF, Lu R. Identification and characterization of the DNA-binding properties of a Zhangfei homologue in Japanese pufferfish, Takifugu rubripes. Biochem Biophys Res Commun. 2006;339(4):1238–1245.
14. Misra V, Rapin N, Akhova O, Bainbridge M, Korchinski P. Zhangfei is a potent and specific inhibitor of the host cell factor-binding transcription factor Luman. J Biol Chem. 2005;280(15):15257–15266.
15. Zhang R, Rapin N, Ying Z, Shklanka E, Bodnarchuk TW, Verge VMK, et al. Zhangfei/CREB-ZF - A Potential Regulator of the Unfolded protein Response. PLoS One. 2013;8(10):e77256.
16. Hogan MR, Cockram GP, Lu R. Cooperative interaction of Zhangfei and ATF4 in transactivation of the cyclic AMP response element. FEBS Lett. 2006;580(1):58–62.
17. Lee JH, Lee GT, Kwon SJ, Jeong J, Ha YS, Kim WJ, et al. CREBZF, a novel Smad8-binding protein. Mol Cell Biochem. 2012;368(1-2):147–153.
18. Akhova O, Bainbridge M, Misra V. The neuronal host cell factor-binding protein Zhangfei inhibits herpes simplex virus replication. J Virol. 2005;79(23):14708–14718.
19. Lopez-Mateo I, Villaronga MA, Llanos S, Belandia B. The transcription factor CREBZF is a novel positive regulator of p53. Cell Cycle. 2012;11(20):3887–3895.
20. Joerger AC, Fersht AR. Structural biology of the tumor suppressor p53. Annu Rev Biochem. 2008;77:557–582.
21. Ciovacco WA, Goldberg CG, Taylor AF, Lemieux JM, Horowitz MC, Donahue HJ, et al. The role of gap junctions in megakaryocyte-mediated osteoblast proliferation and differentiation. Bone. 2009;44(1):80–86.
22. Selvarajah GT, Kirpensteijn J. Prognostic and predictive biomarkers of canine osteosarcoma. Vet J. 2010;185(1):28–35.
23. Fan TM, Charney SC, de Lorimier LP, Garrett LD, Griffon DJ, Gordon-Evans WJ, et al. Double-blind placebo-controlled trial of adjuvant pamidronate with palliative radiotherapy and intravenous doxorubicin for canine appendicular osteosarcoma bone pain. J Vet Intern Med. 2009;23(1):152–60.
24. Tomlin JL, Sturgeon C, Pead MJ, Muir P. Use of the bisphosphonate drug alendronate for palliative management of osteosarcoma in two dogs. Vet Rec. 2000;147(5):129–132.
25. Walter CU, Dernell WS, LaRue SM, Lana SE, Lafferty MH, LaDue TA, et al. Curative-intent radiation therapy as a treatment modality for appendicular and axial osteosarcoma: a preliminary retrospective evaluation of 14 dogs with the disease. Vet Comp Oncol. 2005;3(1):1–7.
26. Brodey RS, Abt DA. Results of surgical treatment in 65 dogs with osteosarcoma. J Am Vet Med Assoc. 1976;168(11):1032–1035.
27. Kurzman ID, MacEwen EG, Rosenthal RC, Fox LE, Keller ET, Helfand SC, et al. Adjuvant therapy for osteosarcoma in dogs: results of randomized clinical trials using combined liposome-encapsulated muramyl tripeptide and cisplatin. Clin Cancer Res. 1995;1(12):1595–1601.
28. Dow S, Elmslie R, Kurzman I, MacEwen G, Pericle F, Liggitt D. Phase I study of liposome-DNA complexes encoding the interleukin–2 gene in dogs with osteosarcoma lung metastases. Hum Gene Ther. 2005;16(8):937–946.
29. Paoloni M, Davis S, Lana S, Withrow S, Sangiorgi L, Picci P, et al. Canine tumor cross-species genomics uncovers targets linked to osteosarcoma progression. BMC Genomics. 2009;10:625.
30. Kaufman RJ, Scheuner D, Schroder M, Shen X, Lee K, Liu CY, et al. The unfolded protein response in nutrient sensing and differentiation. Nat Rev Mol Cell Biol. 2002;3(6):411–421.
31. Meusser B, Hirsch C, Jarosch E, Sommer T. ERAD: the long road to destruction. Nat Cell Biol. 2005;7(8):766–772.
32. Lai E, Teodoro T, Volchuk A. Endoplasmic reticulum stress: signaling the unfolded protein response. Physiology. 2007;22:193–201.

33. Mendoza S, Konishi T, Dernell WS, Withrow SJ, Miller CW. Status of the p53, Rb and MDM2 genes in canine osteosarcoma. Anticancer Res. 1998;18(6A):4449–4453.

34. van Leeuwen IS, Cornelisse CJ, Misdorp W, Goedegebuure SA, Kirpensteijn J, Rutteman GR. P53 gene mutations in osteosarcomas in the dog. Cancer Lett. 1997;111(1–2):173–178.

35. Johnson AS, Couto CG, Weghorst CM. Mutation of the p53 tumor suppressor gene in spontaneously occurring osteosarcomas of the dog. Carcinogenesis. 1998;19(1):213–217.

36. Kanaya N, Yazawa M, Goto-Koshino Y, Mochizuki M, Nishimura R, Ohno K, et al. Anti-tumor effect of adenoviral vector-mediated p53 gene transfer on the growth of canine osteosarcoma xenografts in nude mice. J Vet Med Sci. 2011;73(7):877–883.

37. Yazawa M, Setoguchi A, Hong SH, Uyama R, Nakagawa T, Kanaya N, et al. Effect of an adenoviral vector that expresses the canine p53 gene on cell growth of canine osteosarcoma and mammary adenocarcinoma cell lines. Am J Vet Res. 2003;64(7):880–888.

38. Fu HL, Shao L, Wang Q, Jia T, Li M, Yang DP. A systematic review of p53 as a biomarker of survival in patients with osteosarcoma. Tumour Biol. 2013;34(6):3817–3821.

39. Sagartz JE, Bodley WL, Gamblin RM, Couto CG, Tierney LA, Capen CC. p53 tumor suppressor protein overexpression in osteogenic tumors of dogs. Vet Pathol. 1996;33(2):213–221.

40. Loukopoulos P, Thornton JR, Robinson WF. Clinical and pathologic relevance of p53 index in canine osseous tumors. Vet Pathol. 2003;40(3):237–248.

41. O'Donoghue LE, Rivest JP, Duval DL. Polymerase chain reaction-based species verification and microsatellite analysis for canine cell line validation. J Vet Diagn Invest. 2011;23(4):780–785.

11

Inter-observer agreement of canine and feline paroxysmal event semiology and classification by veterinary neurology specialists and non-specialists

Rowena MA Packer[1], Mette Berendt[2], Sofie Bhatti[3], Marios Charalambous[4], Sigitas Cizinauskas[5], Luisa De Risio[6], Robyn Farquhar[7], Rachel Hampel[1], Myfanwy Hill[1], Paul JJ Mandigers[8], Akos Pakozdy[9], Stephanie M Preston[1], Clare Rusbridge[10], Veronika M Stein[11], Fran Taylor-Brown[1], Andrea Tipold[11] and Holger A Volk[1]*

Abstract

Background: Advances in mobile technology mean vets are now commonly presented with videos of paroxysmal events by clients, but the consistency of the interpretation of these videos has not been investigated. The objective of this study was to investigate the level of agreement between vets (both neurology specialists and non-specialists) on the description and classification of videos depicting paroxysmal events, without knowing any results of diagnostic workup. An online questionnaire study was conducted, where participants watched 100 videos of dogs and cats exhibiting paroxysmal events and answered questions regarding: epileptic seizure presence (yes/no), seizure type, consciousness status, and the presence of motor, autonomic and neurobehavioural signs. Agreement statistics (percentage agreement and kappa) calculated for each variable, with prevalence indices calculated to aid their interpretation.

Results: Only a fair level of agreement ($\kappa = 0.40$) was found for epileptic seizure presence. Overall agreement of seizure type was moderate ($\kappa = 0.44$), with primary generalised seizures showing the highest level of agreement ($\kappa = 0.60$), and focal the lowest ($\kappa = 0.31$). Fair agreement was found for consciousness status and the presence of autonomic signs ($\kappa = 0.21–0.40$), but poor agreement for neurobehavioral signs ($\kappa = 0.16$). Agreement for motor signs ranged from poor ($\kappa = \leq 0.20$) to moderate ($\kappa = 0.41–0.60$). Differences between specialists and non-specialists were identified.

Conclusions: The relatively low levels of agreement described here highlight the need for further discussions between neurology experts regarding classifying and describing epileptic seizures, and additional training of non-specialists to facilitate accurate diagnosis. There is a need for diagnostic tools (e.g. electroencephalogram) able to differentiate between epileptic and non-epileptic paroxysms.

Keywords: Seizure, Epilepsy, Canine, Feline, Video, Paroxysmal event, Agreement, Kappa

* Correspondence: hvolk@rvc.ac.uk
[1]Department of Clinical Science and Services, Royal Veterinary College, Hertfordshire, UK
Full list of author information is available at the end of the article

Background

Diagnosing and appropriately treating canine epilepsy requires accurate epileptic seizure detection and description of seizure semiology, the detailed observations of physical signs during a seizure episode indicative of an alteration in neurological state. Seizure semiology is a simple and cost-effective tool in the understanding of a seizure disorder and attempting to localise the epileptic focus. As such, veterinary neurology specialists and first opinion practitioners require a detailed semiologic description of paroxysmal events to confidently diagnose canine epilepsy and categorise the type of seizures experienced. Semiologic descriptions are often obtained from the family or caregivers of human epilepsy patients, relying on common terms for ictal symptoms [1]; however, video-EEG (electroencephalogram) monitoring is the preferred method for the diagnosis and classification of seizures due to its increased reliability [2]. In veterinary medicine such methods are not widely available, and have doubtful reliability, and thus it is of high importance to establish the accuracy and consistency of observational reports. These reports may come from the owners of affected dogs; however, due to the acute-onset, unpredictable and highly stressful nature of a seizure event, the reliability of these reports may be significantly reduced. Many owners now have access to mobile technology such as smart phones and tablet computers with video-recording capabilities, facilitating the recording of these events, which can later be presented to their veterinary surgeon. This was demonstrated in a recent study of the video-sharing website YouTube, where many owners uploaded videos of their dog's seizure activity either seeking advice from viewers (2/3rd) or to show to their veterinarian (1/3rd) [3]. The consistency of the interpretation of these videos by different vets is therefore an area of importance. If agreement between vets in the classification of videos of paroxysmal events is low, then vets should ensure that videos are not used in isolation of other clinical data such as signalment, history and other diagnostics to diagnose epileptic seizures.

Aims

This study aimed to investigate the level of agreement between vets (both recognised neurology specialists and non-specialists) on the description of videos depicting paroxysmal events without knowing the results of diagnostic workup. As the aim was limited to evaluating the phenotype of the event only, the observers were blinded to any additional history, diagnostics or treatment outcome for all animals. Finding good agreement between observers allows judgements to be made by different observers with some confidence in their consistency, whereas finding poor agreement between observers can highlight deficiencies in classification systems, which

may indicate a need for refinement of definitions, or improved training of observers. The level of agreement between veterinary observers has important practical implications, for example, high agreement between observers is essential in multicentre clinical trials. Thus, this study aimed to highlight areas where further discussion is required, to improve consistency between neurologists diagnosing seizure disorders.

The focus of this study was on the initial perception of whether a paroxysmal event was a seizure or not, and if so, what type of seizure was present. As seizure type is likely predicted by the semiology of the event, the level of agreement between observers over (i) the quality of consciousness in the patient, in addition to (ii) the presence of 13 motor signs, (iii) three autonomic signs and (iv) three neurobehavioural signs was investigated. As this was a novel study, the aspects of seizure semiology investigated were intentionally broad as not to exclude potentially useful characteristics, that if demonstrated to show high concordance between observers could be useful predictors of seizure type.

In addition this study sought to detect differences in the reporting of seizure semiology and classification of seizure type between specialists and non-specialists, to investigate whether there is an effect of additional training upon semiologic description. Finally, this study sought to identify which observer-perceived seizure characteristics predict reported seizure type. If the characteristics used by observers to predict certain seizure types are not highly agreed upon then this could lead to unreliable classification of seizure type.

Hypotheses

H1. There are high levels of agreement between veterinary observers for the prediction of seizure presence and seizure type.

H2. There are high levels of agreement between veterinary observers for the classification of (i) consciousness status, and the presence of (ii) motor signs, (iii) autonomic signs and (iv) neurobehavioural signs.

H3. There are differences in the classification of seizure presence and type, and reporting of seizure semiology between veterinary neurology specialists and non-specialists.

H4. Observer-reported seizure semiology will differentiate between primary generalised seizures, focal seizures, and focal seizures with secondary generalisation.

Methods

A questionnaire was hosted on SurveyMonkey© in April 2014, with 10 senior neurology specialists (9 Diplomates of the European College of Veterinary Neurology (ECVN) and 1 associate ECVN member), and 5 Royal College of Veterinary Surgeon (RCVS) registered non-specialist veterinary surgeons invited to participate. One hundred videos of dogs and cats (sourced: 15 videos from one of the authors and 85 uploaded to YouTube©) exhibiting paroxysmal events were provided. Videos that were initially sourced from YouTube© were identified using the search term "dog seizure" or "cat seizure". All videos on YouTube are constantly shuffled by the website's confidential search algorithms. To randomise video selection, every 5th video was selected for analysis; however, the following exclusion criteria were applied: only one video per uploader, very poor quality videos, professional videos, advertisements, photographic collages, videos not showing domestic dogs or cats, and videos with text overlying the footage. The resultant 85 YouTube©-sourced videos and 15 author-sourced videos were provided to participants at the start of the study.

Participants were requested to watch all 100 videos and initially answer the following questions:

(1) Is what you see in the video an epileptic seizure?
(2) If you think it is NOT an epileptic seizure, what term would you use to describe the episode?

Participants were allowed to view the videos as often as they wished and were allowed to review the video as they were answering the survey. If the participant responded that they believed it was *not* an epileptic seizure they were instructed to move on to the next video. If participants responded that the video did indeed show an epileptic seizure, they were requested to categorise what the seizure type was best classified as (focal, focal with secondary generalisation or primary generalised). Participants were then requested to further characterise the epileptic seizure based on the presence and type of motor signs, autonomic signs and neurobehavioural signs and quality/status of consciousness, which were listed as tick boxes with the option to select as many as believed to apply (Additional file 1). This study was approved by the Royal Veterinary College Ethics and Welfare Committee.

Statistical analysis

Hypothesis 1 and 2: are there high levels of agreement between veterinary observers for the prediction of seizure presence and type, the classification of consciousness status, and the presence of motor, autonomic and neurobehavioural signs?

Agreement statistics were calculated using Minitab version 17. Raw percentage (%) agreement, the percentage of the total number of observations for each variable where there is agreement was calculated for each

variable across all videos, with the mean and 95% CI reported for each variable. Percentage agreement should not be solely relied upon however, as it does not take into account chance agreement, and thus to be more stringent, Fleiss' kappa (κ) for more than 2 observers was calculated for each variable in the questionnaire to determine which aspects of a seizure were agreed upon between observers [4].

This study compared observers equally against one another, rather than against an objective method or a trained individual and thus no 'gold standard' was used to compare ratings with. Good agreement was indicated by % agreements close to 100 and by κ values close to 1. In line with Benbir et al. (2013), concordance was rated as 'poor' for κ values ≤ 0.2; 'fair' if κ were in the range 0.21–0.40; 'moderate' for 0.41–0.60; 'good' for 0.61–0.80; and 'excellent' if κ exceeded 0.81. This was an exploratory study to see which aspects of a seizure were most or least agreed upon, and thus a minimum threshold of κ was not set. As a guide, the minimum threshold for κ is often arbitrarily set at $\kappa \leq 0.4$ [5].

A limitation of the kappa statistics is that the magnitude of κ is a function of the prevalence of the trait measured by a question as well as the number of discordant responses [6,7] and thus a skewed distribution of data lowers the κ coefficient. In near-homogenous populations, evidence for agreement above chance levels is difficult to identify, resulting in low κ values. To aid the interpretation of κ values and % agreement for each variable, the prevalence index (PI) for multiple observers [8] was calculated using the following formula:

$$PI = \frac{R_1 - R_2}{N_n}$$

PI = The absolute difference between the number of ratings in categories 1 and 2 (R_1 and R_2, respectively), divided by the number of subjects (N) multiplied by the number of ratings per subject (n).

Where high κ and % agreement values are achieved (and are of a similar magnitude), PI may not need to be consulted; however, if κ is low, or if the κ and % agreement values disagree, the PI can aid in the interpretation of this result. For example, if the % agreement is high but κ is low, this result is inconclusive due to the PI being too high, rather than due to clear inconsistency between observers. Where κ is low, but % agreement is correspondingly low, this is due to inconsistency between observers, and the variable should be considered unreliable. Such occurrences are highlighted in the results.

Table 1 Inter-observer agreement of seizure presence, type and consciousness status

Variable	Mean % agreement (95% CI)	PI	Category	κ	SE (κ)	Z	p
Is this an epileptic seizure?	29% (19-40%)	0.4	Yes	0.40	0.01	35.12	<0.001
What type of epileptic seizure?	18% (10-28%)	0.47	Focal seizure	0.31	0.01	27.36	<0.001
		0.86	Focal seizure with secondary generalisation	0.53	0.01	45.63	<0.001
		0.27	Primary generalised seizure	0.60	0.01	51.93	<0.001
			Overall	0.44	0.01	62.08	<0.001
Is the dog conscious?	9% (3-19%)	0.72	Conscious (No impairment)	0.45	0.01	39.92	<0.001
		0.38	Impairment in consciousness	0.20	0.01	15.16	<0.001
		0.48	Unconscious	0.54	0.01	41.99	<0.001
			Overall	0.39	0.01	42.59	<0.001

(κ = kappa, PI = prevalence index, SE = standard error).

Hypothesis 3: are there differences in the classification of seizure presence and type, and reporting of seizure semiology between veterinary neurology specialists and non-specialists?

The influence of experience and training was investigated by analysing associations between observer type (specialist *vs.* non-specialist) and seizure type/characteristics, using IBM SPSS v19. The binomial dependent variable was neurology specialist or non-specialist, and the independent variables were seizure presence, type, consciousness status and the presence of motor (13), autonomic (3) and behavioural (3) signs. Associations were screened at the univariate level using Chi-squared analysis for categorical variables. If significant variables were identified they were taken forwards to a binary mixed model, where video number and observer were included as random effects to control for these sources of non-independence.

Hypothesis 4: does observer-reported seizure semiology differentiate between primary generalised seizures, focal seizures, and focal seizures with secondary generalisation?

Multinomial mixed model analyses were carried out in IBM SPSS v19 to determine which factors influenced the choice of seizure type. Three dependent variables were used in the multinomial models: primary generalised seizures, focal seizures, and focal seizures with secondary generalisation. Independent variables in the model were the observer-perceived consciousness status, and presence of thirteen motor, three autonomic and three neurobehavioural signs. All independent factors were first tested at the univariable level using Chi-squared analysis to identify significant factors for inclusion in the multinomial model, with $P < 0.2$ considered for inclusion. A backward stepwise model building strategy was used, selecting models based on fit, as determined by the Akaike information criterion (AIC) statistic, significance

Table 2 Inter-observer agreements of motor signs present in epileptic seizures

Variable	Mean % agreement (95% CI)	PI	κ	SE (κ)	Z	p
Does the dog show motor signs?	73% (63-83%)	0.92	0.06	0.01	4.84	<0.001
Were movements more present on the left?	77% (67-86%)	0.88	0.28	0.01	24.59	<0.001
Were movements more present on the right?	67% (56-77%)	0.86	0.07	0.01	6.05	<0.001
Was the head turned to the side?	63% (51-73%)	0.84	0.14	0.01	11.95	<0.001
Were there running movements?	59% (48-70%)	0.40	0.58	0.01	50.27	<0.001
Were there rhythmic jerks around the mouth?	46% (35-57%)	0.40	0.44	0.01	38.35	<0.001
Was there rhythmic pelvic limb movements?	39% (28-50%)	0.12	0.56	0.01	48.79	<0.001
Are there rhythmic thoracic limb movements?	35% (25-46%)	0.17	0.55	0.01	48.02	<0.001
Was there oral movement (lip smacking)?	34% (24-45%)	0.20	0.35	0.01	30.43	<0.001
Was there stiffening of the pelvic limbs?	28% (19-39%)	0.42	0.37	0.01	33.80	<0.001
Was there stiffening of the thoracic limbs?	25% (16-36%)	0.01	0.39	0.01	34.09	<0.001
Were movements equal between both sides?	18% (10-28%)	0.04	0.37	0.01	32.00	<0.001
Are the eyes open?	5% (1-12%)	0.16	0.17	0.01	15.13	<0.001

(κ = kappa, PI = prevalence index, SE = standard error).

Table 3 Inter-observer agreement of autonomic and neurobehavioural signs in epileptic seizures

Variable	Mean % agreement (95% CI)	PI	κ	SE (κ)	Z	p
Does the dog show autonomic signs?	10% (4-18%)	0.09	0.28	0.01	24.35	<0.001
Did the dog salivate?	53% (42-64%)	0.51	0.64	0.01	55.24	<0.001
Did the dog urinate?	92% (83-97%)	0.97	0.17	0.01	14.89	<0.001
Did the dog defecate?	99% (93-100%)	0.99	−0.01	0.01	−0.07	0.5298
Does the dog show neurobehavioral signs?	4% (1-10%)	0.15	0.16	0.01	14.09	<0.001
Did the dog show fear/anxiety?	22% (13-32%)	0.61	0.15	0.01	12.66	<0.001
Did the dog show aggression?	86% (76-92%)	0.96	0.17	0.01	14.48	<0.001
Did the dog appear to hallucinate?	65% (54-75%)	0.89	0.13	0.01	11.48	<0.001

(κ = kappa, , PI = prevalence index, SE = standard error).

of terms included (P ≤ 0.05 was considered significant), and maximisation of the correct percentage classification of cases. Multicollinearity was initially avoided via examining the associations between all nominal independent variables to detect any high levels of association. If found, the variable that resulted in better model fit was selected for the final model. All models were also checked for collinearity via inspection of the standard errors of the regression coefficients to see if they were inflated which would signify multicollinearity was a problem in that model.

Results

To allow for statistical analysis, all videos must have been rated by an equal number of observers, and thus 17 of the 100 videos were excluded from the analysis due to missing data, and all ratings from 1 observer were excluded due to their low response rate to the questions. In total 1162 ratings were made of 83 videos by the remaining 14 independent observers.

Hypothesis 1 and 2: are there high levels of agreement between veterinary observers for the prediction of seizure presence and type, the classification of consciousness status, and the presence of motor, autonomic and neurobehavioural signs?

Epileptic seizure presence and type

When questioned on whether the paroxysmal events in the videos represented epileptic seizures, 72% of responses to all videos reported they thought the event was a seizure; however, there was a fair level of agreement ($\kappa = 0.40$) with on average only 29% (95% CI 19-40%) agreement between observers as to whether it was a seizure or not for each video (Table 1). Overall agreement of seizure type was moderate ($\kappa = 0.44$), with on average only 18% agreement between observers across videos. The most common seizure type reported from the videos was primary generalised (36% of all ratings), with the highest level of agreement ($\kappa = 0.60$) of all types. The lowest level of agreement was for focal seizures ($\kappa = 0.31$).

Consciousness status

Very low% agreement was achieved regarding the consciousness status of the dog, with on average 9% agreement between observers as to whether the dog was conscious during the paroxysmal events (Table 1). The poorest agreement was achieved for impairment in consciousness ($\kappa = 0.20$), versus moderate levels of agreement for unconscious ($\kappa = 0.54$).

Motor signs

When questioned on whether the paroxysmal events in the videos showed motor signs, 96% of responses to all videos reported they thought motor signs were present, with on average 73% agreement between observers as to whether motor signs were present (Table 2). As the PI was exceptionally high for this variable, with a homogenous sample dominated by 'yes' responses, the κ is artificially lowered to a level of poor agreement ($\kappa = 0.06$). The highest levels of agreement for individual signs, as determined by κ values, were whether there were running movements, whether there were rhythmic pelvic limbs movements and whether there were rhythmic thoracic limb movements (moderate agreement). The lowest levels of agreement as determined by κ values were for whether the eyes were open, whether the head was turned to the side and whether movements were more present on the right side. The latter two variables had high PIs and thus the sample population may be too homogenous to interpret these results.

Autonomic signs

When questioned on whether the paroxysmal events in the videos showed autonomic signs, 55% of responses to all videos reported they thought autonomic signs were present; however, % agreement was low with on average just 10% agreement between observers and a 'fair' κ value ($\kappa = 0.28$) (Table 3). There was good agreement as to whether the dog salivated in the video ($\kappa = 0.64$), but poor κ values for urination or defecation. There were high PIs for both urination and defecation owing to their rarity of reporting (1.4% and 0.1% of all ratings, respectively), and thus despite high % agreement (both with on average over 90% agreement between observers), their κ values were low and thus the reliability of these signs is inconclusive.

Neurobehavioural signs

When questioned on whether the paroxysmal events in the videos showed neurobehavioral signs, over half of responses reported that they were present (58%); however, % agreement was again very low with average agreement of just 4% across all videos and a poor κ value. κ values for all three neurobehavioural signs were poor; however % agreement was high for aggression and hallucination and thus their κ was artificially lowered due to the homogeneity of the sample and the rarity of their reporting (2% and 5% of all ratings, respectively). Fear and anxiety was reported in nearly a fifth of ratings (19%); however had both a poor κ and % agreement, thus indicating low levels of agreement of its presence.

Hypothesis 3: are there differences in the classification of seizure presence and type, and reporting of seizure semiology between veterinary neurology specialists and non-specialists?

Chi-squared analyses revealed significant differences in seizure semiology and classification between specialists and non-specialists. Specialists were less likely to report what they saw in the videos as a seizure than non-specialists (68% vs. 75%; p = 0.008). When questioned on what this was if *not* a seizure, specialists were more likely to report a movement disorder (53% vs. 43%; p = 0.047) and pain associated behaviour (3% vs. 0%; p = 0.047) than non-specialists. Specialists were less likely to report a seizure as focal (34% *vs.* 42%; p = 0.011), more likely to report impaired consciousness (47% *vs.* 37%; p = 0.003) and less likely to report unconsciousness (32% *vs.* 45%; p < 0.001) than non-specialists. With regard to motor signs, specialists were less likely to report the eyes as open (48% *vs.* 76%; p < 0.001), oral movement (36% *vs.* 47%; p = 0.001), rhythmic jerks around the mouth (28% *vs.* 34%; p = 0.031), stiffening of the thoracic limbs (46% *vs.* 56%; p = 0.003), rhythmic pelvic limb movements (41% *vs.* 50%; p = 0.005) or that movements were equal on each side (44% *vs.* 55%; p = 0.001) than non-specialists. There was no difference in the reporting of autonomic signs between specialists and non-specialists. The only difference in the reporting of neurobehavioural signs was that specialists were more likely to report aggression than non-specialists (5% *vs.* 1%; p < 0.001). There were differences in the perception of duration, with non-specialists less likely to report short episodes of only seconds (5% vs. 9%; p = 0.005) or less than 1 minute (27% *vs.* 45%; p < 0.001) than specialists. When a binary mixed model analysis was attempted to determine

which factors were associated with the observer being a specialist or a non-specialist, no factors were found to be significantly associated when video number and observer were included as random effects.

Hypothesis 4: does observer-reported seizure semiology differentiate between primary generalised seizures, focal seizures, and focal seizures with secondary generalisation?

At the univariate level, Chi-squared analysis identified several factors associated with the classification of seizure type including the presence of motor (p < 0.001), autonomic (p < 0.001) and neurobehavioural (p = 0.009) signs. Multinomial mixed models identified seven factors significantly associated with reported seizure types: oral movement, stiffening of thoracic limbs, rhythmic thoracic limb movements, running movements, equal movements on each side, salivation, hallucination (Table 4 and Additional file 2: Table S1).

Reports of oral movements were associated with classification as a focal seizure, with reports of their absence decreasing the likelihood of a report of a focal seizure 0.45 fold *vs.* a primary generalised seizure (p = 0.008). Reports of thoracic limb stiffening were associated with classification of primary generalised seizures, with their absence increasing the likelihood of classification as a focal seizure 7.83 fold *vs.* a primary generalised seizure (p < 0.001), and decreasing the likelihood of classification as a focal seizure with secondary generalisation 0.19 fold *vs.* a focal seizure (p < 0.001). Reports of rhythmic thoracic limb movements were also associated with classification of primary generalised seizures, with their absence increasing the likelihood of classification as a focal seizure 3.7 fold *vs.* a primary generalised seizure (p < 0.001). Reports of running movements were associated with classification as a primary generalised seizures and focal seizures with secondary generalisation, with their absence increasing the likelihood of classification as a focal seizure 9.75 fold *vs.* a primary generalised seizure (p < 0.001). In addition, the absence of running movements decreased the likelihood of classification as a focal seizure with secondary generalisation 0.17 fold vs. a focal seizure (p = 0.004). Reports of equal movements on each side of the body were associated with classification as primary generalised seizures, with reports of unequal movements increasing the likelihood of classification as a focal seizure 4.70 fold *vs.* a primary generalised seizure (p < 0.001) and increasing the likelihood of classification as a focal seizure with secondary generalisation 2.37 fold *vs.* primary generalised seizures (p = 0.034).

Reports of salivation were associated with the classification of primary generalised seizures, with reports of absence of salivation increasing the likelihood of classification as a focal seizure 2.69 fold *vs.* a primary

Table 4 Multinomial mixed model analysis of which observer perceived seizure characteristics predict reported seizure type

Risk factor		Focal vs. primary generalised				Focal with secondary generalisation vs. primary generalised				Focal with secondary generalisation vs. focal			
		OR	95% CI	t	p	OR	95% CI	t	p	OR	95% CI	t	p
Oral movement	No	0.45	0.25-0.81	−2.64	0.008	0.50	0.23-1.09	−1.74	0.082	0.98	0.44-2.20	−0.04	0.966
	Yes					ref							
Stiffening of thoracic limbs	No	7.82	4.39-13.96	6.98	<0.001	1.07	0.50-2.27	0.17	0.868	0.19	0.08-0.41	−4.21	<0.001
	Yes					ref							
Rhythmic thoracic limb movements	No	3.70	1.88-7.27	3.80	<0.001	1.85	0.73-4.68	1.31	0.191	0.64	0.24-1.65	−0.93	0.352
	Yes					ref							
Running movements	No	9.75	3.60-26.42	4.48	<0.001	1.49	0.58-3.85	0.82	0.409	0.17	0.05-0.56	−2.89	0.004
	Yes					ref							
Equal movements on each side	No	4.70	2.61-8.47	5.15	<0.001	2.37	1.07-5.27	2.13	0.034	0.78	0.34-1.79	−0.60	0.551
	Yes					ref							
Salivation	No	2.69	1.29-5.61	2.63	0.009	1.19	0.45-3.17	0.35	0.730	0.43	0.16-1.18	−1.64	0.102
	Yes					ref							
Hallucination	No	0.24	0.07-0.86	−2.19	0.029	0.37	0.07-2.08	−1.13	0.260	2.44	0.47-12.7	1.06	0.290
	Yes					ref							

(κ = kappa, SE = standard error, OR = odds ratio, *ref* = reference category).

generalised seizure (p = 0.009). Finally, reports of hallucination were associated with the classification of focal seizures, with reports of absence of hallucination decreasing the likelihood of classification as a focal seizure 0.24 fold *vs.* a primary generalised seizure (p = 0.029).

There was overlap in the prediction of seizure type for three aspects of seizure semiology, where their presence increased the likelihood of two seizure types. Stiffening of the thoracic limbs was associated with reports of a primary generalised seizure (rather than a focal seizure), but also reports of a focal seizure with secondary generalisation (rather than a focal seizure) (Table 4; Additional file 2: Table S1). Running movements were associated with reports of a primary generalised seizure (rather than a focal seizure), but also reports of a focal seizure (rather than a focal seizure with secondary generalisation). Finally, equal movements on each side of the body were associated with reports of a primary generalised seizure (rather than a focal seizure AND rather than a focal seizure with secondary generalisation).

Discussion

Hypothesis 1 and 2: are there high levels of agreement between veterinary observers for the prediction of seizure presence and type, the classification of consciousness status, and the presence of motor, autonomic and neurobehavioural signs?

Prior to this study, no data were available in the literature regarding inter-observer agreement for paroxysmal event semiology between vets. Contrary to our initial hypotheses of high levels of agreement between veterinary observers for the prediction of seizure presence, type and description of seizure semiology, this study has demonstrated that there was only fair-moderate inter-observer agreement in the description of seizure semiology between a cohort of veterinary neurology specialists and non-specialists as ascertained by κ analysis and percentage agreement, with prevalence indices to aid interpretation. No variables achieved excellent agreement, and the only variable to achieve good agreement was whether the dog salivated or not, followed by whether the seizure type was primary generalised, which nearly missed good agreement. Few of the variables showed poor agreement; however, neurobehavioural signs were the least agreed upon domain with consistently poor agreement ratings. There was on average only 29% agreement between observers as to whether a video represented a seizure event or not, achieving a κ value of just 0.4, a value that is commonly stated as the minimum threshold for reliability [5]. This suggests that in isolation, observing videos of paroxysmal events may be an unreliable way to diagnose a seizure, thus highlighting the importance of detailed history taking, physical examination and diagnostic testing in determining whether an epileptic seizure has occurred.

Similar studies have been carried out in human medicine, and parallels can be made with the results of this study [2]. Impairment of consciousness was the least agreed upon consciousness status category in this study, as has been demonstrated previously in a human epilepsy study [2]. That study also demonstrated that head turning was less well agreed upon than other variables in humans, which in this study only showed poor agreement. In comparison to that study, agreement between veterinarians is much lower than between human neurologists, for example concordance between two human neurologists was classed as good to excellent (using the same scale) for all 23 questions posed; however, it must be noted that in the human epilepsy study, raters were aware that the paroxysm was an epileptic seizure which may have improved agreement on aspects of semiology. Despite this, the relatively low agreement between veterinarians described by this study may justify further discussions between experts regarding semiologic descriptions, and further training to non-specialists, to improve levels of agreement.

One of the poorest areas of agreement was regarding the consciousness status of the dog, with particularly poor agreement for option 'impairment in consciousness'. In the authors' collective experiences, impairment in consciousness is often interpreted and reported by the observer when dogs are standing with a blank stare and apparently being incapable of recognizing owner/surroundings, for example they do not respond to commands, but it have been argued that impairment of consciousness cannot be objectively assessed in dogs [9]. Assessment of consciousness during epileptic seizures is generally not a simple topic; it is individually different, not always global, and "pieces" of consciousness (perception, cognition, responsiveness, memory function, motor performance) can be altered [10]. The oversimplification with categorization into conscious and unconscious was eliminated in the last human classification; however recognition of impairment remained an important point [1]. In animals, the responsiveness by motor function is the main (if not the only part) of consciousness which can be evaluated.

Classification of seizure type has implications for future multicentre treatment studies, as some medications used may have better effects on certain seizure types, so agreement here is of high importance. Focal seizures were the least agreed upon seizure type, which may be due to the complex array of signs that may be reported during them, including a variety of motor, postural, autonomic and behavioural signs [9]. One study has shown that neurobehavioral and autonomic signs are not uncommon in dogs and indicated that motor signs are not necessarily the most dominant clinical expression of a focal seizure [9]. Hallucination was thought to be associated with focal seizures in this study, a sign that may be potentially difficult to confidently and reliably recognise.

Hypothesis 3: are there differences in the classification of seizure presence and type, and reporting of seizure semiology between veterinary neurology specialists and non-specialists?

As hypothesised, differences were seen in the classification of seizure presence and type, and reporting of seizure semiology between veterinary neurology specialists and non-specialists. These differences were limited to the univariate level, which may be due to the low sample size, particularly for non-specialists (n = 5). This has never been studied before and thus further study with a larger, balanced sample size of specialists and non-specialists may be warranted to confirm these results. At the univariate level, specialists were less likely to report what they saw in the videos as an epileptic seizure than non-specialists, which may be due to their experience of other, less common paroxysmal events (without seizure activity) that non-specialists may not recognise (e.g. specialists were more likely to report the paroxysmal event as a movement disorder than non-specialists such as idiopathic head bobbing, episodic falling, cramping syndrome), or may be more experienced in recognising more subtle signs (e.g. specialists were more likely to report pain associated behaviour than non-specialists) and thus categorising the episodes as non-seizure events. Reporting of motor, autonomic and neurobehavioral signs were similar between specialists and non-specialists, with the exception of several motor variables that non-specialists were more likely to report. It would be expected that the specialists would be more accurate than non-specialists owing to their training and experience, so it is possible that these were 'false positives' by the non-specialists rather than under recognition by the specialists. Specialists were more likely to report the presence of aggression than non-specialists, which may be due to the recognition of more subtle signs of aggression e.g. changes in body posture or facial expression rather than overt signs such as snarling or growling; however, as individual signs indicating aggression were not requested it is not possible to infer the cause of this difference. In a previous study of experienced and inexperienced people describing dog behaviour, observers showed little agreement when classifying aggression [11], so it is possible that additional training in this area from behavioural experts may be useful.

Hypothesis 4: does observer-reported seizure semiology differentiate between primary generalised seizures, focal seizures, and focal seizures with secondary generalisation?

Only seven of the nineteen studied aspects of seizure semiology significantly differentiated between seizure type: oral movement, stiffening and rhythmic movement of the thoracic limbs, running movements, movements equally on both sides, salivation and hallucination. With regard to the five motor signs: oral movement, stiffening of the forelimbs and equal movements on each side only achieved fair kappa values, while rhythmic thoracic limb movements achieved moderate agreement and running movements almost reached good agreement, Salivation achieved a good level of agreement; however, hallucination had poor agreement. As observers use these aspects of semiology most prominently to differentiate between seizure type, emphasis should be made to train observers to recognise these characteristics to improve agreement for those with poorer levels of achievement. Factors that did not differentiate between any of the three seizure types may be considered less useful in the categorisation of seizure type in the future; however, due to this being a novel study, further data should be gathered before these criteria are discarded. When classifying seizure type, of the seven significant variables, those that are associated with only one seizure type may be considered most valuable, for example hallucination was only associated with focal seizures, in contrast to running movements which were associated with both primary generalised seizures and focal seizures with secondary generalisation, thus requiring further inquiry to differentiate.

Statistical limitations

There were limitations to the statistics performed in this study, as in near-homogenous populations, evidence for agreement above chance levels is difficult to identify, resulting in low κ values [4]. Some variables in this study suffered from this problem, as reflected in very high prevalence indices (PI), meaning that the interpretation of their corresponding κ value was limited, with low κ values but high% agreement values reflecting inconclusive statistics rather than genuinely poor agreement. In future studies, to avoid this problem, a more balanced population should be initially selected; with approximately equal numbers of subjects in each category e.g. 50% of videos show seizures and 50% of videos show non-seizure paroxysmal episodes. To facilitate this, a gold standard observer would be required to determine the designation of each video; for example, a specialist not participating in the study, using videos of patients that had been diagnosed with epilepsy following full work up that had evidence of response to anticonvulsive treatment. Establishing an accepted gold standard may still be challenging due to the varying beliefs of neurology specialists. For example, some neurologists believe that Spike's disease (Canine Epileptoid Cramping Syndrome) is a focal seizure, while others believe it is a movement disorder. Balancing the subjects in each category e.g. for the presence of each motor, neurobehavioral and autonomic sign may not be feasible for such a large sample.

Due to the presence of missing data, a direct comparison of agreement between the two sub-groups, specialists and non-specialists could not be carried out. This was due to agreement statistics requiring an equal amount of observers to rate an equal amount of videos, resulting in videos being removed from the analyses when missing data was present for that video. As different missing data was present, and thus different videos removed for specialists and non-specialists, this would not be a direct comparison. The alternative approach of analysing how these groups compared in their ratings was instead carried out.

Video limitations

The variable quality of the videos used in this study due to their unstandardized online source may have influenced observers' abilities to report on the features of the episodes. Recent studies have successfully used YouTube© videos to study neurological and behavioural problems in dogs [3,12], and its capacity to facilitate large-scale studies may counterbalance this limitation. This also reflects a real-life clinical situation where video quality is likely to vary between owners and between seizures e.g. those that happen in poor light conditions. A further limitation of using owner-recorded videos is that owners may not have video recording equipment tohand when the seizure episode begins. This is particularly problematic when observers are differentiating between primary generalised and secondary generalised seizures, as missing the beginning of a secondary generalised seizure may lead observers to erroneously classify it as a primary generalised seizure.

Limitations of experience categorisation

A further limitation of this study was the designation of 'specialist' vs. 'non-specialist', which may not capture the differences in experience between the veterinarians involved. All of the specialists had undergone extensive years of training in neurology; however, years as a specialist since this initial training was not considered, with additional years of experience potentially improving diagnostic accuracy. Some specialists may also have a clinical and/or research focus in epilepsy further increasing their experience. In addition, although classed as 'non-specialists', those veterinarians involved in this study had an interest in veterinary neurology and may have seen more relevant cases, making them different from other first opinion practitioners. As such, experience is more of a spectrum than a binomial trait. Whether the non-specialists were representative of all first opinion veterinarians or referral veterinarians of another specialism is also debatable as individual details were not requested here, and as such further study with a larger sample size may be needed to improve how representative these results are. A further limitation related to the observers was the amount of time participating veterinarians had available to view and rate the videos may have impacted upon their responses.

Information required to supplement videos of paroxysmal events

An important limitation of our study (similarly in daily veterinary practice) is the lack of reliable method for the differentiation between epileptic and non-epileptic paroxysms. The current definition of epileptic seizure is "a transient occurrence of signs and/or symptoms due to abnormal excessive or synchronous neuronal activity in the brain" [13]. For a definitive diagnosis, the epileptic activity should be recorded, which is especially important in cases with unclear episodes. Advance in the veterinary EEG diagnostic is required. Video-EEG studies, more commonly used as a diagnostic tool in human neurology, could be used more widely in veterinary medicine to aid characterisation of episodes beyond what can be observed on a video alone. This additional information could potentially improve inter-observer agreement. A recent veterinary video-EEG study diagnosed a juvenile Chihuahua with subtle myoclonic absences with perioral myoclonia and head twitching [14]. The patient had been admitted for evaluation of what was suspected to be focal seizures, with a four-month history of recurrent episodes of head and nose twitching, associated with intermittent hind limb jerking and suspected staring for a duration of a few seconds. The author confirmed bilateral generalized synchronous 4 Hz spike-and-wave complexes on ictal EEG time locked with the episodes. The case represents the first confirmed absence seizure in dog. Without video-EEG the epileptic origin could only have been speculated [14].

In daily veterinary practice, some additional information is usually available that may be helpful for the assessment whether the paroxysmal event is of epileptic origin or not. This includes breed, age of onset, pre and postictal signs, precipitating event, duration of the event, occurrence of the event during daytime, laboratory results, neuroimaging findings and response to antiepileptic therapy. These data were not investigated (except breed) in the present study; however, it should be borne in mind that these results and the level of agreement could have been influenced by their inclusion.

Further study

Further exploration of this area could include an inter-observer agreement study of seizure-episode videos between owners and neurologists to investigate the accuracy of reports they are provided with. In a study of human epilepsy [2], high concordance between physicians and caregivers was observed. This was not anticipated by the authors; with differences in training and experience expected to lead to reduced concordance. The authors speculated that because of long disease duration and high seizure frequency in the majority of patients, most caregivers are likely to have experienced several seizure episodes first-hand, and thus their increased familiarity with the condition would increase the similarity of their ratings with physicians. This could be investigated in veterinary patients, with owners with differing levels of experience of canine epilepsy (e.g. newly diagnosed vs. longer-term cases) and between owners of dogs experiencing different seizure phenotypes (e.g. high vs. low frequency, clustering etc.). If good concordance is seen between vets and owners, then greater confidence may be given to owner descriptions for those cases where videos are not provided.

Conclusion

In conclusion, this study has demonstrated that there were relatively low levels of agreement of seizure presence, type and semiologies reported by veterinary neurology specialists and non-specialists, highlighting the need for ongoing debate regarding the descriptive terminology used for seizure semiology in veterinary medicine, and the need for further training in focussed areas. Although the use of videos to diagnose seizure activity may be increasingly common, the results presented here demonstrate that it should not be solely relied upon, with existing diagnostics always supplementing videos, and new diagnostics such as EEG more widely used for more objective, definitive diagnoses.

Additional files

> **Additional file 1: Questionnaire hosted on SurveyMonkey®**
> **(repeated by each observer for 100 videos).**
>
> **Additional file 2: Table S1.** Simplified schematic of significant associations between seven aspects of seizure semiology and observer-reported seizure type (adapted from Table 4). Yellow cells signify aspects of seizure semiology that were deemed to be associated with focal seizures, blue for primary generalised seizures, and red focal seizures with secondary generalisation.

Abbreviations
ECVN: European College of Veterinary Neurology; RCVS: Royal College of Veterinary Surgeon; PI: Prevalence index; CI: Confidence interval; SE: Standard error; EEG: Electroencephalogram.

Competing interests
The authors declare that they have no competing interests.

Authors' contributions
RMAP and HAV designed, analysed and drafted the manuscript of this study. MB, SB, MC, SC, LDR, RF, RH, MH, PM, AP, SMP, CR. VMS, FTB and AT completed the online questionnaire and contributed to the manuscript of this study. All authors read and approved the final manuscript.

Acknowledgements
The paper was internally approved for publication (manuscript ID: CSS_00847). This study was not financially supported by any organization or grant.

Author details

[1]Department of Clinical Science and Services, Royal Veterinary College, Hertfordshire, UK. [2]Department of Veterinary Clinical and Animal Sciences, Faculty of Health and Medical Sciences, University of Copenhagen, Frederiksberg, Denmark. [3]Department of Small Animal Medicine and Clinical Biology, Faculty of Veterinary Medicine, Ghent University, Ghent, Belgium. [4]Cornell University College of Veterinary Medicine, Ithaca, New York, USA. [5]The Referral Animal Neurology Hospital "Aisti", Vantaa, Finland. [6]Animal Health Trust, Lanwades Park, Newmarket, UK. [7]Fernside Veterinary Centre, Hertfordshire, UK. [8]Department of Clinical Sciences of Companion Animals, Utrecht University, Utrecht, The Netherlands. [9]University Clinic for Small Animals, Clinical Department for Companion Animals and Horses, University of Veterinary Medicine, Vienna, Austria. [10]School of Veterinary Medicine, Faculty of Health & Medical Sciences, University of Surrey, Surrey, UK. [11]Department of Small Animal Medicine and Surgery, University of Veterinary Medicine Hannover, Buenteweg 9, 30559 Hannover, Germany.

References

1.   Berg AT, Berkovic SF, Brodie MJ, Buchhalter J, Cross JH, Van Emde BW, et al. Revised terminology and concepts for organization of seizures and epilepsies: Report of the ILAE Commission on Classification and Terminology, 2005–2009. Epilepsia. 2010;51(4):676–85.

2.   Benbir G, Demiray DY, Delil S, Yeni N. Interobserver variability of seizure semiology between two neurologist and caregivers. Seizure. 2013;22(7):548–52.

3.   Preston SM, Shihab N, Volk HA. Public perception of epilepsy in dogs is more favorable than in humans. Epilepsy Behav. 2013;27(1):243–6.

4.   Hoehler FK. Bias and prevalence effects on kappa viewed in terms of sensitivity and specificity. J Clin Epidemiol. 2000;53(5):499–503.

5.   Sim J, Wright CC. The Kappa Statistic in Reliability Studies: Use, Interpretation, and Sample Size Requirements. Phys Ther. 2005;85(3):257–68.

6.   Byrt T, Bishop J, Carlin JB. Bias, prevalence and kappa. J Clin Epidemiol. 1993;46(5):423–9.

7.   Sargeant JM, Martin SW. The dependence of kappa on attribute prevalence when assessing the repeatability of questionnaire data. Prev Vet Med. 1998;34(2–3):115–23.

8.   Burn CC, Weir AAS. Using prevalence indices to aid interpretation and comparison of agreement ratings between two or more observers. Vet J. 2011;188(2):166–70.

9.   Berendt M, Gredal H, Alving J. Characteristics and phenomenology of epileptic partial seizures in dogs: similarities with human seizure semiology. Epilepsy Res. 2004;61(1–3):167–73.

10.   Blumenfeld H. Consciousness and epilepsy: why are patients with absence seizures absent? Prog Brain Res. 2005;150:271–86.

11.   Tami G, Gallagher A. Description of the behaviour of domestic dog (Canis familiaris) by experienced and inexperienced people. Appl Animal Behav Sci. 2009;120(3–4):159–69.

12.   Burn CC. A Vicious Cycle: A Cross-Sectional Study of Canine Tail-Chasing and Human Responses to It, Using a Free Video-Sharing Website. Plos One. 2011;6(11):e26553.

13.   Fisher RS, van Emde BW, Blume W, Elger C, Genton P, Lee P, et al. Epileptic seizures and epilepsy: definitions proposed by the International League Against Epilepsy (ILAE) and the International Bureau for Epilepsy (IBE). Epilepsia. 2005;46(4):470–2.

14.   Poma R, Ochi A, Cortez MA. Absence seizures with myoclonic features in a juvenile Chihuahua dog. Epileptic Disord. 2010;12(2):138–41.

12

Oral antigen exposure in newborn piglets circumvents induction of oral tolerance in response to intraperitoneal vaccination in later life

J Alex Pasternak[1], Siew Hon Ng[1], Rachelle M Buchanan[1], Sonja Mertins[2], George K Mutwiri[1], Volker Gerdts[1] and Heather L Wilson[1]*

Abstract

Background: We previously determined that newborn piglets orally gavaged with Ovalbumin (OVA) responded to systemic OVA re-exposure with tolerance; if adjuvants were included in oral vaccine, piglets responded with antibody-mediated immunity (Vet Immunol Immunopathol 161(3–4):211–21, 2014). Here, we will investigate whether newborn piglets gavaged with a vaccine comprised of OVA plus unmethylated CpG oligodeoxynucleotides (CpG; soluble component; OVA/CpG) combined with OVA plus CpG encapsulated within polyphosphazene microparticles (MP; particulate component) responded with systemic and mucosal immunity. To monitor the response to systemic antigen re-exposure, piglets were i.p.-immunized with OVA plus Incomplete Freund's Adjuvant (IFA) one month later.

Results: Newborn piglets (n = 5/group) were gavaged with a combined soluble and particulate vaccine consisting of OVA (0.5-0.05 mg) plus 50 µg CpG and 0.5 mg OVA plus 50 µg CpG encapsulated within a polyphosphazene MP (0.5 mg) referred to as OVA/CpG + MP. Control piglets were gavaged with saline alone. Piglets were i.p. immunized with 10 mg OVA (or saline) in IFA at four weeks of age and then euthanized at eight weeks of age. We observed significantly higher titres of serum anti-OVA immunoglobulin (Ig) IgM, IgA, IgG, IgG1, IgG2 and IgG in piglets immunized with 0.05 mg OVA/CpG + MP relative to saline control animals. Thus, a single oral exposure at birth to a combined soluble and particulate OVA vaccine including adjuvants can circumvent induction of oral tolerance which impacts response to i.p. vaccination in later life. Further, piglets gavaged with 0.05 mg OVA/CpG + MP generated significant anti-OVA IgG and IgG1 titres in lung compared to saline control piglets but results were comparable to titres measured in parenteral control piglets. Peripheral blood mononuclear cells (PBMCs) *ex vivo*-stimulated with OVA showed markedly decreased production of IL-10 cytokine after 72 hours relative to animal-matched cells incubated with media alone. No production of IFN-γ was observed from any groups.

Conclusion: Newborn piglets gavaged with low dose soluble and particulate OVA plus CpG ODN and polyphosphazene adjuvants produced antigen-specific antibodies in serum and lung after systemic re-exposure in later life. These data indicate circumvention of oral tolerance but not induction of oral immunity.

Keywords: Piglets, Neonate, Ovalbumin, Oral, Tolerance

* Correspondence: heather.wilson@usask.ca
[1]Vaccine and Infectious Disease Organization (VIDO), University of Saskatchewan, 120 Veterinary Road, Saskatoon, SK S7N 5E3, Canada
Full list of author information is available at the end of the article

Background

If exposure to an antigen by the oral route fails to promote an oral immune response, any subsequent re-exposure (even by a systemic route) results in suppression of immunity; this process is known as oral tolerance. Oral tolerance is a major suppressive immunological process designed to prevent local and peripheral overreaction to innocuous antigens [1,2]. Commensal bacteria are critically required for proper gut-associated lymphoid tissue (GALT) development and induction of oral tolerance [3,4]. Mucosal dendritic cells (DCs) play an active role in inducing oral tolerance through mechanisms which require retinoic acid, vitamin D, interleukin (IL)-10, Transforming growth factor (TGF)-β, and indoleamine-2,3,-dioxygenase [5-9]. In the mesenteric lymph nodes (MLNs), T regulatory (Treg) cells undergo differentiation and home back to the inductor site to induce and/or maintain antigen-specific oral tolerance [8]. Several physical barriers prevent antigen/pathogen contact with GALT and subsequent penetration of the gut wall making targeted induction of oral immunity a significant challenge [10,11]. The gut of the newborn piglet is uniquely designed to be semi-permeable or 'leaky' for a limited time to allow colostrum-derived cells, antibodies, and other macromolecules such as albumin, cytokines, antimicrobial peptides and many other bioactive products to be passively transferred to the piglets. These maternally-derived cells and macromolecules traverse the gut wall then enter into the vasculature where they play a variety of roles including passive immunity against disease [12-15]. 'Gut closure' occurs within a few days after birth in ruminants [16] and pigs [17], but it does not occur until after weaning (two weeks of age) in rats and mice [18-20]. In humans, a considerable amount of 'gut-closure' occurs both before birth and within a few days after birth but it may in fact take up to two years to reach the same level of impermeability that is observed in the adult gut [21,22]. Once across the gut wall, antigens may be able to interact with DCs within the subepithelial dome which can then present antigens to T cells within isolated lymphoid follicles and/or Peyer's Patches to promote induction of oral immunity rather than being taken up by tolerogenic mucosal DCs which promote oral tolerance [23,24]. Despite the overwhelming propensity to respond to an oral antigen with tolerance, oral vaccines are highly sought because of their ease of administration. They are needle-free and therefore present reduced risk of transmitting infections and less need for qualified personnel to administer the vaccine. Moreover, an estimated 90% of all pathogens invade through mucosal surfaces, therefore mucosal immunity (induced by mucosal vaccines) offer the potential to control pathogens at their point of entry.

Previous work from our lab showed that rat pups and lambs orally vaccinated starting the day after birth with multiple doses of soluble ovalbumin (OVA; without adjuvants) responded with immunity to subsequent intraperitoneal (i.p.) immunization [25,26]. In contrast, we showed that newborn piglets orally immunized within six hours after birth with single bolus of soluble OVA then boosted through the i.p. route one month later showed significantly lower anti-OVA immunoglobulin (Ig) A titres and a strong trend towards lower anti-OVA IgM, IgG1, IgG2 and IgG titres relative to the i.p. control group indicating induction of oral tolerance [27]. These data showed agreement with Haverson et al [28] who demonstrated that newborn piglets orally vaccinated once with OVA induced classical oral tolerance following a systemic challenge by showing reduced specific systemic IgG responses. When we included unmethylated oligonucleotides containing CG oligodeoxynucleotides (CpG ODNs) and soluble polyphosphazene in the oral vaccine administered at birth, the response to i.p. immunization one month later was induction of immunity (i.e. increased serum anti-OVA IgA, IgM, IgG1, IgG2 and IgG titres relative to piglets immunized with OVA alone) [27]. Clearly the components of the oral vaccine administered at birth impacted the response to the booster immunization one month later.

Factors contributing to induction of oral tolerance include: the host's immunological maturity at time of exposure, the timing and the frequency of exposure, and the nature of the antigen [29-32]. We established that a single bolus of soluble OVA with CpG ODN and polyphosphazene adjuvants administered the day after birth induced oral immunity in piglets [27]. Our next step will be to establish whether inclusion of the antigen in a particulate form promotes oral immunity and whether the response could be observed at distal mucosal sites. To test this hypothesis, conventionally reared neonatal piglets were gavaged within six hours after birth with 0.5 mg or 0.05 mg OVA plus CpG ODN in a soluble form as well as OVA plus CpG ODN encapsulated within a polyphosphazene microparticle (MP) [33-35]. Systemic and mucosal antibody titres and *ex vivo* cytokine production are assessed to determine antibody-mediated and cell-mediated immunity.

Results

Explanation of vaccination procedure

Piglets were gavaged with a two-part vaccine consisting of soluble OVA (0.5 mg or 0.05 mg) with 50 µg soluble CpG 2395 (which together make up the soluble components of the vaccine; OVA/CpG) as well as a MP encapsulating 0.5 mg OVA + 50 µg CpG 2395 (which comprised the particulate part of the vaccine). These vaccines will be referred to as 0.5 mg OVA/CpG + MP and 0.05 mg OVA/CpG + MP. The experimental time-line is detailed in Figure 1. Piglets were gavaged at less than six hours of age when their gut would be semi-permeable with the idea that both the soluble OVA/CpG and the OVA and CpG ODN within the MP would cross the leaky gut wall. Polyphosphazene-based MPs are water-soluble and would then dissolve over time to re-lease the encapsulated OVA and CpG ODN thus acting like a prime-boost [36,37]. Piglets were bled three days after birth, day seven after birth, and weekly thereafter (Figure 1, grey arrows specify bleed times). Piglets were i.p. immunized with 10 mg OVA (or saline) plus Incomplete Freund's Adjuvant (IFA) at 28 days of age and all piglets were euthanized at 49 days of age. The i.p. control group received a saline gavage but piglets were boosted with the i.p. vaccination (OVA + IFA) to act as our primary i.p. vaccine control group.

Newborn piglets vaccinated by oral gavage responded with significant serum anti-OVA IgM, IgA, and IgG1, IgG2 and IgG production after re-exposure by the i.p. route

The definition for oral tolerance is that oral exposure to antigen which is subsequently encountered via a sys-temic route triggers reduced immune responses (such as antibody production) relative to animals exposed to anti-gen systemically without prior oral exposure [38]. Previ-ous work in our laboratory showed that animals orally immunized six hours after birth with 5 mg or 0.05 mg OVA responded to i.p. immunization at one month of age with oral tolerance, not oral immunity [27]. There-fore these groups (OVA alone without adjuvants) were not repeated here. In the current trial, when we assessed the serum antibody titres in the piglets prior to weaning (less than day 21) for all groups, we observed negligible

anti-OVA antibodies of any isotype indicating that the sows did not pass any interfering OVA-specific passive immunity to the piglets (data not shown). Even one week after weaning (Figure 2, day 28), all isotypes of pig-let serum anti-OVA antibodies titres were negligible sug-gesting that oral gavage at birth with 0.5 mg or 0.05 mg OVA/CpG + MP alone did not promote antibody-mediated immunity. On day 42, which was two weeks after the i.p. booster immunization, we observed a sig-nificant increase in serum anti-OVA IgM (Figure 2A; $p < 0.05$), IgA (Figure 2B; $p < 0.05$), IgG1 (Figure 2D; $p < 0.05$), and IgG2 (Figure 2E; $p < 0.05$) titres in the i.p. control group relative to the saline control group. The group gavaged with 0.05 mg OVA/CpG + MP showed sig-nificant induction of anti-OVA IgM (Figure 2A; $p < 0.05$), IgA (Figure 2B; $p < 0.01$), IgG (Figure 2C; $p < 0.05$), IgG1 (Figure 2D; $p < 0.01$), and IgG2 (Figure 2E; $p < 0.01$) relative to the saline control group suggesting that prior oral ex-posure to low dose OVA circumvented induction of oral tolerance. The animals gavaged with ten-fold higher dose of soluble OVA (0.5 mg OVA/CpG + MP) showed a strong trend towards increased anti-OVA antibody production relative to the saline control group but the data were not statistically significant.

On day 49, serum titres from animals within the i.p. control group showed a significant increase in anti-OVA IgG1 antibodies (Figure 2D; $p < 0.05$) relative to the sa-line control group. In contrast, the group gavaged with 0.05 mg OVA/CpG + MP showed significantly more anti-OVA IgM (Figure 2A; $p < 0.05$), IgA (Figure 2B; $p < 0.05$), IgG1 (Figure 2D; $p < 0.01$), and IgG2 (Figure 2E; $p < 0.01$) titres than what was observed in the saline con-trol group. The group gavaged at birth with 0.5 mg OVA/CpG + MP showed significantly more anti-OVA

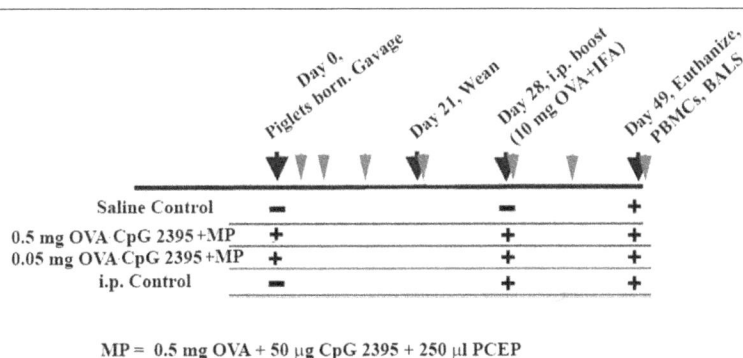

MP = 0.5 mg OVA + 50 µg CpG 2395 + 250 µl PCEP

Figure 1 Description and timeline of immunization protocol. Piglets (n = 5/group) were gavaged with ovalbumin (OVA) (0.05 mg or 0.5 mg) + 50 µg unmethylated oligonucleotides containing CG oligodeoxynucleotides (CpG 2395) as a soluble vaccine as well as with 0.5 mg OVA + 50 µg CpG 2395 within a 0.5 mg PCEP polyphosphazene microparticles (MP). Gavages took place within six hours of birth. The negative control (saline) group and the i.p. control group were gavaged with saline. With the exception of the saline control group, the remaining groups were i.p. immunized at four weeks of age with 10 mg OVA in Incomplete Freunds' Adjuvant (IFA). At eight weeks of age, piglets were euthanized and lung lavages were harvested. Blood was obtained on day three, day seven and then weekly (grey arrows). At time of death, blood was drawn for PBMC isolation.

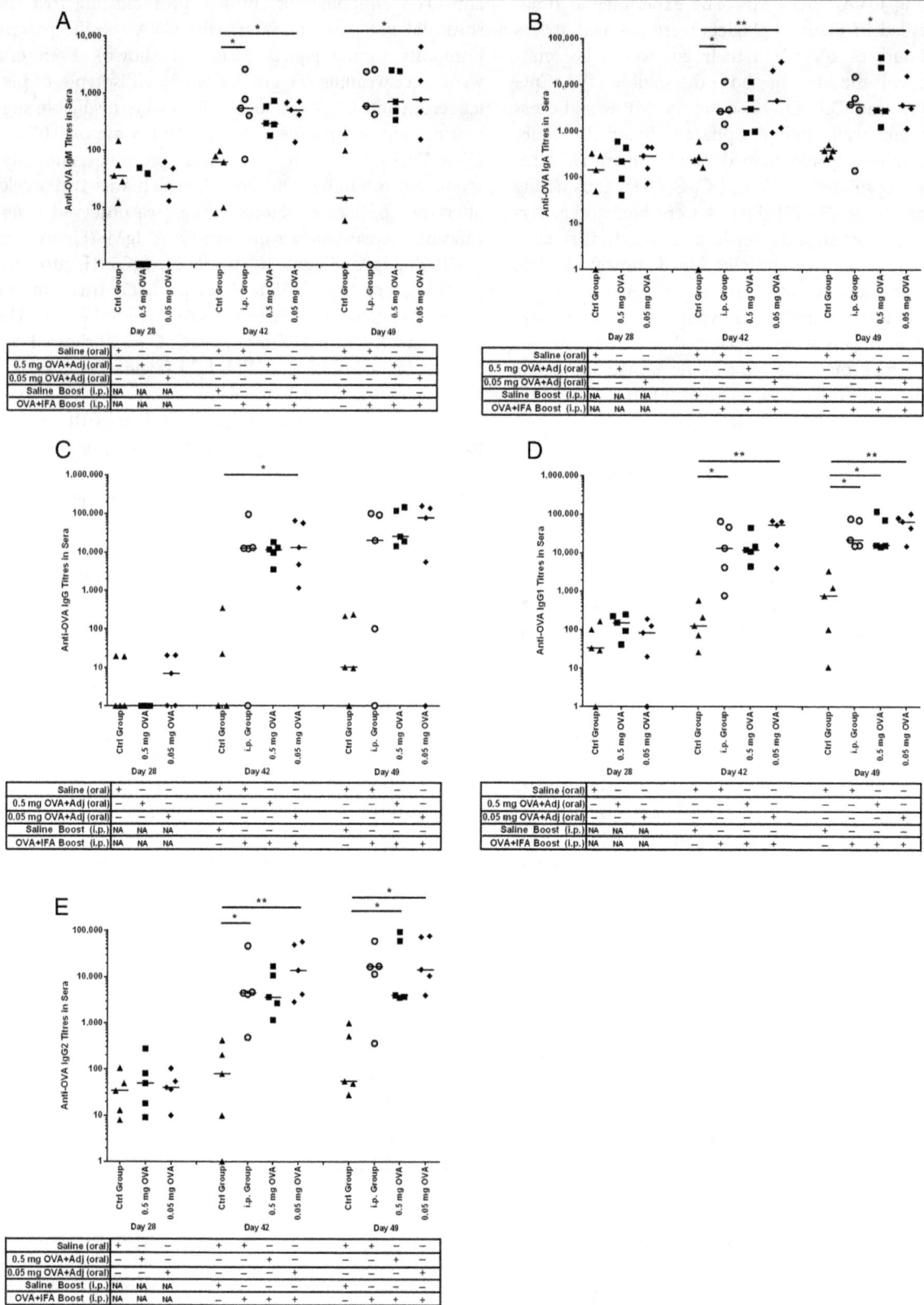

Figure 2 (See legend on next page.)

(See figure on previous page.)
Figure 2 OVA-specific antibody-mediated immune responses in serum from newborn piglets gavaged with OVA then i.p. immunized with OVA at four weeks of age. Piglets (n = 5/group) were gavaged and i.p. immunized as described in Figure 1. Control newborn piglets were not gavaged or immunized with OVA. We measured serum anti-OVA IgM (**A**), IgA (**B**), IgG (**C**), IgG1 (**D**) and IgG2 (**E**) production on day 28, day 42 and day 49 after birth. Each data point represents an individual animal and median values are indicated by horizontal lines. *p < 0.05., **p < 0.01.

IgG1 (Figure 2D; p < 0.05), and IgG2 (Figure 2E; p < 0.05) antibodies compared to the saline control group, but the other isotypes did not. Thus, unlike our previous data which showed that piglets orally vaccinated with soluble OVA alone induced oral tolerance [27], data from the current trial shows that piglets orally vaccinated with 0.5 mg or 0.05 mg OVA/CpG + MP showed significant induction of anti-OVA antibodies in serum indicating circumvention of oral tolerance.

Newborn piglets vaccinated orally with low dose OVA/CpG + MP responded with significant anti-OVA IgG1 and IgG titres in lung lavage after re-exposure by the i.p. route

According to the 'Common Mucosal Immune System' theory, antigen-sensitized precursor B and T lymphocytes generated at one mucosal site (i.e. such as the gut) can be detected at anatomically remote and functionally distinct compartments (such as the respiratory mucosa) [39-45]. After 49 days, the pigs were euthanized and bronchoalveolar lavage was collected. Piglets gavaged with saline but injected with OVA and IFA by the i.p. route alone (i.e. the i.p. control group) failed to trigger significant anti-OVA IgM (Figure 3A), IgA (Figure 3B), IgG (Figure 3C), IgG1 (Figure 3D), or IgG (Figure 3E) titres relative to the saline control group. Newborn piglets gavaged with 0.05 mg OVA/CpG + MP had very low titres of anti-OVA IgM (Figure 3A), IgA (Figure 3B), and IgG2 (Figure 3E) but the titres for anti-OVA IgG (Figure 3C, p < 0.05) and IgG1 (Figure 3D; p < 0.05) were statistically higher than the saline control group. Collectively, these results suggest that oral exposure to OVA/CpG + MP triggered low level mucosal immunity at a distal site.

Neonatal piglets gavaged with OVA/CpG + MP did not respond with induction of OVA-specific cell-mediated immunity

Finally, we sought to determine whether neonatal piglets orally gavaged with 0.5 mg or 0.05 mg OVA/CpG + MP developed cell-mediated immunity as measured by IFN-γ (Type 1 T-helper cell (Th1)) cytokines and IL-10 (Th2 cytokines). Peripheral blood mononuclear cells (PBMCs) were collected at eight weeks of age and they were restimulated *ex vivo* with OVA or media for 72 hours before the supernatants were collected and antibody titres were assessed. PBMCs did not show OVA-specific

induction of IFN-γ for any group except in the presence of the mitogen Concanavalin A (data not shown). Interestingly, we observed a decrease in production of the anti-inflammatory cytokine IL-10 relative to unstimulated (media control) cells in all groups including the saline control groups. These data indicate that oral gavage of newborn piglets did not promote cell-mediated immunity as measured at 8 weeks of age.

Discussion

Because the vast majority of infectious agents enter the body through mucosal routes, it is reasonable to assume that mucosal immunity which combats the infectious agent prior to colonization and penetration would be much more effective than systemic immunity. But it has proven very challenging to design effective oral subunit vaccine without the use of very strong mucosal adjuvants such as cholera toxin [46,47]. The majority of clinically approved oral vaccines for use in pigs are live attenuated viruses or bacteria (www.vetvac.org/index.php). One may speculate that in order to trigger an immune response instead of tolerance, the pathogen must traverse the gut wall and/or penetrate the epithelial cells lining the gut wall. If this is the case, it is understandable that subunit vaccines that lack strong adjuvants such as cholera toxin should fail to promote immunity [48]. However, such adjuvants cause significant side effects and are therefore not in clinical use. Due to the inherent risk of attenuated pathogen vaccines reverting to virulence, live attenuated vaccines against pathogens such as Porcine Reproductive and Respiratory Virus are not recommended for use in seronegative herds and are therefore a reactive vaccine instead of a proactive vaccine [49-51].

Previous work in our lab showed that oral administration of soluble OVA in rat pups or lambs starting immediately after birth was sufficient to promote oral immunity or at minimum prevented induction of oral tolerance [25,26]. In contrast, our research with piglets showed that soluble OVA administered immediately after birth triggered induction of oral tolerance [27]. However, if CpG ODN and polyphosphazene adjuvants were included in the soluble oral vaccine, there was instead evidence of induction of serum antibody-mediated immunity in response to systemic re-exposure in later life [27]. In the current study, we investigated whether oral immunization with a mixture of soluble and particulate OVA plus CpG ODN and polyphosphazene adjuvants could promote oral

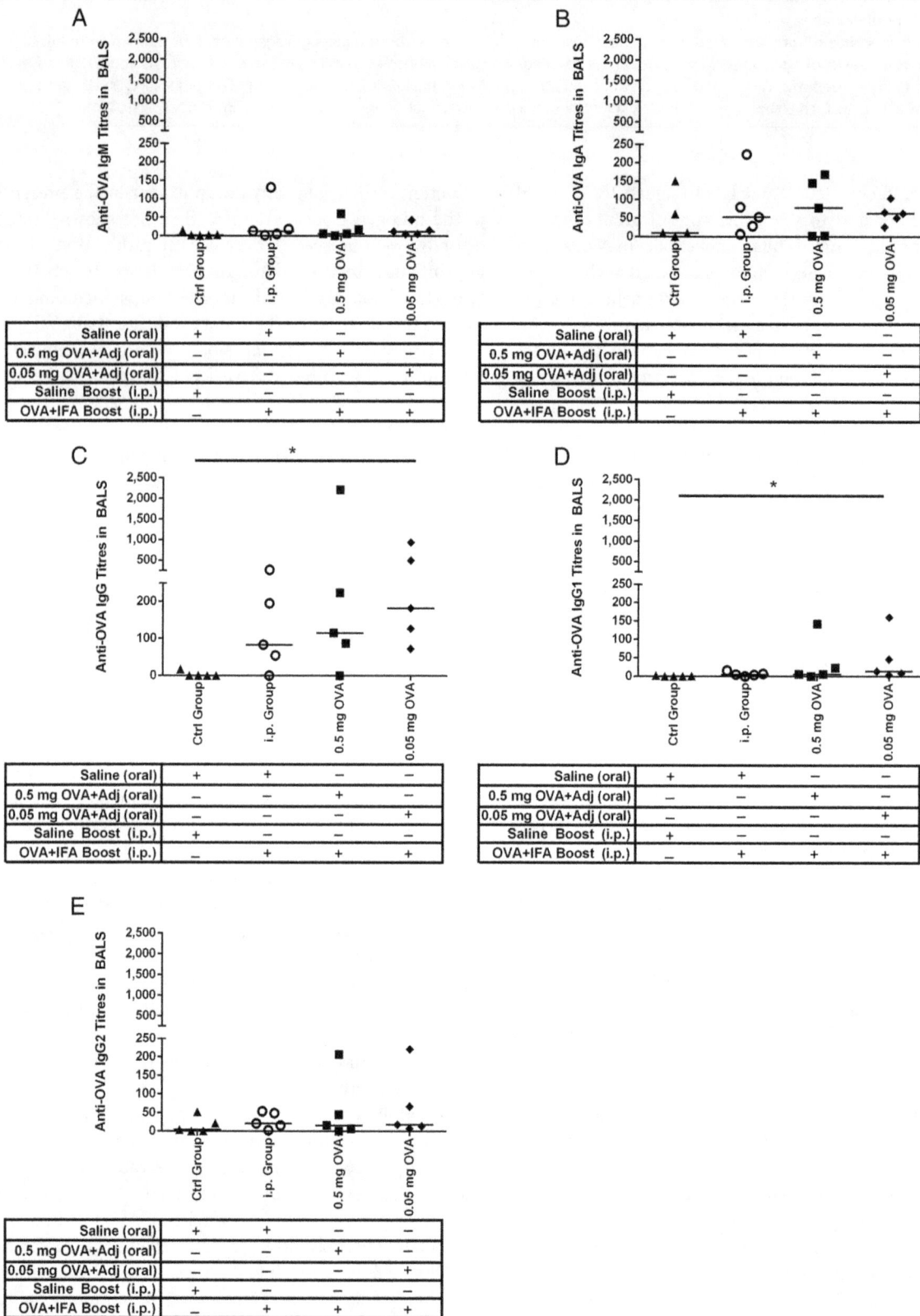

Figure 3 (See legend on next page.)

Oral antigen exposure in newborn piglets circumvents induction of oral tolerance in response to intraperitoneal...

113

(See figure on previous page.)
Figure 3 OVA-specific antibody-mediated immune responses in lung washes from newborn piglets gavaged with OVA then i.p. immunized with OVA at four weeks of age. Piglets (n = 5/group) were gavaged and i.p. immunized as described in Figure 1. Control newborn piglets were not gavaged or immunized with OVA. Lung lavages were collected four weeks post i.p. immunization and OVA-specific serum IgM (**A**), IgA (**B**), IgG (**C**), IgG1 (**D**), and IgG2 (**E**) titres were measured. ELISA titres are expressed as the reciprocal of the highest dilution resulting in a reading of two standard deviations above the negative control. Each data point represents an individual animal and median values are indicated by horizontal lines. *p < 0.05, **p < 0.01.

immunity. We determined that systemic anti-OVA antibody-mediated immune responses were induced in newborn piglets gavaged once on the day of birth with 0.5 mg or 0.05 mg OVA/CpG + MP and subsequently boosted with OVA and IFA by the i.p. route one month later. If oral tolerance to OVA had been induced instead, re-exposure to the antigen by i.p. injection should have resulted in a reduction of serum anti-OVA antibody titres as observed in [27]. Anti-OVA IgG and IgG1 titres in lung lavages were significantly induced in piglets gavaged at birth with 0.05 mg OVA/CpG + MP indicating induction of mucosal antibody-mediated immunity at a distal mucosal site. IgG has not traditionally been recognized as a major mucosal immunoglobulin, however there is growing evidence that oral vaccines can elevate local and systemic IgG titres [52,53] and that IgG antibodies may play a role in passive transfer of luminal antigens across the gut wall using FcRN [54]. Therefore, our data shows that vaccination of newborn piglets with a joint soluble and particulate subunit vaccine triggered systemic antibody-mediated immunity which contrasts with what is reported in older piglets orally vaccinated with soluble antigens or newborn piglets gavaged with OVA alone [27,52].

Results from our lab showed that oral vaccination of newborn lambs with OVA produced minimal cell-mediated immunity as established by IFN-γ expression and lymphocyte proliferation in *ex vivo* stimulated splenocytes [26]. Similarly, *ex vivo*-stimulated mLN cells from rat pups gavaged with OVA after birth failed to produce significantly higher IFN-γ titres relative to cells from pups gavaged after birth with saline [25]. In the current study, we gavaged piglets with soluble and particulate OVA plus polyphosphazene and CpG ODN, the latter of which is known to promote IFN-γ production [55]. Despite inclusion of CpG ODN in the oral piglet vaccine, IFN-γ production was negligible suggesting that oral immunization of newborns may not induce significant cell-mediated immunity.

Further studies must be undertaken to clarify the precise dose, vaccine formulation and timing of exposure required for induction of cellular immunity as well as including direct measurements of mucosal immunity. Experiments are underway to elucidate the kinetics of gut permeability and the impact this has on the mechanisms

of antigen uptake and where antigen presentation to lymphocytes occurs (i.e. in the Peyer's patches, isolated lymphoid follicles, or mesenteric lymph nodes). Should early life oral vaccination consistently circumvent induction of oral tolerance and/or promote oral immunity, it will have important implications for protecting against infectious diseases in the very young and it may reduce the number of carriers of disease-producing organisms within a herd.

Conclusions
In the present study, we determined that low dose OVA/CpG + MP circumvented induction of oral tolerance with comparable serum anti-OVA antibodies relative to the animals gavaged with 0.05 mg OVA/CpG + MP relative to the i.p. control animals. There was a trend towards induction of mucosal immunity but the results were not statistically significant. These results are intriguing and should be studied further to establish whether it may be advisable to proactively orally vaccinate newborn piglets to prevent induction of oral tolerance to ensure that the they can respond appropriately to parenteral vaccines in later life.

Methods
Immunization procedure
This work was approved by the University of Saskatchewan's Animal Research Ethics Board, and adhered to the Canadian Council on Animal Care guidelines for humane animal use. Pregnant Landrace-cross sows were housed at VIDO with *ad libitum* access to standard feed and water. Piglets were randomly assigned to treatment groups. We gavaged piglets with a single bolus of saline or 0.5 mg or 0.05 mg OVA (Sigma-Aldrich Canada Ltd, Oakville, ON, Canada) plus 50 µg CpG 2395 (soluble components; 5'- TCGTCGTTTTCGGCGCGC GCCG -3' phosphorothioate oligodeoxy-nucleotide from Merial Limited (Lyon, France)), as well as the particulate component comprised of 0.5 mg OVA + 50 µg CpG 2395 + 500 µg poly [di(sodiumcarboxylatoethylphenoxy)-phosphazene] (PCEP) (synthesized by Idaho National Laboratory (Idaho Falls, ID, USA). (These doses were extrapolated from a successful oral vaccination with OVA in lambs and weight adjusted [26]). Microparticles were formulated as detailed in [34]. A total volume of

10 mL was administered via gavage using soft Nalgene Tubing with a monojet catheter tip (Fisher Scientific Ltd., Ottawa, ON) gently inserted into the back of the throat. Piglets were bleed on day three and day seven and then weekly until day 49 (Grey arrows, Figure 1). All blood samples were collected using Ethylenediaminetetraacetic acid (EDTA) Vacutainers (BD Biosciences-Canada, Mississauga, ON), centrifuged (4547 × g) and serum stored at −20°C until antibody titres were measured. At four weeks age, piglets were i.p.-injected with 10 mg OVA plus IFA (Sigma-Aldrich). To generate the parenteral control group, piglets received saline by oral gavage and they were i.p. immunization with OVA plus IFA at four weeks as indicated above. This route was used because it is considered relevant for stimulating the mucosal tissues [56,57]. On day 49, piglets were euthanized using 2 mL/10 lb body weight with Pentobarbital Sodium Injection (240 mg/mL; Euthanyl, Bimeda-MTC Animal Health Inc., Cambridge, ON). Lung lavages were obtained at the end of the trial (Eight weeks; Figure 1). The lung lavage was kept on ice until centrifuged at 400 × g at 4°C for 10 min, then cells were washed twice with cold PBS, counted, and suspended to a final concentration of 4×10^6 cells/mL in 10% complete Roswell Park Memorial Institute (RPMI) medium (Gibco; Life Technologies, Burlington, Ontario), supplemented with 0.2 mM L-glutamine, 0.1 mM HEPES, 0.05 mg/mL gentamicin, 0.02 mM 2-mercaptoethanol (Sigma-Aldrich for all), and 10% heat inactivated horse serum (Gibco; Life Technologies). Cells were stored at -20°C until used for cytokine ELISAs. Endotoxin concentration in OVA was determined to be 8,000 U/ml using the Limulus Amebocyte Lysate enzymatic assay QCL-1000 (Lonza Group Ltd, Basel, Switzerland) according to the manufacturer's instructions.

Serum and lung lavages ELISA

To measure OVA-specific antibody titres, blood sera and lung lavages was obtained as indicated above and ELISAs were performed as previously described [33]. Immunolon II microtiter plates (Dynex Technology Inc., Chantilly, VA, USA) were coated overnight at 4°C with OVA at 500 μg/ml in carbonate coating buffer (15 mM Na_2CO_3, 35 mM $NaHCO_3$, pH 9.6; Sigma-Aldrich) and 100 μL of antigen added to each well. Wells were washed six times with distilled H_2O. Pig serum or lavage samples were diluted as appropriate in Tris-buffered saline plus 0.05% Tween (Sigma-Aldrich) then they were added to the wells at 100 μL/well and incubated for two hours at room temperature (RT). Wells were washed again with distilled H_2O and mouse anti-porcine IgA (Ab Serotec, Raleigh, NC, #MCA 638, 1/300), mouse anti-porcine IgG1 (Ab Serotec, #MCA 635, 1/600), mouse anti-porcine IgG2 (Ab Serotec, #MCA 636, 1/300),

or mouse anti-porcine IgM (Ab Serotec, #MCA 637, 1/100) were added to the wells in a 100 μL volume and incubated for one hour at RT. Wells were washed again with dH_2O and goat anti-mouse IgG (H + L) alkaline phosphatase conjugated (KPL, Gaithersburg, MD, USA, #075-1806, 1/5000) was added to each well at 100 μL/well followed by incubation for one hour at room temperature (RT). One hundred microlitres of goat anti-porcine IgG alkaline phosphatase conjugated (KPL, Gaithersburg, MD, USA, #15-14-06, 1/5000) to each well was used for total IgG detection. Wells were washed six times in dH_2O before di(Tris) p-nitrophenyl phosphate (PNPP; Sigma-Aldrich) was diluted 1 mg/mL in PNPP substrate buffer (1 mM of $MgCl_2$, 200 mM of Tris-HCl, pH 9.8; Sigma-Aldrich) and 100 μL/well was added to the wells. The reaction was allowed to develop for 60 min before absorbance was read as optical density (OD) at 405 nm in a Microplate Reader (Bio-Rad Laboratories, CA, USA). Results were reported as titres which are the reciprocal of the highest dilution that gave a positive OD reading. A positive titre was defined as an OD reading that was at least two times greater than the values for a negative sample.

PBMC Isolation and Bioplex Cytokine Assays

PBMCs were isolated following the protocol described by Buchanan et al [58]. Stimulation of PBMCs were performed in 96-well, round-bottom plates (Nunc, Naperville, Ill., USA) using AIM-V® medium supplemented with 10% fetal bovine serum (Invitrogen, Burlington, ON), 2 mM L-glutamine, 50 μM 2-mercaptoethanol and 10 μg/mL polymyxin B sulfate (Sigma-Aldrich for all) as described before [12]. For each treatment, 5×10^5 cells were cultured for 72 h in triplicate wells with media alone or 20 μg/ml OVA in 200 μL total volume. Culture supernatants were harvested and stored at −20°C until assayed for IL-10 and IFN-γ using Bioplex Cytokine Assay.

Bioplex bead coupling was performed as per the manufacturer's instructions. The reagents were as follows: Coating antibody: monoclonal anti-swine IL-10 (Invitrogen ASC0104), Detection antibody: monoclonal anti-swine IL-10 biotin (Invitrogen ASC9109), Standard: recombinant swine IL-10 (Invitrogen PSC0104) and Coating antibody: monoclonal anti-swine IFN-γ (Fisher Scientific Ltd, ENMP700), Detection antibody: monoclonal anti-swine IFN-γ (Fisher Scientific Ltd,ENPP700; biotinylated in-house), Standard: recombinant swine IFN-γ (Ceiba Geigy). The multiplex assay was carried out in a 96 well Grenier Bio-One Fluotrac 200 96 F black (VWR CanLab Mississauga, ON, #82050-754) which allows washing and retention of the Luminex beads. The porcine IFN-γ and porcine IL-10 protein standards were added to the wells at 50 μl per well at an initial concentration of 2000 pg/mL and 5000 pg/ml, respectively followed by two-fold dilutions to make a standard curve. The PBMC supernatants were prediluted 1:3 and added to the wells at 50 μL per well. The two beadsets conjugated with the IFN-γ and IL-10 antigens were vortexed for 30 s followed by sonication for another 30 s to ensure total bead dispersal. The bead density was adjusted to 1200 beads per μl in PBS-BN (1x PBS + 1% BSA (Sigma-Aldrich) + 0.05% sodium azide (Sigma-Aldrich), pH 7.4) and 1 μL of each beadset was added to 49 μl of the PBSA + 1% New Zealand Pig Serum (Sigma-Aldrich P3484) + 0.05% sodium azide (Sigma-Aldrich) which was then added to each well. The plate was sealed with plate sealer (Fisher Scientific Ltd, #12565491) and covered with foil lid. The plate was agitated at 800 rpm for one hour at room temperature. After one hour incubation with serum, the plate was washed using the Bio-Plex ProII Wash Station (Bio-Rad Laboratories; soak 20 s, wash with 150 μL PBST three times). A 50 μL cocktail consisting of porcine IFN-γ (Fisher Scientific Ltd, (Endogen); 1/300 (which was biotinylated in-house) and biotinylated porcine IL-10 (Invitrogen; 0.5 μg/mL) was added to each well. The plate was again sealed, covered and agitated at 800 rpm for 30 minutes at room temperature then washed again as indicated above. A 50 μL volume of Streptavidin R-Phycoerythrin (RPE) (diluted

to 5 μg/mL; Cedarlane, Burlington, ON; # PJRS20) was added to each well. The plate was again sealed, covered and agitated at 800 rpm for 30 minutes at room temperature and washed as indicated above. A 100 μL volume of 1 × Tris-EDTA was added to each well and then the plate was vortexed for 5 minutes before reading on the Luminex100 xMAP™ instrument (Luminex, Toronto, ON) following the manufacturer's instructions and as described in [59]. The instrument was set up to read beadsets in regions 43 and 28 for IFN-γ and IL-10, respectively. A minimum of 60 events per beadset were read and the median value obtained for each reaction event per beadset. For all samples the multiplex assay mean fluorescent intensity (MFI) data was corrected for subtracting the background levels.

Statistical analysis

The outcome data from this study were not normally distributed and therefore, differences among experimental groups were tested using Kruskal-Wallis analysis and medians were compared using Dunn's test. In Figure 4, significance was determined using Mann-Whitney test. Differences were considered significant if $p < 0.05$. All statistical analyses and graphing were formed using GraphPad Prism 5 software (GraphPad Software, San Diego, CA).

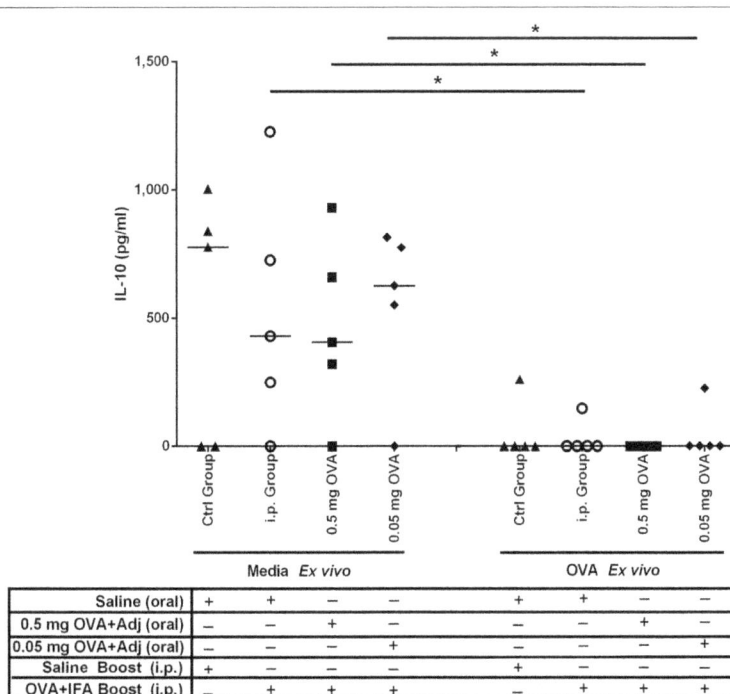

	Media *Ex vivo*				OVA *Ex vivo*			
	Ctrl Group	i.p. Group	0.5 mg OVA	0.05 mg OVA	Ctrl Group	i.p. Group	0.5 mg OVA	0.05 mg OVA
Saline (oral)	+	+	−	−	+	+	−	−
0.5 mg OVA+Adj (oral)	−	−	+	−	−	−	+	−
0.05 mg OVA+Adj (oral)	−	−	−	+	−	−	−	+
Saline Boost (i.p.)	+	−	−	−	+	−	−	−
OVA+IFA Boost (i.p.)	−	+	+	+	−	+	+	+

Figure 4 OVA-specific cytokine production by PBMCs from piglets gavaged with OVA subunit vaccine then i.p. immunized with OVA/IFA at four weeks of age. Piglets (n = 5/group) were gavaged and i.p. immunized as described in Figure 1. IL-10 production was measured from PBMCs obtained four weeks post i.p. immunization. PBMCs were re-stimulated with OVA or media ex vivo. After 72 hours, the supernatants were collected and measured by BioPlex assay. Each data point represents an individual animal and median values are indicated by horizontal lines.

Abbreviations

BALs: Bronchoalveolar lavage; CMI: Cell-mediated immune response; DCs: Dendritic cells; PNPP: di(Tris) p-nitrophenyl phosphate; ELISA: Enzyme-linked immunosorbent assays; GALT: Gut-associated lymphoid tissues; h: hour; IL: Interleukin; IFA: Incomplete Freund's Adjuvant; i.p: intraperitoneal; Ig: Immunoglobulin; IFLs: Isolated lymphoid follicles; MW: Molecular Weight; MFI: Mean fluorescent intensity; MLN: Mesenteric lymph node; MP: Microparticle; OVA: Ovalbumin; OD: Optical density; PBMC: Peripheral blood mononuclear cell; RPE: R-Phycoerythrin; RT: Room temperature; SIgA: Secretory IgA; StDev: Standard deviation; Th: T-helper cell; Treg: T regulatory cell; TBST: Tris-buffered saline with Tween 20; VIDO: Vaccine & Infectious Disease Organization.

Competing interests

The authors declare that they have no competing interests.

Authors' contributions

JAP performed the immunizations and coordinated the animal experiments. HLW conceived of and designed the experiments. JAP and HLW jointly wrote the manuscript. SN, RMB and SM performed the laboratory experiments. GKM and VG were responsible for the design of the particulate vaccine component. All authors read and approved the final version.

Acknowledgments

We gratefully acknowledge financial support from the Alberta Livestock and Meat Agency, Ontario Pork and the Saskatchewan Agriculture Development Fund (Saskatchewan Ministry of Agriculture and the Canada-Saskatchewan Growing Forward bi-lateral agreement). We would like to thank the members of the Animal Care Group at VIDO for their excellent expertise as well as Donna Dent, Dr. Andrea Ladinig and Dr. John Harding for their excellent technical assistance with the BioPlex assays. We are grateful to Merial Limited for synthesis of CpG 2395 and Idaho National Laboratory for synthesis of PCEP. HLW is an adjunct professor in the Department of Biochemistry and the School of Public Health at the University of Saskatchewan. GKM is a professor at School of Public Health at the University of Saskatchewan. VG is a professor of Veterinary Microbiology at the University of Saskatchewan. This manuscript is published with the permission of the Director of VIDO as journal series no. 701.

Author details

[1]Vaccine and Infectious Disease Organization (VIDO), University of Saskatchewan, 120 Veterinary Road, Saskatoon, SK S7N 5E3, Canada. [2]Current address: Klinikum der Universität zu Köln, Institut für Medizinische Mikrobiologie, Immunologie und Hygiene, Goldenfelsstraße 19-21, 50935 Köln, Germany.

References

1. Faria AMC, Maron R, Ficker SM, Slavin AJ, Spahn T, Weiner HL. Oral tolerance induced by continuous feeding: enhanced up-regulation of transforming growth factor-beta/interleukin-10 and suppression of experimental autoimmune encephalomyelitis. J Autoimmun. 2003;20(2):135–45.
2. Faria AMC, Weiner HL. Oral tolerance. Immunol Rev. 2005;206(1):232–59.
3. Wannemuehler MJ, Kiyono H, Babb JL, Michalek SM, Mcghee JR. Lipopolysaccharide (Lps) Regulation of the Immune-Response - Lps Converts Germ-Free Mice to Sensitivity to Oral Tolerance Induction. J Immunol. 1982;129(3):959–65.
4. Sudo N, Sawamura SA, Tanaka K, Aiba Y, Kubo C, Koga Y. The requirement of intestinal bacterial flora for the development of an IgE production system fully susceptible to oral tolerance induction. J Immunol. 1997;159(4):1739–45.
5. Kushwah R, Hu J. Role of dendritic cells in the induction of regulatory T cells. Cell Biosci. 2011;1(1):20.
6. Worbs T, Bode U, Yan S, Hoffmann MW, Hintzen G, Bernhardt G, et al. Oral tolerance originates in the intestinal immune system and relies on antigen carriage by dendritic cells. J Exp Med. 2006;203(3):519–27.
7. Alpan O, Rudomen G, Matzinger P. The role of dendritic cells, B cells, and M cells in gut-oriented immune responses. J Immunol. 2001;166(8):4843–52.
8. Roncarolo MG, Levings MK, Traversari C. Differentiation of T regulatory cells by immature dendritic cells. J Exp Med. 2001;193(2):F5–9.
9. Tezuka H, Ohteki T. Regulation of intestinal homeostasis by dendritic cells. Immunol Rev. 2010;234(1):247–58.
10. Pasetti MF, Simon JK, Sztein MB, Levine MM. Immunology of gut mucosal vaccines. Immunol Revs. 2011;239(1):125–48.
11. Medina E, Guzmán CA. Modulation of immune responses following antigen administration by mucosal route. FEMS Immunol Med Microbiol. 2000;27(4):305–11.
12. Nguyen TV, Yuan L, Azevedo MS, Jeong KI, Gonzalez AM, Saif LJ. Transfer of maternal cytokines to suckling piglets: in vivo and in vitro models with implications for immunomodulation of neonatal immunity. Vet Immunol Immunopathol. 2007;117(3–4):236–48.
13. Lecce JG, Matrone G. Porcine neonatal nutrition: the effect of diet on blood serum proteins and performance of the baby pig. J Nutr. 1960;70:13–20.
14. Nechvatalova K, Kudlackova H, Leva L, Babickova K, Faldyna M. Transfer of humoral and cell-mediated immunity via colostrum in pigs. Vet Immunol Immunopathol. 2011;142(1–2):95–100.
15. Bandrick M, Ariza-Nieto C, Baidoo SK, Molitor TW. Colostral antibody-mediated and cell-mediated immunity contributes to innate and antigen-specific immunity in piglets. Dev Comp Immunol. 2014;43(1):114–20.
16. Stott GH, Marx DB, Menefee BE, Nightengale GT. Colostral immunoglobulin transfer in calves I. Period of absorption. J Dairy Sci. 1979;62(10):1632–8.
17. Jensen AR, Elnif J, Burrin DG, Sangild PT. Development of intestinal immunoglobulin absorption and enzyme activities in neonatal pigs is diet dependent. J Nutr. 2001;131(12):3259–65.
18. Halliday R. The absorption of antibodies from immune sera by the gut of the young rat. Proc R Soc Lond B Biol Sci. 1955;143(912):408–13.
19. Appleby P, Catty D. Transmission of immunoglobulin to foetal and neonatal mice. J Reprod Immunol. 1983;5(4):203–13.
20. Wenzl HH, Schimpl G, Feierl G, Steinwender G. Time course of spontaneous bacterial translocation from gastrointestinal tract and its relationship to intestinal microflora in conventionally reared infant rats. Dig Dis Sci. 2001;46(5):1120–6.
21. Vukavic T. Timing of the gut closure. J Pediatr Gastroenterol Nutr. 1984;3(5):700–3.
22. Brandtzaeg P, Nilssen DE, Rognum TO, Thrane PS. Ontogeny of the mucosal immune system and IgA deficiency. Gastroenterol Clin North Am. 1991;20(3):397–439.
23. Lorenz RG, Newberry RD. Isolated lymphoid follicles can function as sites for induction of mucosal immune responses. Ann N Y Acad Sci. 2004;1029:44–57.
24. Cesta MF. Normal Structure, Function, and Histology of Mucosa-Associated Lymphoid Tissue. Tox Pathol. 2006;34(5):599–608.
25. Buchanan R, Tetland S, Wilson HL. Low dose antigen exposure for a finite period in newborn rats triggers mucosal immunity rather than tolerance in later life. PLoS ONE. 2012;7(12):e51437.
26. Buchanan R, Mertins S, Wilson H. Oral antigen exposure in extreme early life in lambs influences the magnitude of the immune response which can be generated in later life. BMC Vet Res. 2013;9:160. doi:10.1186/1746-6148-9-160.
27. Pasternak JA, Ng SH, Wilson HL. A single, low dose oral antigen exposure in newborn piglets primes mucosal immunity if administered with CpG oligodeoxynucleotides and polyphosphazene adjuvants. Vet Immunol Immunopathol. 2014;161(3–4):211–21.
28. Haverson K, Corfield G, Jones PH, Kenny M, Fowler J, Bailey M, et al. Effect of Oral Antigen and Antibody Exposure at Birth on Subsequent Immune Status. Int Arch Allergy Imm. 2009;150(2):192–204.
29. Strobel S, Ferguson A. Immune responses to fed protein antigens in mice. 3. Systemic tolerance or priming is related to age at which antigen is first encountered. Pediatr Res. 1984;18(7):588–94.
30. Miller A, Lider O, Abramsky O, Weiner HL. Orally administered myelin basic protein in neonates primes for immune responses and enhances experimental autoimmune encephalomyelitis in adult animals. Eur J Immunol. 1994;24(5):1026–32.
31. Tobagus IT, Thomas WR, Holt PG. Adjuvant costimulation during secondary antigen challenge directs qualitative aspects of oral tolerance induction, particularly during the neonatal period. J Immunol. 2004;172(4):2274–85.
32. Strobel S. Immunity induced after a feed of antigen during early life: oral tolerance v. sensitisation. Proc Nutr Soc. 2001;60(4):437–42.
33. Wilson HL, Kovacs-Nolan J, Latimer L, Buchanan R, Gomis S, Babiuk L, et al. A novel triple adjuvant formulation promotes strong, Th1-biased immune responses and significant antigen retention at the site of injection. Vaccine. 2010;28(52):8288–99.

34. Garlapati S, Eng NF, Wilson HL, Buchanan R, Mutwiri GK, Babiuk LA, et al. PCPP (poly[di(carboxylatophenoxy)-phosphazene]) microparticles co-encapsulating ovalbumin and CpG oligo-deoxynucleotides are potent enhancers of antigen specific Th1 immune responses in mice. Vaccine. 2010;28(52):8306–14.

35. Awate S, Wilson HL, Lai K, Babiuk LA, Mutwiri G. Activation of adjuvant core response genes by the novel adjuvant PCEP. Mol Immunol. 2012;51(3–4):292–303.

36. Mutwiri G, Benjamin P, Soita H, Townsend H, Yost R, Roberts B, et al. Poly[di(sodium carboxylatoethylphenoxy) phosphazene] (PCEP) is a potent enhancer of mixed Th1/Th2 immune responses in mice immunized with influenza virus antigens. Vaccine. 2007;25(7):1204–13.

37. Mutwiri G, Bowersock TL, Babiuk LA. Microparticles for oral delivery of vaccines. Expert Opin Drug Deliv. 2005;2(5):791–806.

38. Mowat AM. The regulation of immune responses to dietary protein antigens. Immunol Today. 1987;8(3):93–8.

39. Wilson HL, Obradovic MR. Evidence for a common mucosal immune system in the pig. Mol Immunol. 2014. doi: 10.1016/j.molimm.2014.09.004.

40. McNeilly TN, McClure SJ, Huntley JF. Mucosal immunity in sheep and implications for mucosal vaccine development. Sm Ruminant Res. 2008;76(1–2):83–91.

41. McGhee JR, Xu-Amano J, Miller CJ, Jackson RJ, Fujihashi K, Staats HF, et al. The common mucosal immune system: from basic principles to enteric vaccines with relevance for the female reproductive tract. Reprod Fertil Dev. 1994;6(3):369–79.

42. Mestecky J. The common mucosal immune system and current strategies for induction of immune responses in external secretions. J Clin Immunol. 1987;7(4):265–76.

43. Brandtzaeg P. Regionalized immune function of tonsils and adenoids. Immunol Today. 1999;20(8):383–4.

44. Czerkinsky C, Holmgren J. Topical immunization strategies. Mucosal Immunol. 2010;3(6):545–55.

45. Bourges D, Chevaleyre C, Wang C, Berri M, Zhang X, Nicaise L, et al. Differential expression of adhesion molecules and chemokines between nasal and small intestinal mucosae: implications for T- and sIgA+ B-lymphocyte recruitment. Immunology. 2007;122(4):551–61.

46. Foss DL, Murtaugh MP. Mucosal immunogenicity and adjuvanticity of cholera toxin in swine. Vaccine. 1999;17(7–8):788–801.

47. Verdonck F, De Hauwere V, Bouckaert J, Goddeeris BM, Cox E. Fimbriae of enterotoxigenic Escherichia coli function as a mucosal carrier for a coupled heterologous antigen. J Control Release. 2005;104(2):243–58.

48. Kabir S. Cholera vaccines: the current status and problems. Rev Med Microbiol. 2005;16(3):101–16.

49. Botner A, Strandbygaard B, Sorensen KJ, Have P, Madsen KG, Madsen ES, et al. Appearance of acute PRRS-like symptoms in sow herds after vaccination with a modified live PRRS vaccine. Vet Rec. 1997;141(19):497–9.

50. Storgaard T, Oleksiewicz M, Botner A. Examination of the selective pressures on a live PRRS vaccine virus. Arch Virol. 1999;144(12):2389–401.

51. Hu J, Zhang C. Porcine reproductive and respiratory syndrome virus vaccines: current status and strategies to a universal vaccine. Transbound Emerg Dis. 2014;61(2):109–20.

52. Delisle B, Calinescu C, Mateescu MA, Fairbrother JM, Nadeau E. Oral immunization with F4 fimbriae and CpG formulated with carboxymethyl starch enhances F4-specific mucosal immune response and modulates Th1 and Th2 cytokines in weaned pigs. J Pharm Pharm Sci. 2012;15(5):642–56.

53. Snoeck V, Huyghebaert N, Cox E, Vermeire A, Vancaeneghem S, Remon JP, et al. Enteric-coated pellets of F4 fimbriae for oral vaccination of suckling piglets against enterotoxigenic Escherichia coli infections. Vet Immunol Immunopathol. 2003;96(3–4):219–27.

54. Snoeck V, Peters IR, Cox E. The IgA system: a comparison of structure and function in different species. Vet Res. 2006;37(3):455–67.

55. Cowdery JS, Chace JH, Yi AK, Krieg AM. Bacterial DNA induces NK cells to produce IFN-gamma in vivo and increases the toxicity of lipopolysaccharides. J Immunol. 1996;156(12):4570–5.

56. Sheldrake RF, Husband AJ, Watson DL. Origin of antibody-containing cells in the ovine mammary gland following intraperitoneal and intramammary immunisation. Res Vet Sci. 1988;45(2):156–9.

57. Husband AJ, McDowell GH. Local and systemic immune responses following oral immunization of foetal lambs. Immunology. 1975;29(6):1019–28.

58. Buchanan RM, Popowych Y, Arsic N, Townsend HG, Mutwiri GK, Potter AA, et al. B-cell activating factor (BAFF) promotes CpG ODN-induced B cell activation and proliferation. Cell Immunol. 2011;271(1):16–28.

59. Anderson S, Wakeley P, Wibberley G, Webster K, Sawyer J. Development and evaluation of a Luminex multiplex serology assay to detect antibodies to bovine herpes virus 1, parainfluenza 3 virus, bovine viral diarrhoea virus, and bovine respiratory syncytial virus, with comparison to existing ELISA detection methods. J Immunol Methods. 2011;366(1–2):79–88.

13

Fatal disease associated with Swine *Hepatitis E virus* and *Porcine circovirus 2* co-infection in four weaned pigs in China

Yifei Yang[1†], Ruihan Shi[1†], Ruiping She[1*], Jingjing Mao[1], Yue Zhao[1], Fang Du[1], Can Liu[1], Jianchai Liu[2], Minheng Cheng[1], Rining Zhu[1], Wei Li[1], Xiaoyang Wang[1] and Majid Hussain Soomro[1]

Abstract

Background: In recent decades, *Porcine circovirus 2* (PCV2) infection has been recognized as the causative agent of postweaning multisystemic wasting syndrome, and has become a threat to the swine industry. *Hepatitis E virus* (HEV) is another high prevalent pathogen in swine in many regions of the world. PCV2 and HEV are both highly prevalent in pig farms in China.

Case presentation: In this study, we characterized the HEV and PCV2 co-infection in 2–3 month-old piglets, based on pathogen identification and the pathological changes observed, in Hebei Province, China. The pathological changes were severe, and general hyperemia, hemorrhage, inflammatory cell infiltration, and necrosis were evident in the tissues of dead swine. PCR was used to identify the pathogen and we tested for eight viruses (HEV, *Porcine reproductive and respiratory syndrome virus*, PCV2, *Classical swine fever virus*, *Porcine epidemic diarrhea virus*, *Transmissible gastroenteritis coronavirus*, *Porcine parvovirus* and *Pseudorabies virus*) that are prevalent in Chinese pig farms. The livers, kidneys, spleens, and other organs of the necropsied swine were positive for HEV and/or PCV2. Immunohistochemical staining showed HEV- and PCV2-antigen-positive signals in the livers, kidneys, lungs, lymph nodes, and intestine.

Conclusion: HEV and PCV2 co-infection in piglets was detected in four out of seven dead pigs from two pig farms in Hebei, China, producing severe pathological changes. The natural co-infection of HEV and PCV2 in pigs in China has rarely been reported. We speculate that co-infection with PCV2 and HEV may bring some negative effect on pig production and recommend that more attention should be paid to this phenomenon.

Keywords: Weaned pigs, *Hepatitis E virus*, *Porcine circovirus 2*, Co-infection, High mortality

Background

The rapid development of the pig industry in China accompanies with outbreaks of epidemic diseases in recent years. *Hepatitis E virus* (HEV) has been identified on pig farms in many regions of the world, including China [1-3]. HEV seropositivity rates of 76.6% and 90% have been reported in pig herds of large-scale and family-scale farms in China, respectively [4]. Increasing evidence indicates that HEV can infect both humans and animal [5]. To date, most studies of HEV based on prevalence surveys, and research into HEV-associated mortality during natural infection was limited. Mao et al. reported that co-infection with HEV and *Porcine reproductive and respiratory syndrome virus* (PRRSV) could lead to high mortality in swine [6], and they speculated that co-infection with HEV and other pathogens could cause serious disease. It has been demonstrated that HEV and *Porcine circovirus 2* (PCV2) could cause infectious hepatitis, but swine naturally co-infected with HEV and PCV2 in China has rarely been reported [3,7,8]. PCV2 infection occurs in many countries and poses a considerable threat to the swine industry [9]. Although the recently research showed that infection of PCV2 could be effectively reduced by utilizing PCV2 vaccine [10], prevention of PCV2 in the pig production should be paid more attention. In the

* Correspondence: sheruiping@126.com
†Equal contributors
[1]Laboratory of Animal Pathology and Public Health, College of Veterinary Medicine, China Agricultural University; Key Laboratory of Zoonosis of Ministry of Agriculture, China Agricultural University, Beijing 100193, China
Full list of author information is available at the end of the article

present study, pathogen identification and the observation of pathological changes demonstrated a natural co-infection with HEV and PCV2 in the swine on two pig farms in Hebei Province, China. This discovery may provide a new perspective for clinical research.

Case presentation

Medical history and clinical symptoms

From November to December 2013, an outbreak of an unknown disease occurred at two small-scale pig farms (103 pigs in farm A and 101 pigs in farm B), operating for a short time in Hebei Province, China. All of the piglets fed in both pig farm A and B were aged 2–3 months. Pig farm A reported the deaths of 93 piglets (mortality rate was 90.3%), and pig farm B the deaths of 90 pigs (mortality rate was 89.1%). The affected animals on both farms presented with symptoms of fever, dyspnea, diarrhea, and anorexia. In pig farm A, the veterinary administrated timicosin and doxycycline to treat the pigs. And in pig farm B, florfenicol was administrated. However, the swine did not respond to antibiotic treatment.

Sampling and pathological changes

Necropsies were performed on seven dead piglets: three from farm A (pigs 1, 2, and 3) and four from farm B (pigs 4, 5, 6, and 7). The tissues examined included the liver, spleen, lung, kidney, heart, intestine, and lymph nodes. All tissues used for histological examination were fixed in 2.5% (w/v) glutaraldehyde–polyoxymethylene solution for 48 h. The fixed tissues were routinely processed, embedded in paraffin, sectioned (4 μm thickness), and stained with hematoxylin and eosin. Portions of the liver, spleen, kidney, brain and lung tissues were used for pathogen detection and stored at −80°C until required.

Gross lesions

Seven dead piglets were necropsied and diagnosed. Scattered hemorrhagic spots were observed on the surface of the skin (Figure 1A). The right ventricle was dilated so that the ratio of the transverse/longitudinal diameters was increased (Figure 1B). Hyperemia, hemorrhage, and necrosis were present in large local areas of the lung (Figure 1C). A transparent gelatinous exudate was observed in the trachea (Figure 1D). The liver was enlarged and the surface was a dark red color (Figure 1E). It was difficult to strip the kidney capsule, and all the kidneys showed varying degrees of enlargement (Figure 1F). The lymph nodes and spleens were swollen to varying degrees (Figure 1G, H). Hemorrhage and infarction were observed in the spleen (Figure 1H). The mesenteric lymph nodes were enlarged and hyperemic (Figure 1I).

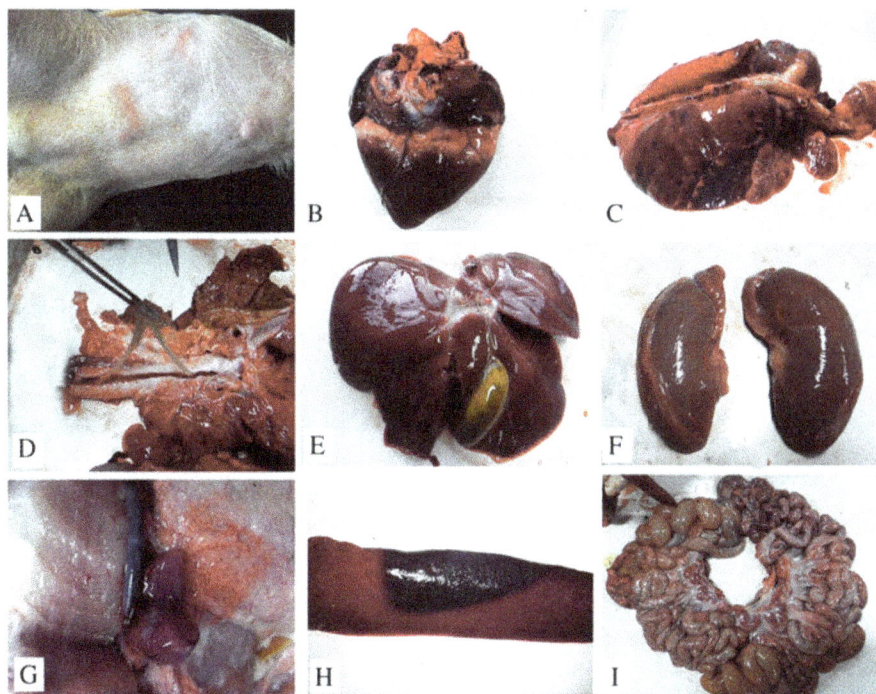

Figure 1 Necropsy observations. (A) Hemorrhage in the skin. **(B)** Dilated right ventricle of the heart. **(C, D)** Lung with hemorrhage, hyperemia, necrosis, and tracheal exudate. **(E)** Dark red and swollen liver. **(F)** Enlarged kidneys. **(G)** Clearly swollen lymph node. **(H)** Enlarged spleen, with infarction. **(I)** Enlarged mesenteric lymph nodes.

Histological lesions

The pathological changes in various tissues were determined with microscopy. The lesions observed in the lung, liver, heart, kidney, lymph node, spleen and intestinal tract tissues were similar in all the pigs necropsied. The heart lesions were characterized as viral myocarditis (Figure 2A). The epicardium was predominantly infiltrated by lymphocytes, with a small number of neutrophils (Figure 2B). Granular myocardial degeneration, edema, and lymphocyte and neutrophil infiltration in the myocardium were observed (Figure 2C). A hepatic examination revealed features characteristic of hepatitis in a number of liver samples, including congestion, vacuolization, and necrosis, (Figure 2E). Lymphocyte and neutrophil infiltration, particularly in the portal area, was clearly observed (Figure 2F). Examination of the lungs demonstrated large areas of hyperemia, hemorrhage, and lymphocyte and neutrophil infiltration, with very little normal histological structure. The bronchioles contained exfoliated alveolar epithelial cells and pink liquid exudate (Figure 2G,H). Enlargement of the glomerulus and focal lymphocyte infiltration were observed in the kidneys. The renal tubule epithelial cells showed granular degeneration and necrosis, and congestion and hemorrhage were present in the kidneys. The renal tubule epithelial cells shed off from the basilar membrane. The glomerulus contained albuminoid droplets of exudate (Figure 2I,J). The organs of immune system were severely underdeveloped, and malformed splenic white pulp was responsible for the reduced numbers of lymphocytes (Figure 2D). Poorly developed lymph nodes were also evident. The majority of capillaries were expanded and hyperemia was present. The lymphoid nodules were smaller than normal, resulting from fibrosis, necrosis, and lymphocyte depletion (Figure 2K, L). Examination of the intestine revealed necrosis, and coagulation of the intestinal villi. The submucosal layer was exposed due to the loss of mucosal layer. Epithelial cell shedding and secretion from the intestinal glands into the gut cavity were increased (Figure 2M, N). The main pathological changes observed in the various organs of the seven necropsied pigs are summarized in Table 1.

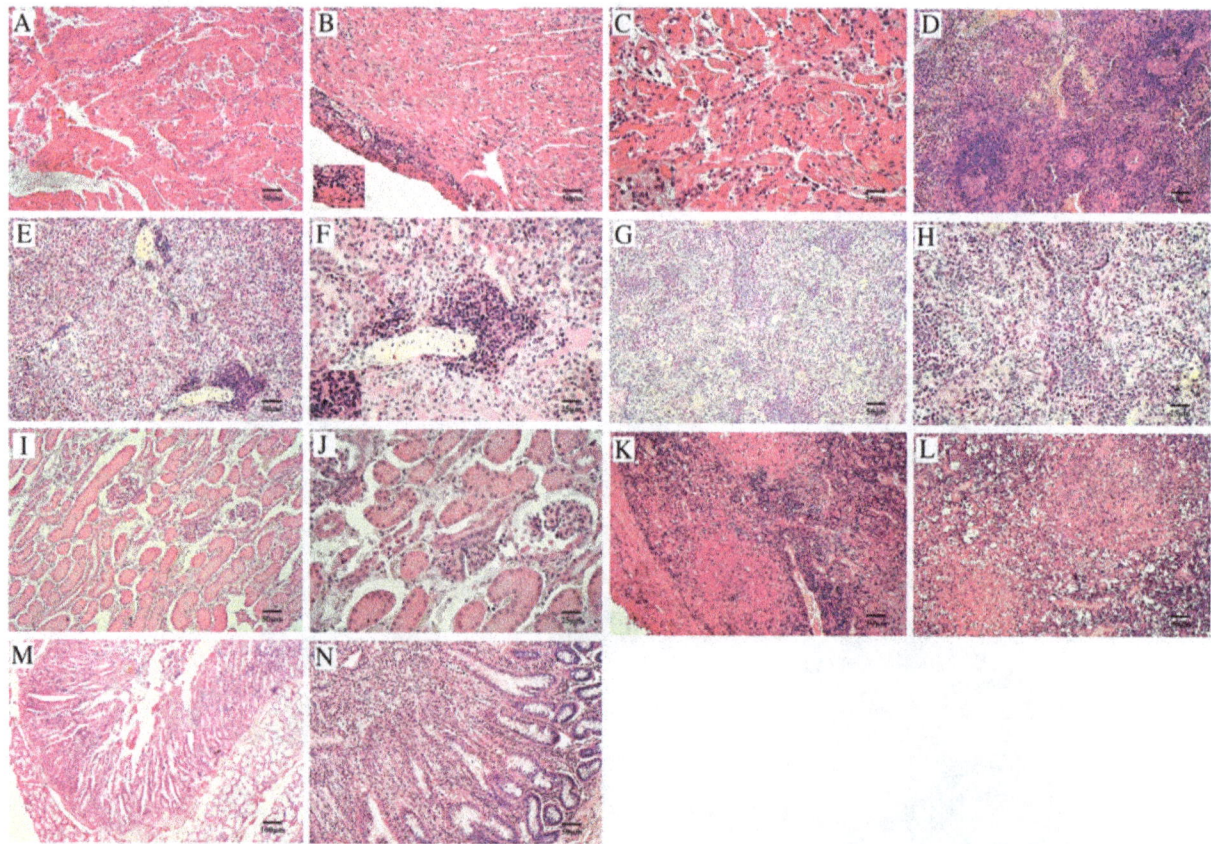

Figure 2 Histological lesions in multiple organs. Pathological changes were characterized by hemorrhage, hyperemia, inflammatory infiltration, and necrosis. **(A, B, C)** Myocarditis. **(D)** Dysplasia of the lymphoid follicles in the spleen. **(E, F)** Liver displaying hepatic necrosis and lymphocyte infiltration. **(G, H)** Lung with extensive lymphocyte infiltration, hemosiderosis, hemorrhage, and shed alveolar epithelial cells within the bronchioles and alveoli. **(I, J)** Necrosis and degeneration in the kidney. **(K, L)** Dysplasia, fibrosis, lack of lymphocytes, and necrosis in a lymph node. **(M, N)** Coagulation, necrosis, and abruption of the intestinal villi.

Table 1 Main pathological changes in the organs of the seven pigs necropsied

Organ	Pathological changes	Pig farm A			Pig farm B			
		1 HEV+ PCV+	2 HEV+ PCV-	3 HEV+ PCV+	4 HEV+ PCV+	5 HEV+ PCV+	6 HEV- PCV+	7 HEV- PCV+
Liver	Degeneration	+	+	+	+	+	+	+
	Edema	+	+	-	+	+	+	-
	Congestion	+	+	+	+	+	+	+
	Hemorrage	-	+	-	-	-	+	-
	Necrosis	+	+	+	+	+	+	+
	Inflammation	+	+	+	+	+	+	+
	Fibrosis	-	-	-	-	-	-	-
Heart	Degeneration	+	+	+	+	+	+	+
	Edema	+	-	+	-	+	+	+
	Necrosis	+	+	-	-	+	+	
	Inflammation	+	+	-	+	-	-	+
Lung	Degeneration	+	+	+	+	+	+	+
	Congestion	+	+	+	+	+	+	+
	Hemorrage	+	+	+	+	+	+	+
	Necrosis	+	+	+	+	+	+	+
	Inflammation	+	+	+	+	+	+	+
	Exfoliation of alveolar epithelial cells	+	+	-	+		+	+
Kidney	Degeneration	+	+	+	+	+	+	+
	Edema	+	+	+	+	+	+	+

Pathogen detection

PCR was used to detect any viruses in the liver, lung, spleen, brain and kidney samples (Table 1). Viral pathogens responsible for suspicious diseases in swine were investigated: HEV, PCV2, *Classical swine fever virus* (CSFV), *Porcine epidemic diarrhea virus* (PEDV), *Transmissible gastroenteritis coronavirus* (TGEV), *Pseudorabies virus* (PRV), *Porcine parvovirus* (PPV), and PRRSV. PCV2 was detected in the livers of six of the seven pigs (GenBank accession nos. KJ534661, KJ534662, KJ534659, KJ534658, KJ534663, and KJ534660) (Figure 3A) and five of the seven pig livers were HEV positive (GenBank accession nos. KJ123761, KM024042, KJ141160, KJ534657, and KJ534656) (Figure 3B).

A phylogenetic analysis based on the 348-nt open reading frame (ORF) 2 of HEV was used to establish the genetic relatedness of the strains isolated in this study to representative isolates of the four HEV genotypes. Isolates CHN-HB-HD-L1, CHN-HB-HD-L2, HB-L3, CHN-HB-HD-L4, and CHN-HB-HD-L5 were identified as genotype 4, and were most closely related to swCH25 (AY594199), CHN-SD-sHEV (KF176351), HE-JA2 (AB220974) (Figure 4). A phylogenetic analysis based on the 494-nt ORF2 of PCV2 was used to establish the genetic relatedness of the strains isolated in

this study to PCV2 strains isolated globally, including in China. The HBHD-L1, HBHD-L3, HBHD-L4, HBHD-L5, HBHD-L6, and HBHD-L7 (Figure 5) isolates were closely related to genotype PCV2d strains HNF911 (KJ680361), SD-ZB2 (KJ511876), WSEC11 (KJ680353), GXYQ12 (KJ680367), TDBS12 (KJ680354). Other tissues were also tested using PCR. The liver, spleen, kidney, lung, and brain of pig No. 1, 2, 3, 4, and 5 were positive for HEV RNA and these tissues were PCV2 DNA positive in pig No. 1, 3, 4, 5, 6, and 7. The co-infection rate for HEV and PCV2 was 57.1% (4/7). The livers, lungs, kidneys, and spleens of the necropsied pigs were negative for PEDV, TGEV, CSFV, PRRSV, PRV, and PPV.

Immunohistochemistry

Immunohistochemical (IHC) staining confirmed the presence of HEV and PCV2 antigens in several tissues and organs. HEV antigen was detected in the livers, kidneys, lung, intestine and lymph nodes of all five HEV-positive swine (pig No.1, 2, 3, 4, 5). Granular or diffuse positive staining was seen in the hepatic sinusoid and the cytoplasm of hepatocytes (Figure 6A). The nuclei and cytoplasm of the renal tubular epithelial cells (Figure 6B) and lung cells (Figure 6C) were positive for HEV antigen. The staining for HEV antigen in

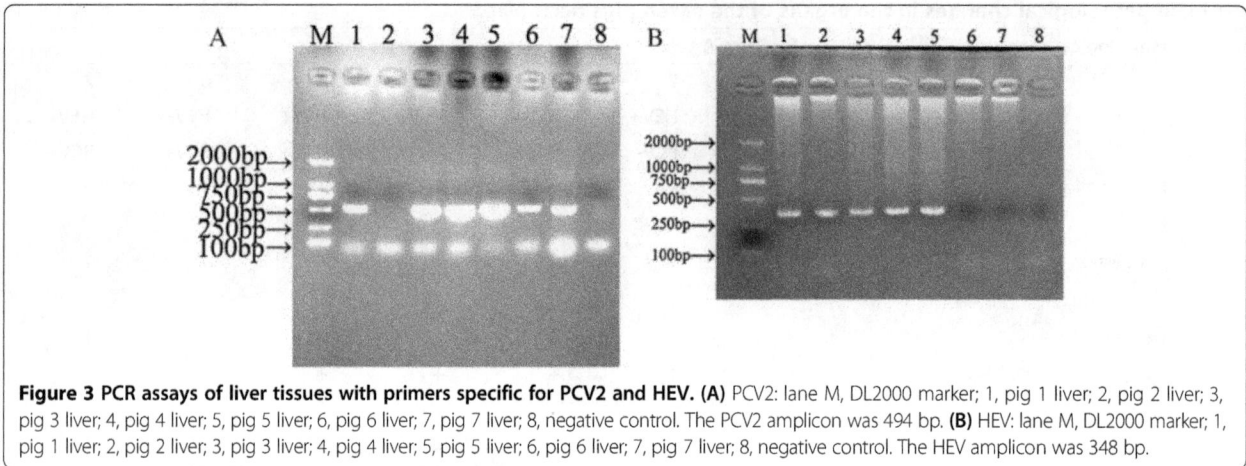

Figure 3 PCR assays of liver tissues with primers specific for PCV2 and HEV. (A) PCV2: lane M, DL2000 marker; 1, pig 1 liver; 2, pig 2 liver; 3, pig 3 liver; 4, pig 4 liver; 5, pig 5 liver; 6, pig 6 liver; 7, pig 7 liver; 8, negative control. The PCV2 amplicon was 494 bp. **(B)** HEV: lane M, DL2000 marker; 1, pig 1 liver; 2, pig 2 liver; 3, pig 3 liver; 4, pig 4 liver; 5, pig 5 liver; 6, pig 6 liver; 7, pig 7 liver; 8, negative control. The HEV amplicon was 348 bp.

the lymph nodes was intense in the lymphocytes and macrophages (Figure 6D). The staining for HEV antigen in the intestinal tissue was intense in the lamina propria and gut-associated lymphoid tissue (Figure 6E). The negative control is shown in Figure 7. HEV antigen was negative in the two HEV RNA negative swine (pig No.6 and 7).

The lungs, livers, kidneys, lymph nodes, and intestine were tested for PCV2 antigen with IHC staining. The tissue distribution of the PCV2 antigen was similar in all PCV2 DNA positive pigs (pig No.1, 3, 4, 5, 6, 7). In the liver, PCV2 antigen was detected within the hepatocytes and Küpffer cells (Figure 8A); in the kidneys, the positive

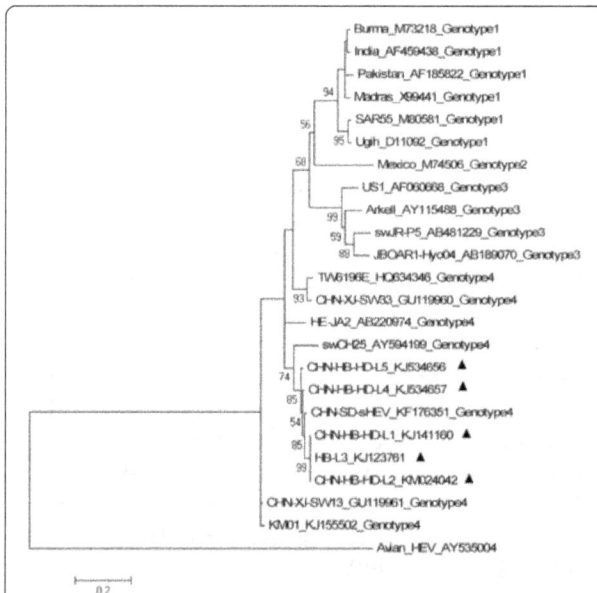

Figure 4 Phylogenetic analysis based on HEV ORF2 (304 nt, the primers not included) showing the genetic relationships between the isolates identified in this study and isolates from across China and other countries. A neighbor-joining tree was constructed with bootstrap values calculated from 1,000 replicates. The isolates used for the comparative analysis were HEV genotype 4 strains CHN-SD-sHEV (KF176351), CHN-XJ-SW13 (GU119961), HE-JA2 (AB220974), KM01 (KJ155502), TW6196E (HQ634346), CHN-XJ-SW33 (GU119960), swCH25 (AY594199), genotype 3 strains swJR-P5 (AB481229), Arkell (AY115488), JBOAR1-Hyo04 (AB189070), genotype 2 strain Mexico (M74506), genotype 1 strain India (AF459438), Madras (X99441), Pakistan (AF185822), SAR55 (M80581), Ugih (D11092), US1 (AF060668), Burma (M73218), and Avian HEV (AY535004).

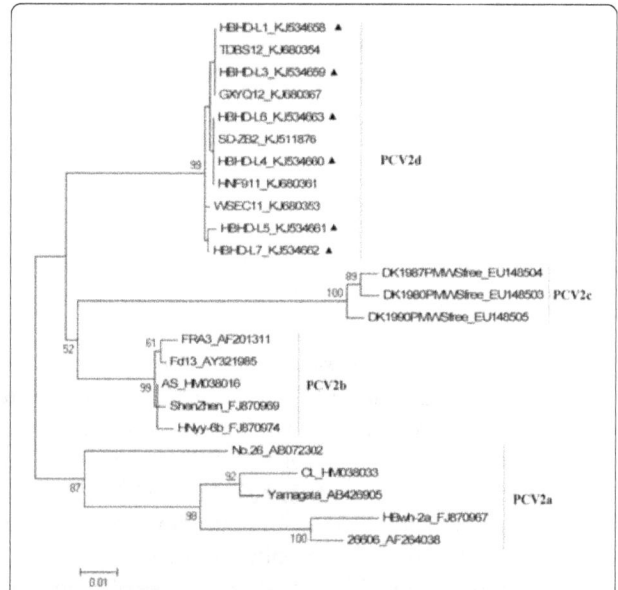

Figure 5 Phylogenetic analysis based on PCV2 ORF2 (451 nt, the primers not included) showing the genetic relationships between the isolates identified in this study and isolates from across China or other countries. A neighbor-joining tree was constructed with bootstrap values calculated from 1,000 replicates. The isolates used for the comparative analysis were genotype PCV2d strains HNF911 (KJ680361), SD-ZB2 (KJ511876), WSEC11 (KJ680353), GXYQ12 (KJ680367), TDBS12 (KJ680354), DK1990PMWSfree (EU148505), genotype PCV2c strains DK1987PMWSfree (EU148504), DK1980PMWSfree (EU148503), genotype PCV2b strains AS (HM038016), ShenZhen (FJ870969), HNyy-6b (FJ870974), FRA3 (AF201311), Fd13 (AY321985), genotype PCV2a strains CL (HM038033), HBwh-2a (FJ870967), 26606 (AF264038), Yamagata (AB426905), and No. 26 (AB072302).

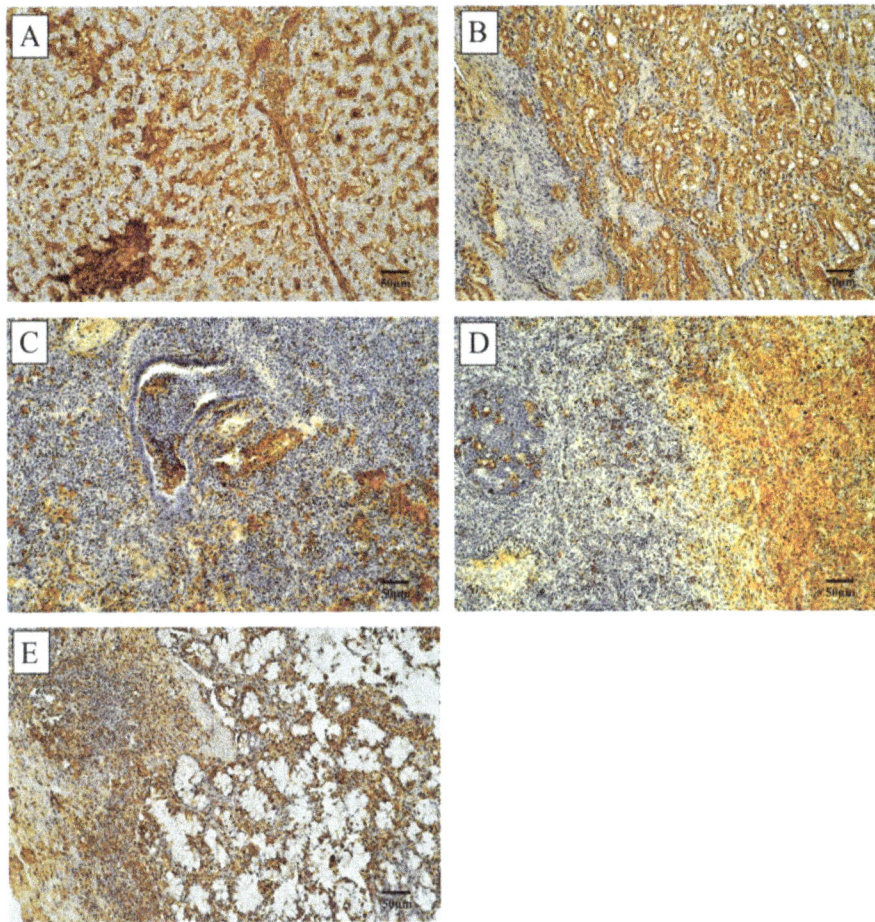

Figure 6 Detection of HEV antigen in different organs of the dead swine. (A) Positive HEV signal in the liver. **(B)** Positive HEV signal in the kidney. **(C)** Positive HEV signal in the lung. **(D)** Positive HEV signal in a lymph node. **(E)** Positive HEV signal in the intestine.

signals were in the tubular epithelial cells (Figure 8B); and for the lungs, PCV2-antigen positive signals were in the alveolar and septal macrophages, and fibroblast-like cells in the lamina propria of the airways (Figure 8C). PCV2 antigen was intense in the lymphocytes and macrophages in the lymph nodes (Figure 8D), and the mucous layer and lamina propria of the intestine (Figure 8E). The negative control is shown in Figure 7. PCV2 antigen was negative in the PCV2 DNA negative pig (pig No.2).

Conclusions

Hepatitis E virus infections are a major cause of acute hepatitis in developing countries, and because of the zoonotic transmission of HEV, they are also an emerging health problem in industrialized countries. Swine are considered to be a major reservoir of the HEV transmitted to humans [3,11]. Four main genotypes have been identified in HEV. Genotypes 1 and 2 have only been found in humans, whereas genotypes 3 and 4 have been recovered from both humans and pigs [12]. Smith et al. recently proposed a taxonomic scheme, which divided the family

Hepeviridae into the genera Orthohepevirus (all mammalian and avian hepatitis E virus (HEV) isolates) and Piscihepevirus (cutthroat trout virus) [13]. The livers of pigs naturally infected or intravenously inoculated with HEV display focal lymphocytic infiltration and swollen, vacuolated hepatocytes [14]. The livers of the seven pigs investigated in the present study had significant lymphocytic infiltration in the portal area, and large localized areas of fibrosis, necrosis, and vacuolization. IHC staining showed that the ORF2 protein of HEV was distributed across multiple organs, particularly in the liver and kidneys. This result was not unexpected because the liver is the target organ of HEV, and the kidney plays an integral role in maintaining extracellular fluid homeostasis. The previous study also demonstrates that HEV has been found in liver and kidney after experimental infection in domestic pigs [15]. A PCR assay specific for HEV ORF2 confirmed that the pigs were HEV positive. Isolates CHN-HB-HD-L1, CHN-HB-HD-L2, HB-L3, CHN-HB-HD-L4, and CHN-HB-HD-L5 were shown to belong to genotype 4, the most prevalent HEV genotype in China.

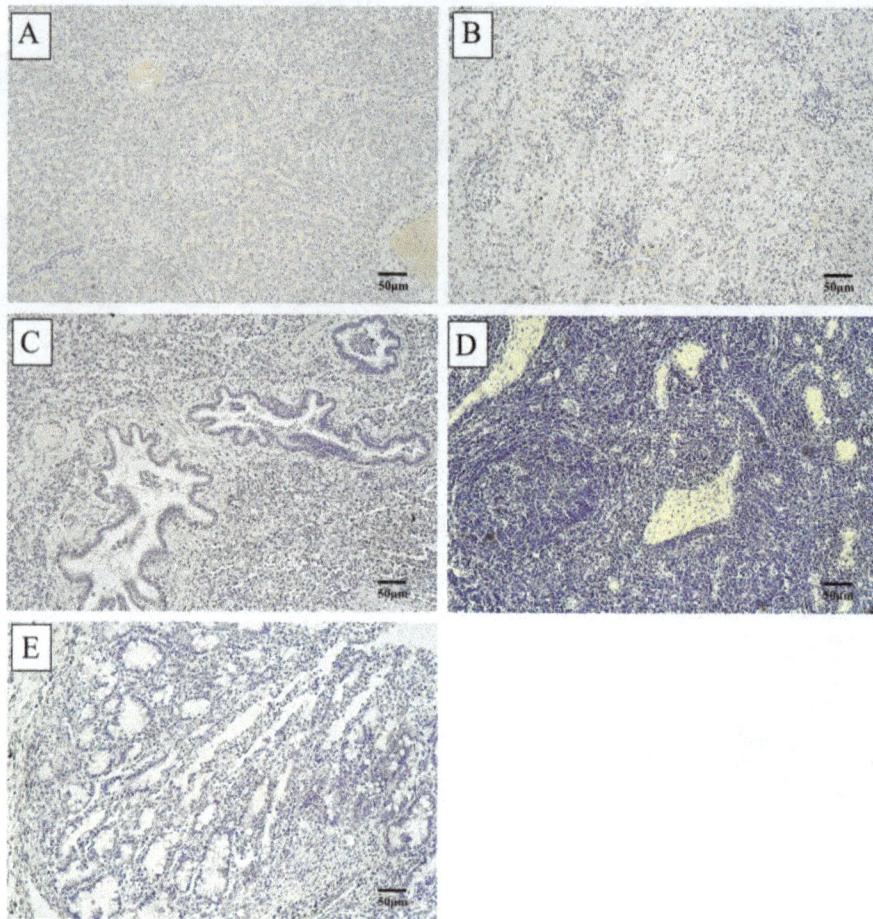

Figure 7 Negative controls for IHC analysis of different tissues. **(A)** Liver. **(B)** Kidney. **(C)** Lung. **(D)** Lymph node. **(E)** Intestine.

According to Smith et al. [13], the HEV strains isolated in our case were classified to Orthohepevirus A.

PCV2 is the primary causative agent of PMWS which was first described in Canada in 1991 [16]. In recent years, PMWS has become a serious economic problem for the swine industry in China. According to the data from a prevalence survey, more than 67.1% of piglet stool samples were PCV2 positive [17]. The disease predominantly affects pigs between 5 and 15 weeks of age and is characterized by growth retardation, diarrhea, dyspnea, jaundice, and enlargement of the inguinal lymph nodes. In our study, infected swine aged 2–3 months displayed clinical symptoms consistent with previous reports of the disease [9].

In this study, the clinical and pathological changes observed were consistent with typical PCV2 infection. Hemorrhage, hyperemia, edema, necrosis, and lymphocyte infiltration were observed in all organs, most notably the lungs. Histological changes consistent with lobar pneumonia were also evident in the lungs, and normal lung histology was rarely seen. The alveolar walls were thickened, with substantial lymphocyte, erythrocyte,

and exudate infiltration. Exfoliated alveolar epithelial cells and pink liquid exudate were observed within the bronchioles. PCV2 has a small, nonenveloped icosahedral virion, and a single-stranded circular DNA genome, 1,767–1,768 nt in length. The genome has two major ORFs encoded in the antisense direction [18]. Isolates HBHD-L1, HBHD-L3, HBHD-L4, HBHD-L5, HBHD-L6, and HBHD-L7 recovered in this study were closely related to the genotype PCV2d strains HNF911 (KJ680361), SD-ZB2 (KJ511876), WSEC11 (KJ680353), GXYQ12 (KJ680367), TDBS12 (KJ680354) (Figure 4). The genotype PCV2d represented a novel genotype and a shift from PCV2a to PCV2b as the predominant genotype in China in recent years [19]. A genetic analysis, combined with the observed pathological changes, indicated that the PCV2 isolates detected in this study were probably high prevalent in China [20]. IHC staining of tissues for the ORF2 protein of PCV2 revealed that the antigen was observed in the lungs, liver, lymph node, intestine and kidneys, further evidence of PCV2 infection.

Further pathological changes typical of PCV2 infection were observed in this study. Significant immune-system-

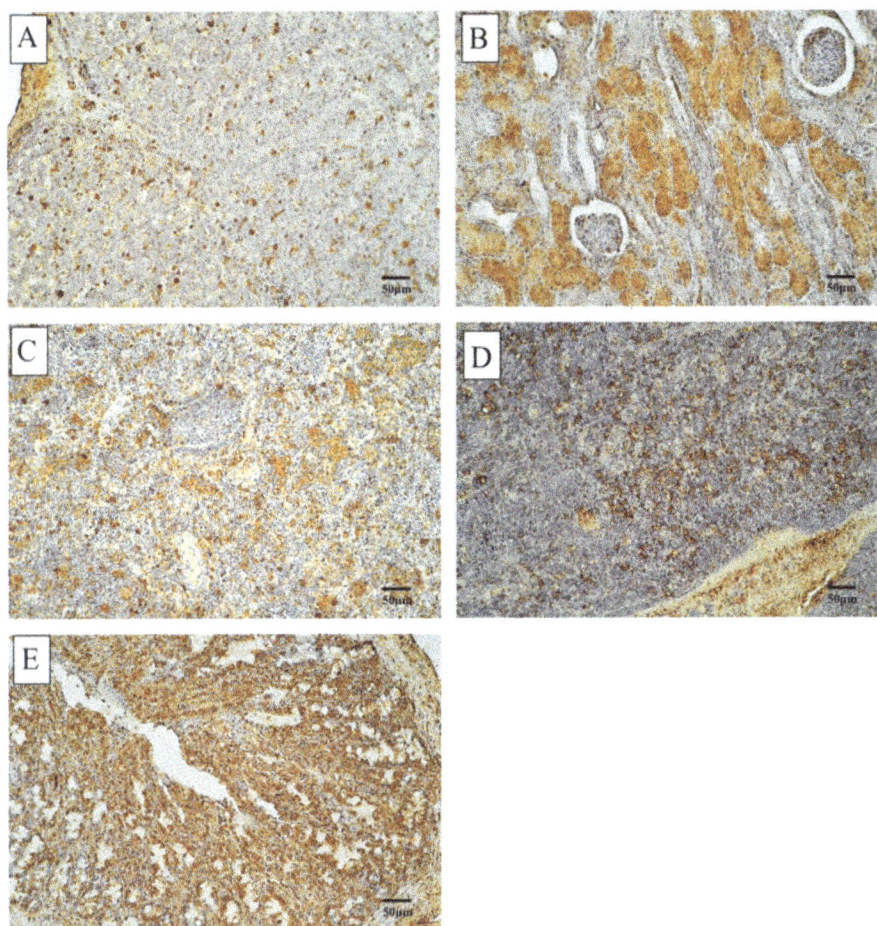

Figure 8 **Detection of PCV2 antigen in different organs of the dead swine.** (**A**) Positive PCV2 signal in the liver. (**B**) Positive PCV2 signal in the kidney. (**C**) Positive PCV2 signal in the lung. (**D**) Positive PCV2 signal in a lymph node. (**E**) Positive PCV2 signal in the intestine.

organ dysplasia was apparent, with the characteristic histopathological findings of lymphoid depletion and histiocytic replacement in the lymphoid tissues. Combined with the positive PCV2 ORF2 signals in lymph node in IHC, these results suggest that the systemic immune function of these pigs had been disrupted.

IHC staining for HEV and PCV2 antigens revealed a diffuse labeling pattern in the intestine, with the greatest reactivity observed in the cytoplasm of cells in the mucous layer and lamina propria. This observation is consistent with the viral invasion pathways. The transmission of HEV occurs via the fecal–oral route, so HEV may invade the animal through the intestinal mucous layer, with infection progressing to the lamina propria. We have investigated the mucosal immunity in the intestines of rabbits [21] and gerbils (data not shown) experimentally infected with HEV, and both studies demonstrated a strong HEV ORF2 positive signals in intestinal. In the present study, naturally infected swine exhibited significant necrosis of the intestinal epithelial cells and also showed HEV ORF2 positive signals in intestine. Therefore,

HEV invasion of the intestine may proceed rapidly and widely, consistent with the diffuse labeling pattern observed in the intestine in this study.

We also tested for other suspicious pathogens in this study. According to the medical history, the sick piglets failed to respond to antibiotic treatment (timicosin and doxycycline in pig farm A, and florfenicol in pig farm B), indicating that bacterial infection was unlikely. PRRSV, CSFV, PEDV, TGEV, PRV, and PPV are high prevalent in swine in China and across the globe. Although infections with these viruses may present with similar clinical symptoms, including fever, diarrhea, depressed, and decrease of feed intake. PCR confirmed that all seven pigs were negative for these viruses.

Presence of signs and lesions such as lymphoid depletions, hepatitis, nephritis, etc. resemble the microscopic characteristic of PMWS. Nevertheless, no typical microscopic lesions such as granulomatous inflammation or intracytoplasmic inclusion bodies were observed in lymphoid tissue, liver, spleen, and other tissues [22]. The mortality associated with PCV2 infection is generally around 10% (range 4%–20%), but can reach 50% [23]. In our case, seven pigs were detected and the pathogens had been identified. However, the true reason for the high mortality in the whole pig farm A and B still need more exploring. The occurrence of this disease may not be only a matter of PMWS caused by PCV2 infection. The previous study showed swine HEV infection can be a significant factor to the development of hepatitis regardless of the PMWS status [8]. In addition, J. Ellis [24] claimed that the severity of hepatic lesions in PCV-2 infected pigs may be enhanced by co-infection with swine hepatitis E virus. It may indicate that the significance of HEV is hardly negligent. Further investigation about the mechanistic basis for the pathogenesis of the clinical syndrome that associated with PCV2 and HEV co-infection needs to be conducted.

HEV infection in humans and animals is common, but the natural occurrence of HEV and PCV2 co-infection in pigs in China, reported here, has rarely been seen. The experimental infection of domestic pigs with HEV did not cause death [25]. Therefore, the HEV-infected swine observed in this study requires further investigation. Based on these results, we believe that considerable attention should be directed towards co-infections of HEV and PCV2 in swine.

According to the comparison of histopathological changes between these cases in Table 1, no specific characteristics are demonstrated, which is really thought-provoking. It is very significant to explore the reasons for the similar pathological changes in the HEV and/or PCV2 infected pigs. In order to reveal the mechanism for the similar pathological changes in the HEV and/or PCV2 infected pigs, further tests about HEV and PCV2 co-infection, single HEV infection and single PCV2 infection in pigs have been in the planning. We hope to reveal the mechanism of the similar pathological changes and also discover the similarity and differences between the natural cases and the experimental infected pigs. To our best knowledge, theses following reasons are speculated to explain the similar pathological changes: a) the individual differences in pigs. Different pigs may have different reaction to the attack of the viruses; b) pig No.2 may once have been infected with PCV2 and then PCV2 were neutralized by the antibody. But lesions in the tissues hadn't recovered when it died; c) HEV is RNA virus without envelope. It may have degraded in tissues in pig No.6 and 7 before testing. d) the complicate in natural infected cases.

In conclusion, co-infection of HEV and PCV2 were identified in four out of seven dead weaned pigs from two pig farms in China. Severe pathological changes and high mortality were observed in the infected animals. Our results indicate that co-infection with HEV and PCV2 may bring some negative effect on the swine industry in China, and this phenomenon requires further investigation. What's more, further research is required to demonstrate the role of co-infection of HEV and PCV2 in swine and whether these two viruses exert a synergistic effect.

Materials and methods

Consent

Written informed consent was obtained from the owners of the two farms for the publication of this report and any accompanying images.

Determination of pathogen

According to the gross and histopathological lesions, eight suspected viruses were detected. Total RNA and DNA were extracted from liver, lung, kidney, brain, and spleen specimens using the UltraPure™ RNA Kit and the General AllGen Kit (CWBIO, Beijing, China), according to the manufacturers' instructions. The extracted RNA

Table 2 Sequences of primers used in the PCR assays

Primer	Sequence 5'-3'	Reference
PRRSV ORF7 gene		[26]
PRRSV-F	CCAAATAACAACGGCAAGCA	
PRRSV-R	ATGCTGAGGGTGATGCTGTGA	
PCV2 ORF2 gene		[27]
PCV2.S4	CACGGATATTGTAGTCCTGGT	
PCV2.A4	CCGCACCTTCGGATATACTGTC	
HEV ORF2 gene		[3]
HEV- externer primer	AATTATGCYCAGTAYCGRGTTG	
HEV- externer primer	CCCTTRTCYTGCTGMGCATTCTC	
HEV- interner primer	GTWATGCTYTGCATWCATGGCT	
HEV- interner primer	AGCCGACGAAATCAATTCTGTC	
CSFV E2 gene		[28]
E2- externer primer	GCATCAACCAYKGCATTCC	
E2- externer primer	GTCTGTGTGGGTRATTAAGTTCCCTA	
E2- interner primer	CTRGTRACTGGGGCACAAGG	
E2- interner primer	ACCAGCRGCGAGTTGYTCTG	
PEDV S gene		[29]
P1	TTCTGAGTCACGAACAGCCA	
P2	CATATGCAGCCTGCTCTGAA	
TGEV S gene		[29]
T1	GTGGTTTTGGTYRTAAATGC	
T2	CACTAACCAACGTGGARCTA	
PRV gB genes		[30]
PRVF	GGGGTTGGACAGGAAGGACACCA	
PRVR	AACCAGCTGCACGCGCTCAA	
PPV NS1 gene		[30]
PPVF	AGTTAGAATAGGATGCGAGGAA	
PPVR	AGAGTCTGTTGGTGTATTTATTGG	

was used in reverse-transcription polymerase chain reaction (PCR) assays to detect HEV, PRRSV, PEDV, TGEV, and CSFV. The extracted DNA was used to detect PCV2, PRV, and PPV. The virus-specific primers used in this study are listed in Table 2. PCR for PRRSV, PEDV, TGEV, CSFV, PCV2, PRV, and PPV, included initial denaturation at 94°C for 5 min, followed by 35 cycles of 94°C for 30 sec, 55°C for 30 sec, and 72°C for 30 sec, with a final extension step at 72°C for 10 min. PCR for HEV included initial denaturation at 95°C for 7 min, followed by 35 cycles of 94°C for 1 min, 42°C for 1 min, and 72°C for 2 min, with a final extension step at 72°C for 10 min. Sterile ddH$_2$O (1 μL) was included as the negative control.

Sequencing and phylogenetic analysis

The PCR products were purified and ligated into the pMD18-T vector (TaKaRa, Dalian, China), and sequenced on an ABI PRISM® 377 DNA Sequencer using reagents from BGI Life Technologies (Beijing, China). The sequences were analyzed with DNAMAN (version 5.2.2; Lynnon Corp., Quebec, Canada). Phylogenetic analyses were performed with the MEGA software (version 4.0; http://www.megasoftware.net) using the neighbor-joining method with 1000 bootstrap replicates.

Immunohistochemistry

Immunohistochemistry was used to detect HEV and PCV2 antigens in the liver, kidney, lymph nodes, intestine and lung. The endogenous enzymatic activity in the tissues was blocked with 5% H$_2$O$_2$. Goat serum was used to block the Fc receptors in the tissues. The primary antibody, monoclonal mouse anti-HEV ORF2 antibody (1:300 dilution; Beijing Protein Institute, Beijing, China), was added to the sections and incubated at 37°C for 2 h. IHC staining was performed with the Histostain™-Plus Kit (ZSGB-BIO, Beijing, China), according to the manufacturer's instructions. The substrate 3,3'-diaminobenzidine tetrahydrochloride (ZSGB-BIO) was applied for 10 min, after which Gill's hematoxylin counterstain was added. A monoclonal mouse anti-PCV2 ORF2 antibody (1:200 dilution; kindly supplied by Dr. Liu Jue, Beijing Municipal Key Laboratory for the Prevention and Control of Infectious Diseases in Livestock and Poultry, Beijing, China) was used to detect PCV2. For the negative controls, the primary antibody was omitted and replaced with phosphate-buffered saline. In another negative control, the primary antibody was replaced with IgG from a normal mouse to demonstrate the specificity of the signal.

Abbreviations

HEV: *Hepatitis E virus*; HE: Hepatitis E; PCV2: Porcine circovirus 2; PRRSV: Porcine reproductive and respiratory syndrome virus; CSFV: Classical swine fever virus; PEDV: Porcine epidemic diarrhea virus; TGEV: Transmissible gastroenteritis coronavirus; PRV: *Pseudorabies virus*; PPV: *Porcine parvovirus*; PMWS: Postweaning multisystemic wasting syndrome.

Competing interests

The authors declare that they have no competing interests.

Authors' contributions

YY, RShi, and RShe designed the study. YY and RShi wrote article. YY, RShi, FD, RN, WL, MC, XW, and MHS performed the laboratory experiments. YY, RShi, CL, JM, YZ, and JL analyzed and interpreted the data. All authors have read, commented upon, and approved the final article.

Acknowledgments

We thank Dr. Liu Jue (Beijing Municipal Key Laboratory for the Prevention and Control of Infectious Diseases in Livestock and Poultry, Beijing, China) for kindly supplying the anti-PCV2 ORF2 antibody for the study.
This work was supported by the National Natural Science Foundation of China (grant nos. 31072110, 31272515). The funders had no role in study design, data collection and analysis, decision to publish, or preparation of the manuscript.

Author details

[1]Laboratory of Animal Pathology and Public Health, College of Veterinary Medicine, China Agricultural University; Key Laboratory of Zoonosis of Ministry of Agriculture, China Agricultural University, Beijing 100193, China. [2]Department of Veterinary Medicine, Laboratory of Animal Histology and Anatomy, College of Agriculture, Hebei University of Engineering, Handan, Hebei 056021, China.

References

1. Xiao P, Li R, She R, Yin J, Li W, Mao J, et al. Prevalence of hepatitis E virus in swine fed on kitchen residue. PLoS One. 2012;7(3):e33480.
2. Martelli F, Toma S, Di Bartolo I, Caprioli A, Ruggeri F, Lelli D, et al. Detection of Hepatitis E Virus (HEV) in Italian pigs displaying different pathological lesions. Res Ve Sci. 2010;88(3):492–6.
3. Meng X-J, Purcell RH, Halbur PG, Lehman JR, Webb DM, Tsareva TS, et al. A novel virus in swine is closely related to the human hepatitis E virus. Proc Natl Acad Sci U S A. 1997;94(18):9860–5.
4. Li W, She R, Wei H, Zhao J, Wang Y, Sun Q, et al. Prevalence of hepatitis E virus in swine under different breeding environment and abattoir in Beijing, China. Vet Microbiol. 2009;133(1):75–83.
5. Lu L, Li C, Hagedorn CH. Phylogenetic analysis of global hepatitis E virus sequences: genetic diversity, subtypes and zoonosis. Rev Med Virol. 2006;16(1):5–36.
6. Mao J, Zhao Y, She R, Xiao P, Tian J, Chen J. One case of swine hepatitis E virus and porcine reproductive and respiratory syndrome virus Co-infection in weaned pigs. Virol J. 2013;10(1):341.
7. Hamel AL, Lin LL, Nayar GP. Nucleotide sequence of porcine circovirus associated with postweaning multisystemic wasting syndrome in pigs. J Virol. 1998;72(6):5262–7.
8. Martin M, Segales J, Huang F, Guenette D, Mateu E, De Deus N, et al. Association of hepatitis E virus (HEV) and postweaning multisystemic wasting syndrome (PMWS) with lesions of hepatitis in pigs. Vet Microbiol. 2007;122(1):16–24.
9. Allan GM, Ellis JA. Porcine circoviruses: a review. J Vet Diagn Invest. 2000;12(1):3–14.
10. Opriessnig T, Gerber PF, Xiao CT, Halbur PG, Matzinger SR, Meng XJ. Commercial PCV2a-based vaccines are effective in protecting naturally PCV2b-infected finisher pigs against experimental challenge with a 2012 mutant PCV2. Vaccine. 2014;32(34):4342–8.
11. Berto A, Backer JA, Mesquita JR, Nascimento MS, Banks M, Martelli F, et al. Prevalence and transmission of hepatitis E virus in domestic swine populations in different European countries. BMC Res Notes. 2012;5(1):190.
12. Ahmad I, Holla RP, Jameel S. Molecular virology of hepatitis E virus. Virus Res. 2011;161(1):47–58.
13. Smith DB, Simmonds P, Jameel S, Emerson SU, Harrison TJ, Meng XJ, et al. Consensus proposals for classification of the family Hepeviridae. J Gen Virol. 2014;95(Pt 10):2223–32.
14. Halbur P, Kasorndorkbua C, Gilbert C, Guenette D, Potters M, Purcell R, et al. Comparative pathogenesis of infection of pigs with hepatitis E viruses recovered from a pig and a human. J Clin Microbiol. 2001;39(3):918–23.

15. Williams TPE, Kasorndorkbua C, Halbur P, Haqshenas G, Guenette D, Toth T, et al. Evidence of extrahepatic sites of replication of the hepatitis E virus in a swine model. J Clin Microbiol. 2001;39(9):3040–6.

16. Ellis J, Hassard L, Clark E, Harding J, Allan G, Willson P, et al. Isolation of circovirus from lesions of pigs with postweaning multisystemic wasting syndrome. Can Vet J. 1998;39(1):44.

17. Li B, Ma J, Liu Y, Wen L, Yu Z, Ni Y, et al. Complete genome sequence of a highly prevalent Porcine Circovirus 2 isolated from piglet stool samples in China. J Virol. 2012;86(8):4716–6.

18. Morozov I, Sirinarumitr T, Sorden SD, Halbur PG, Morgan MK, Yoon K-J, et al. Detection of a novel strain of porcine circovirus in pigs with postweaning multisystemic wasting syndrome. J Clin Microbiol. 1998;36(9):2535–41.

19. Guo LJ, Lu YH, Wei YW, Huang LP, Liu CM. Porcine circovirus type 2 (PCV2): genetic variation and newly emerging genotypes in China. Virol J. 2010;7:273.

20. Wang F, Guo X, Ge X, Wang Z, Chen Y, Cha Z, et al. Genetic variation analysis of Chinese strains of porcine circovirus type 2. Virus Res. 2009;145(1):151–6.

21. Mao J, Zhao Y, She R, Cao B, Xiao P, Wu Q, et al. Detection and Localization of Rabbit Hepatitis E Virus and Antigen in Systemic Tissues from Experimentally Intraperitoneally Infected Rabbits. PLoS One. 2014;9(3):e88607.

22. Chae C. Postweaning multisystemic wasting syndrome: a review of aetiology, diagnosis and pathology. Vet J (London, England : 1997). 2004;168(1):41–9.

23. Gillespie J, Opriessnig T, Meng X, Pelzer K, Buechner-Maxwell V. Porcine circovirus type 2 and porcine circovirus-associated disease. J Vet Intern Med. 2009;23(6):1151–63.

24. Ellis J, Clark E, Haines D, West K, Krakowka S, Kennedy S, et al. Porcine circovirus-2 and concurrent infections in the field. Vet Microbiol. 2004;98(2):159–63.

25. Balayan M, Usmanov R, Zamyatina N, Djumalieva D, Karas F. Experimental hepatitis E infection in domestic pigs. J Med Virol. 1990;32(1):58–9.

26. Le Gall A, Legeay O, Bourhy H, Arnauld C, Albina E, Jestin A. Molecular variation in the nucleoprotein gene (ORF7) of the porcine reproductive and respiratory syndrome virus (PRRSV). Virus Res. 1998;54(1):9–21.

27. Ouardani M, Wilson L, Jette R, Montpetit C, Dea S. Multiplex PCR for detection and typing of porcine circoviruses. J Clin Microbiol. 1999;37(12):3917–24.

28. Chen N, Hu H, Zhang Z, Shuai J, Jiang L, Fang W. Genetic diversity of the envelope glycoprotein E2 of classical swine fever virus: recent isolates branched away from historical and vaccine strains. Vet Microbiol. 2008;127(3):286–99.

29. Zhao J, Shi B-j, Huang X-g, Peng M-y, Zhang X-m, He D-n, et al. A multiplex RT-PCR assay for rapid and differential diagnosis of four porcine diarrhea associated viruses in field samples from pig farms in East China from 2010 to 2012. J Virol Methods. 2013;194(1):107–12.

30. Xu X-G, Chen G-D, Huang Y, Ding L, Li Z-C, Chang C-D, et al. Development of multiplex PCR for simultaneous detection of six swine DNA and RNA viruses. J Virol Methods. 2012;183(1):69–74.

14

Effects of administration of four different doses of *Escherichia coli* phytase on femur properties of 16-week-old turkeys

Marcin R Tatara[1,2*], Witold Krupski[2], Krzysztof Kozłowski[3], Aleksandra Drażbo[3] and Jan Jankowski[3]

Abstract

Background: The enzyme phytase is able to initiate the release of phosphates from phytic acid, making it available for absorption within gastrointestinal tract and following utilization. The aim of the study was to determine effects of *Escherichia coli* phytase administration on morphological, densitometric and mechanical properties of femur in 16-week-old turkeys. One-day-old BUT Big-6 males were assigned to six weight-matched groups. Turkeys receiving diet with standard phosphorus (P) and calcium (Ca) content belonged to the positive control group (Group I). Negative control group (Group II) consisted of birds fed diet with lowered P and Ca content. Turkeys belonging to the remaining groups have received the same diet as group II but enriched with graded levels of *Escherichia coli* phytase: 125 (Group III), 250 (Group IV), 500 (Group V) and 1000 (Group VI) FTU/kg. At the age of 112 days of life, the final body weights were determined and the turkeys were sacrificed to obtain right femur for analyses. Geometric and densitometric properties of femur were determined using quantitative computed tomography (QCT) technique, while mechanical evaluation was performed in three-point bending test.

Results: Phytase administration increased cross-sectional area, second moment of inertia, mean relative wall thickness, cortical bone mineral density and maximum elastic strength decreasing cortical bone area of femur ($P < 0.05$). Reduced dietary Ca and P content decreased final body weight of turkeys by 6.5% ($P = 0.006$). The most advantageous effects of *Escherichia coli* phytase administration on geometric, densitometric and mechanical properties of femur were observed in turkeys receiving 125 and 250 FTU/kg of the diet. Phytase administration at the dosages of 500 and 1000 FTU/kg of the diet improved the final body weight in turkeys.

Conclusions: The results obtained in this study indicate a possible practical application of *Escherichia coli* phytase in turkey feeding to improve skeletal system properties and function.

Keywords: Femur, Turkey, Phytase, Volumetric bone mineral density, Skeletal system

Background

Phosphorus (P) is an essential macro-element involved in physiological functions in mammals and birds, including bone tissue formation, energy metabolism, cellular structure, and egg formation. In plant feedstuffs that are commonly fed to growing and laying poultry species, P is primarily stored as phytate P (phytic acid or its salts known as phytates), and is partly unavailable to birds due to lack of sufficient phytase activity [1,2]. Phytates are considered to be anti-nutrient factors which chelate minerals and react with dietary proteins reducing bioavailability of many nutrients [3]. Phytic acid is known to bind calcium (Ca) and P within gastrointestinal tract limiting their intestinal absorption. The enzyme phytase is able to initiate the release of phosphates from phytic acid, making it available for absorption within gastrointestinal tract and following utilization. Phytase-dependent release of the phosphate groups from phytate eliminates the ability of phytic acid to combine with Ca reducing the decline in mineral intestinal absorption [4]. Poultry species do not produce meaningful quantities of endogenous phytase, the enzyme that can hydrolyse the ester bonds between the phosphate groups

* Correspondence: matatar99@gazeta.pl
[1]Department of Animal Physiology, University of Life Sciences in Lublin, ul. Akademicka 12, 20-950 Lublin, Poland
[2]II Department of Radiology, Medical University of Lublin, ul. Staszica 16, 20-081 Lublin, Poland
Full list of author information is available at the end of the article

and the inositol ring in phytates. Thus, routine supplementation of poultry diets with commercially produced phytases is commonplace [5].

Skeletal system disorders in turkeys, especially concerning long bones of legs, are considered as one of the most important factors influencing final production results and economic profits. Economic costs related to leg weakness due to impaired bone growth and development process are significant and result mainly from increased mortality and decreased body weight gain [6]. Fractures occurring in long bones of legs eliminate locomotory functions and encourage subsequent infections. Epidemiological data have shown that mortality in turkey toms due to bone disorders and leg weakness exceeds 3% of the stock [7]. Experimental studies comparing growing turkeys and chickens have shown the highest growth rate of long leg bones in turkeys reaching even 2 mm per day during the first 10 weeks of development [8]. It was confirmed that leg problems, combined with bone development abnormalities occurrence in poultry may be caused by genetic selection for faster growth rate and higher body weight gain, especially when one considers decreased bone mass to muscle mass ratio with increased body weight. Bones of the pelvic limbs overloaded by extremely heavy muscle mass in combination with centre of gravity destabilized by overgrown breast muscles in meat type turkey toms lead to leg deformities and following fractures [9-12]. Experimental studies showing significantly lower incidence of leg abnormalities in turkeys combined with reduced growth rate and body weight gain prove an insufficient adaptation of the skeletal system to rapid development of high muscle mass in meat-type poultry species [13,14].

Considering importance of P bioavailability in growing meat-type turkeys for proper skeletal development and bone tissue homeostasis maintenance, the aim of the study was to determine morphological, densitometric and mechanical properties of femur obtained from 16-week old male turkeys fed with the diet enriched with four different doses of *Escherichia coli* phytase.

Methods

The study was carried out on the experimental farm (Baldy n. Olsztyn) of the Department of Poultry Science, University of Warmia and Mazury, Olsztyn, Poland. The animal protocol used in this study was approved by the Local Animal Care and Use Committee in Olsztyn, Poland (decision no. 66/2008).

Experimental design

One-day-old BUT Big-6 male turkeys were delivered to the experimental farm from the commercial hatchery (Hatchery Grelavi Co., Kętrzyn, Poland) and randomly assigned to six weight-matched groups. The turkeys were kept on deep litter at a stocking density of 2.5 bird

per m^2 and eight birds were allocated within one pen. The positive control group (Group I or PC group) consisted of turkeys receiving diet with standard phosphorus (P) and calcium (Ca) content at all feeding stages (Table 1) [15]. The negative control group (Group II or NC group) consisted of birds fed diet with lowered P and Ca content (Table 2) [15]. Turkeys belonging to the remaining groups of the experiment received the same diet as group II but enriched with graded levels of *Escherichia coli* phytase (Optiphos, Huvepharma NV, Belgium): 125 (Group III), 250 (Group IV), 500 (Group V) and 1000 FTU/kg (Group VI). At the age of 112 days of life, the turkeys were weighed and sacrificed to obtain right femur for analyses.

Bone analysis

The right femur was isolated and cleaned of all soft tissues to determine weight, length, volumetric bone mineral density (vBMD), and morphometric and mechanical properties of the bone. After isolation, the bone samples were frozen in plastic bags and kept at −25°C until further analyses. Volumetric bone mineral density of each femur was measured with the use of quantitative computed tomography (QCT) technique and Somatom Emotion Siemens apparatus supplied with Somaris/5 VB10B software (Siemens, Erlangen, Germany). Prior to scanning procedure, bones were thawed in bags for 2 hours at room temperature. Raw data acquisition using the scanning procedure lasted approximately 10 minutes for 8 bones representing single experimental group. The measurement of vBMD was performed for the trabecular and cortical bone compartments using 2-mm thick cross-sectional metaphyseal and diaphyseal QCT scans. Volumetric BMD of the trabecular bone (trabecular bone mineral density – Td) of femur was determined in the distal metaphysis of femur at 7% of total bone length, measuring from the distal extremity. Volumetric BMD of the cortical bone (cortical bone mineral density – Cd) was measured on mid-diaphyseal scan placed at 50% of the femur length. Cortical bone area (CBA) was measured automatically at the midshaft of femur. Volume evaluation software (Siemens, Erlangen, Germany) was used to measure the total bone volume (Bvol) and mean volumetric bone mineral density (MvBMD) of each femur. For Bvol and MvBMD measurements, the volume-of-interest was limited by minimum and maximum density of the investigated samples at 0 and 3000 Hounsfield units, respectively. The measurements of Bvol and MvBMD were executed for the whole bone, and results obtained reflect the values determined within all anatomic structures of the investigated bone.

Geometrical properties of each femur were determined on the basis of measurements of horizontal and vertical diameters of the mid-diaphyseal cross-section of the bone obtained from computed tomography multiplanar

Table 1 Composition and calculated nutritive value of the diet supplied in the positive control group (Group I)

Components (%)	Age of birds (weeks)			
	1 – 4	5 – 8	9 – 12	13 – 16
Wheat	15.00	15.00	15.00	15.00
Corn	30.12	35.36	39.41	46.35
Soybean meal	43.34	40.19	37.63	28.23
Potato protein	5.00	3.00	-	-
Soybean oil	1.44	1.10	2.00	-
Animal fat	-	1.10	2.13	5.01
$NaHCO_3$	0.15	0.10	0.10	0.10
Salt	0.21	0.22	0.20	0.15
Limestone	1.68	1.38	1.23	1.12
MCP	2.00	1.55	1.23	1.05
DL-Methionine	0.31	0.34	0.34	0.33
L-Lysine HCl	0.32	0.29	0.29	0.30
L-Threonine	0.07	0.05	0.13	0.08
Premix (vitamins + trace minerals)	0.25[1]	0.25[1]	0.25[2]	0.25[2]
Choline chloride	0.11	0.08	0.07	0.06
Celite	-	-	-	2.00
Energy and nutrient content				
AME_N (MJ/kg)	11.61[3]	12.01[3]	12.62[3]	13.22[3]
Crude protein (g/kg)	280[3]/284[4]	255[3]/257[4]	225[3]/231[4]	190[3]/202[4]
Methionine (g/kg)	7.4[3]	7.2[3]	6.6[3]	6.1[3]
Methionine + Cysteine (g/kg)	11.8[3]	11.3[3]	10.4[3]	9.4[3]
Lysine (g/kg)	18.2[3]	16.1[3]	13.9[3]	11.7[3]
Calcium (g/kg)	12.0[3]/12,8[4]	10.0[3]/10.0[4]	8.5[3]/8.4[4]	7.5[3]/7.8[4]
Total phosphorus (g/kg)	8.8[3]/8.7[4]	7.7[3]/7.4[4]	7.0[3]/6.8[4]	6.0[3]/5.9[4]
Available (Av) phosphorus (g/kg)	6.0[3]	5.0[3]	4.3[3]	3.8[3]

[1]Vitamin and mineral premix - nutrients per kg diet: 12,500 IU vitamin A; 5,000 IU vitamin D_3; 100 IU vitamin E; 4.0 mg vitamin K; 4.5 mg vitamin B_1;15 mg vitamin B_2; 5 mg vitamin B_6; 0.04 mg vitamin B_{12}; 110 mg nicotinic acid; 28 mg pantothenic acid; 3.5 mg folic acid; 0.375 mg biotin; 80 mg iron; 25 mg copper; 160 mg manganese; 160 mg zinc; 2.5 mg iodine; 0.3 mg selenium.
[2]Vitamin and mineral premix - nutrients per kg diet: 9,600 IU vitamin A; 4,800 IU vitamin D_3; 60 IU vitamin E; 3.0 mg vitamin K; 2.0 mg vitamin B_1;12 mg vitamin B_2; 5 mg vitamin B_6; 0.025 mg vitamin B_{12}; 85 mg nicotinic acid; 23 mg pantothenic acid; 2.5 mg folic acid; 0.375 mg biotin; 40 mg iron; 25 mg copper; 120 mg manganese; 120 mg zinc; 2 mg iodine; 0.3 mg selenium.
[3]Calculated; [4]Analyzed [15].

reconstructions. The values of cross-sectional area (A), second moment of inertia (Ix), mean relative wall thickness (MRWT) and cortical index (CI) were estimated.

Mechanical properties of femur were determined using the three-point bending test in Instron 3367 apparatus (Instron, Canton, MA, USA) combined with a computer. The relationship between force perpendicular to the longitudinal axis of the bone and the resulting displacement was presented graphically, and the values of maximum elastic strength (Wy) and the ultimate strength (Wf) were determined. The distance between supports of the bone was set at 40% of total femur length and the measuring head loaded bone samples at the midshaft with a constant speed of 50 mm/min.

Statistical analysis

All data were expressed as means and ± S.E.M. The results obtained were analyzed with a use of one-way analysis of variance (ANOVA) and Statistica software v. 10.0 PL. Statistical significance of the differences of the investigated variables between the groups was determined using post hoc multiple comparisons Duncan's test. For all comparisons, P-value ≤ 0.05 was considered as statistically significant.

Results

Body weight

Initial and final body weights of turkeys are shown in Table 3. At the beginning of the experiment, initial body weights of turkeys from all the groups were not significantly different (P > 0.05). Final body weight of 112-day old

Table 2 Composition and calculated nutritive value of the diet supplied in the negative control group (Group II)

Components (%)	Age of birds (weeks)			
	1 – 4	5 – 8	9 – 12	13 – 16
Wheat	15.00	15.00	15.00	15.00
Corn	31.84	36.86	41.64	48.43
Soybean meal	43.03	39.82	37.20	27.83
Potato protein	5.00	3.00	-	-
Soybean oil	0.93	1.00	2.00	-
Animal fat	-	1.00	1.38	4.31
$NaHCO_3$	0.15	0.10	0.10	0.10
Salt	0.21	0.22	0.20	0.15
Limestone	1.70	1.37	1.18	1.01
MCP	1.09	0.63	0.23	0.18
DL-Methionine	0.31	0.33	0.34	0.32
L-Lysine HCl	0.33	0.29	0.29	0.30
L-Threonine	0.07	0.06	0.13	0.08
Premix (vitamins + trace minerals)	0.25[1]	0.25[1]	0.25[2]	0.25[2]
Choline chloride	0.11	0.08	0.07	0.06
Celite	-	-	-	2.00
Energy and nutrient contents				
AME_N (MJ/kg)	11.62[3]	12.11[3]	12.62[3]	13.22[3]
Crude protein (g/kg)	280[3]/283[4]	255[3]/263[4]	225[3]/238[4]	190[3]/207[4]
Methionine (g/kg)	7.4[3]	7.2[3]	6.6[3]	6.1[3]
Methionine + Cysteine (g/kg)	11.8[3]	11.3[3]	10.4[3]	9.4[3]
Lysine (g/kg)	18.2[3]	16.1[3]	13.9[3]	11.7[3]
Calcium (g/kg)	10.1[3]/10.5[4]	8.0[3]/7.9[4]	6.5[3]/6.3[4]	5.5[3]/5.4[4]
Total phosphorus (g/kg)	6.8[3]/7.0[4]	5.7[3]/5.8[4]	4.8[3]/4.9[4]	4.1[3]/4.1[4]
Available (Av) phosphorus (g/kg)	4.0[3]	3.0[3]	2.1[3]	1.9[3]

[1]Vitamin and mineral premix - nutrients per kg diet: 12,500 IU vitamin A; 5,000 IU vitamin D_3; 100 IU vitamin E; 4.0 mg vitamin K; 4.5 mg vitamin B_1;15 mg vitamin B_2; 5 mg vitamin B_6; 0.04 mg vitamin B_{12}; 110 mg nicotinic acid; 28 mg pantothenic acid; 3.5 mg folic acid; 0.375 mg biotin; 80 mg iron; 25 mg copper; 160 mg manganese; 160 mg zinc; 2.5 mg iodine; 0.3 mg selenium.
[2]Vitamin and mineral premix - nutrients per kg diet: 9,600 IU vitamin A; 4,800 IU vitamin D_3; 60 IU vitamin E; 3.0 mg vitamin K; 2.0 mg vitamin B_1;12 mg vitamin B_2; 5 mg vitamin B_6; 0.025 mg vitamin B_{12}; 85 mg nicotinic acid; 23 mg pantothenic acid; 2.5 mg folic acid; 0.375 mg biotin; 40 mg iron; 25 mg copper; 120 mg manganese; 120 mg zinc; 2 mg iodine; 0.3 mg selenium.
[3]Calculated; [4]Analyzed [15].

turkeys from the negative control group was significantly lower when compared to the values in the positive control group (P = 0.006) and groups V and VI receiving the diet enriched with 500 and 1000 FTU/kg of *Escherichia coli* phytase (P < 0.05).

Bone properties in 112-day-old turkeys
Morphometric, densitometric and mechanical parameters of femur in 112-day old turkeys are shown in Table 4. Bone weight reached significantly higher values in groups V and VI when compared to groups II and IV

Table 3 Initial and final body weight of turkeys from the positive and negative control groups (Group I and Group II), and the groups receiving diet experimentally enriched with 125 (Group III), 250 (Group IV), 500 (Group V) and 1000 (Group VI) FTU/kg of *Escherichia coli* phytase

Investigated parameter	Group I (PC group; n = 8)	Group II (NC group; n = 8)	Group III (n = 8)	Group IV (n = 8)	Group V (n = 8)	Group VI (n = 8)
Initial body weight (g)	59.56 ± 0.71	59.42 ± 0.37	60.04 ± 0.86	59.62 ± 0.73	59.62 ± 0.69	59.42 ± 0.64
Final body weight (g)	14463 ± 680[a]	13525 ± 755[b]	13988 ± 461[ab]	14054 ± 595[ab]	14201 ± 460[a]	14380 ± 563[a]

Values are means ± SEM.
[ab]Statistically significant differences between the groups are indicated with different superscript letters for P ≤ 0.05.

Table 4 Morphometric, densitometric and mechanical properties of femur in 112-day old turkeys from the positive and negative control groups (Group I and Group II), and the groups receiving diet experimentally enriched with 125 (Group III), 250 (Group IV), 500 (Group V) and 1000 (Group VI) FTU/kg of _Escherichia coli_ phytase

Investigated parameter	Group I (PC group; n = 8)	Group II (NC group; n = 8)	Group III (n = 8)	Group IV (n = 8)	Group V (n = 8)	Group VI (n = 8)
Bone weight (g)	37.41 ± 0.91^{ab}	34.44 ± 1.34^{b}	37.89 ± 1.64^{ab}	34.49 ± 0.62^{b}	39.58 ± 1.70^{a}	38.84 ± 0.86^{a}
Bone length (mm)	145.4 ± 1.0^{a}	146 ± 1.15^{a}	145.9 ± 1.1^{a}	146.1 ± 0.9^{a}	149.8 ± 1.7^{b}	148.4 ± 1.0^{ab}
Bone volume (cm^3)	17.27 ± 0.74^{ab}	15.62 ± 1.00^{ab}	17.17 ± 1.13^{ab}	15.20 ± 0.37^{a}	18.06 ± 1.06^{b}	17.52 ± 0.7^{ab}
Cortical bone area (mm^2)	89.0 ± 2.4^{a}	80.75 ± 2.8^{b}	72.6 ± 2.5^{c}	70.3 ± 1.5^{c}	69.5 ± 1.7^{c}	71.3 ± 3.2^{c}
Cross-sectional area (mm^2)	77.1 ± 3.5^{a}	76.3 ± 4.3^{a}	100.2 ± 4.3^{b}	79.5 ± 2.8^{a}	83.7 ± 2.4^{a}	88.7 ± 6.4^{a}
Second moment of inertia (mm^4)	2476 ± 177^{ab}	2029 ± 148^{a}	3338 ± 254^{c}	2269 ± 105^{ad}	2703 ± 133^{bde}	3172 ± 258^{ce}
Mean relative wall thickness	0.213 ± 0.010^{a}	0.234 ± 0.016^{a}	0.269 ± 0.007^{b}	0.220 ± 0.011^{a}	0.217 ± 0.007^{a}	0.206 ± 0.016^{a}
Cortical index	17.5 ± 0.6^{a}	18.8 ± 1.0^{a}	21.1 ± 0.4^{b}	17.9 ± 0.7^{a}	17.8 ± 0.4^{a}	16.9 ± 1.1^{a}
Trabecular bone density (g/cm^3)	0.839 ± 0.028^{ab}	0.844 ± 0.019^{ab}	0.893 ± 0.021^{a}	0.823 ± 0.015^{b}	0.847 ± 0.017^{ab}	0.854 ± 0.015^{ab}
Cortical bone density (g/cm^3)	1.967 ± 0.060^{ab}	1.925 ± 0.040^{a}	2.065 ± 0.037^{bc}	2.145 ± 0.048^{c}	2.135 ± 0.039^{c}	2.091 ± 0.043^{bc}
Mean volumetric bone mineral density (g/cm^3)	1.592 ± 0.019	1.546 ± 0.019	1.556 ± 0.031	1.595 ± 0.023	1.575 ± 0.021	1.543 ± 0.018
Maximum elastic strength (N)	242 ± 14^{a}	305 ± 21^{ab}	330 ± 21^{b}	350 ± 30^{b}	295 ± 11^{ab}	266 ± 26^{a}
Ultimate strength (N)	526 ± 42	576 ± 35	586 ± 28	575 ± 43	569 ± 40	493 ± 44

Values are means ± SEM.
$^{a-e}$Statistically significant differences between the groups are indicated with different superscript letters for $P \leq 0.05$.

($P < 0.05$). Bone length was significantly higher in group V when compared to the values obtained in groups I, II, III and IV ($P < 0.05$). Total bone volume was significantly higher in group V when compared to group IV ($P = 0.04$). Cortical bone area was significantly higher by 9.3% in the positive control group when compared to the negative control group ($P = 0.02$). The values of cortical bone area were significantly decreased in groups III, IV, V and VI when compared to groups I and II ($P < 0.05$). Cross-sectional area was found to be significantly higher in group III when compared to the values of this parameter obtained in all other groups of the experiment ($P \leq 0.05$). Second moment of inertia (Ix) reached the highest value in group III, and that was significantly different than the values in group I, II, IV and V ($P < 0.05$). The value of Ix obtained in group VI was significantly higher when compared to groups I, II and IV ($P \leq 0.01$). Statistically higher value of Ix was found in group V when compared to group II ($P = 0.02$). The values of MRWT and CI reached significantly higher values in group III when compared to all other groups of the experiment ($P < 0.05$). Trabecular bone density was significantly higher by 7.2% in group III when compared to group IV ($P = 0.03$). Volumetric BMD of cortical bone was significantly higher in groups IV and V when compared to the positive and negative control groups ($P < 0.05$). Moreover, Cd values in groups III and VI were significantly higher when compared to the values obtained in the negative control group ($P < 0.05$). Maximum elastic strength of femur was significantly

higher in groups III and IV when compared to the values obtained in groups I and VI ($P \leq 0.05$). The values of the ultimate strength obtained in all the groups of experiment (I – VI) were not found to be significantly different ($P > 0.05$).

Discussion

Numerous techniques may be used for skeletal system quality evaluation in poultry species. Postmortal isolation of bone samples enables macro-morphological evaluation in terms of bone weight, length, thickness of compact and spongy layers, and perimeters and diameters of diaphysis, epiphyses and metaphyses [16]. Microscopic evaluation of histological preparations may be used for investigation of endochondral ossification process in growth plates [17]. Microradiographic imaging of transverse sections of bone shaft is utilized for cortical porosity evaluation and standard radiographic mineral density measurement [18]. Dual-energy X-ray absorptiometry (DEXA) method and digital analysis of radiograms using precise software such as Trabecula® may be applied for both _in vivo_ and _ex vivo_ assessment of bone mineral density, bone mineral content and microarchitectural organization of bone samples [19,20]. As opposed to the mentioned above diagnostic techniques which provide two-dimensional analysis of bone samples, quantitative computed tomography enabling three-dimensional morphological and densitometric analysis of bones was used in this study [21].

Pelvic limb long bones such as femur, tibia and tibiotarsus in bipedal domestic meat-type birds are subjected to significant bending forces in order to withstand loading by body tissues [22-24]. It was reported that incidence of clinical manifestations of metabolic bone disorders such as leg deformations, lameness and bone fractures increases together with higher body weight reaching significant percentage in the breeding flock at final stages of the production cycle [25-30]. Experimental data from morphometric and mechanical studies on turkeys suffering from femoral fractures indicated an insufficient skeletal adaptation to heavy body weight as a causative factor responsible for locomotory function impairments [30]. Radiological analysis of tibiotarsal bone in six-week-old Pekin domestic duck has shown that lowered bone mass was associated with bone deformities and fractures [31,32]. Studies on broiler chickens from 15 different flocks revealed the presence of gross lesions in epiphysis and metaphysis of the proximal and distal femur. Moreover, bone fractures and separation of articular cartilage of the femoral bone head with progressive erosions of the subchondral bone were diagnosed confirming impaired bone formation and mineralization processes during skeletal development [33]. Decreased vBMD in proximal metaphysis between 2nd and 4th week, and in the diaphysis between 2nd and 6th week of posthatching development was observed in male Ross broiler chickens. These observations were associated with decreasing relative bone weight from 1.03% to 0.79% and tibia deformations and fractures occurrence [34]. Negative correlation between body weight and trabeculae number in tibiotarsal bone was found in growing domestic geese together with decreasing relative bone mass between 4th and 16th week of age. The observed negative changes of the trabecular structure combined with intensive body weight gain were suggested to be associated with bone deformities and locomotory impairments in those geese [35]. Femoral fracture incidence was also reported in heavy male turkey breeders at the age of 32–35 weeks [29]. Experimental studies on meat-type turkeys have shown that leg deformities are observed in birds characterized by decreased mechanical endurance and volumetric bone mineral density of tibia and femur [36]. In other studies on turkey model, it was shown that increased volumetric bone mineral density of femur and tibia contributes to higher values of maximum elastic strength and ultimate strength – the parameters representing mechanical endurance of bones [37].

Considering importance of intestinal bioavailability and absorption of phosphorus and its contribution to hydroxyapatite structure within bone tissue, the current study was performed to evaluate effects of administration with four different levels of *Escherichia coli* phytase

on mineral density, morphology and mechanical endurance of femur in 16-week old turkeys. The results obtained in this study have shown that the most beneficial effects of phytase administration to growing turkeys was observed in group III receiving 125 FTU/kg of the diet. In this group, femur was characterized by increased geometric parameters such as cross-sectional area, second moment of inertia, mean relative wall thickness and cortical index when compared to the positive and negative control groups. The observed 5% insignificant increase of the volumetric bone mineral density in cortical bone of the midshaft in these birds was associated with significantly higher maximum elastic strength increased by 36% but cortical bone area decreased by 18.4% when compared to the positive control group. Similar effects of phytase administration on Cd, Wy and CBA of femur was observed in group IV that received 250 FTU/kg of the diet; however, all the differences of these parameters were significant in comparison to the positive control group and reached 9%, 44.6% and 21%, respectively. The effects of phytase administration in the dosage of 500 FTU/kg of the diet improved Cd, length and volume of femur with simultaneous reduction of CBA when compared to the positive control group. It is surprising that the analysis of femur obtained from the turkeys receiving the highest phytase dosage in this experiment has shown increased Ix value only in comparison to the positive control group, with concurrently lower CBA. In the negative control group, excluding significantly decreased value of CBA, the values of the analyzed parameters of femur were not significantly different from those obtained in the positive control group. Thus, simultaneous reduction of calcium and available phosphorus content in the turkey diet has not shown significant effects on morphological, densitometric and mechanical properties of femur. However, reduced dietary calcium and phosphorus content induced a significant decrease of final body weight of turkeys by 6.5%. It is worth to underline that both the initial and final body weights of turkeys administered with *Escherichia coli* phytase (Groups III – VI) were not significantly different from these parameters determined in the positive control group.

The results obtained from femur analyses show similarities with previous report describing effects of *Escherichia coli* phytase administration in the same experimental design on tibia properties [38]. In the previous report, ash content and specific gravity of whole tibia, as well as its maximum bone breaking force were not influenced by phytase administration at four different dosages. These observations correspond with the parameters analyzed for whole femur such as weight, length, total volume, MvBMD and Wf. However, contrary to the data from tibia obtained in the previous study, more detailed analyses of femur have shown positive effects of phytase administration in turkeys on geometric parameters and Cd assessed at the midshaft, and maximum elastic strength [38]. The results obtained in the current study are in accordance with previous experiments on male turkeys where *Escherichia coli* phytase administration at 250, 500, 750 and 1000 U/kg improved ash percentage and percentage of non-phytate phosphorus in middle toe and tibia in comparison to the control group. There were no statistically confirmed differentiated effects of the dosage applied on tibia and toe ash in these birds. However, *Escherichia coli* phytase was more effective when compared to two other commercially available phytases which were administered to turkeys [39]. The differences between the current and the previous study on turkeys results from its diverse phytase administration period and the applied dosages, as well as different age of birds and methodological approach. In the study by Applegate et al. (2003) the phytase administration was performed between 10th and 21st day of life when the experiment was terminated. Furthermore, neither morphometric and densitometric parameters nor mechanical endurance of the bones were analyzed in that experiment [39]. In studies on broiler chickens growing up to 49th day of life, the inclusion of phytase at the dosage of 600 U/kg of diet has not induced significant effects on body, femur and tibia weights, as well as ash content in these bones. Moreover, densitometric analysis of whole body and tibia using DEXA method has not proven any effects of phytase administration on bone mineral density and bone mineral content [40]. The discrepancy of the results obtained in the experiment performed by Angel and colleagues (2006) and in the current study may be explained by different origin, treatment duration and dosage of the administered phytase, as well as age- and species-related differences. Among the mechanisms responsible for the observed beneficial effects of phytase administration on femur properties in this study, the improved health status of intestine and digestion processes, and better mineral absorption may be postulated. This hypothesis was confirmed in studies on turkeys in which phytase administration was associated with more efficient mineral, nitrogen and amino acid metabolism [5,41].

Conclusion

In conclusion, the performed study has shown the most advantageous effects of *Escherichia coli* phytase administration on geometric, densitometric and mechanical properties of femur in turkeys receiving 125 and 250 FTU/kg of the diet. Phytase administration in all the experimental groups was associated with significantly decreased cortical bone area in the midshaft of femur. The reduced dietary calcium and phosphorus content in the diet of the negative control group of turkeys has significantly decreased the final body weight of turkeys by 6.5%. Phytase administration at the dosages of 500

and 1000 FTU/kg of the diet improved final body weight of turkeys in this study.

Abbreviations
P: Phosphorus; Ca: Calcium; QCT: Quantitative computed tomography; vBMD: Volumetric bone mineral density; Td: Trabecular bone mineral density; Cd: Cortical bone mineral density; CBA: Cortical bone area; Bvol: Total bone volume; MvBMD: Mean volumetric bone mineral density; A: Cross-sectional area; Ix: Second moment of inertia; MRWT: Mean relative wall thickness; CI: Cortical index; Wy: Maximum elastic strength; Wf: Ultimate strength; ANOVA: One-way analysis of variance; DEXA: Dual-energy X-ray absorptiometry.

Competing interests
The authors declare that they have no competing interests.

Authors' contributions
MT was responsible for morphological, densitometric and mechanical evaluation of bones and data interpretation. WK was responsible for radiological evaluation of femur with the use of quantitative computed tomography technique and data interpretation. KK was responsible for the concept and experimental design of the study, conduction all of the experimental procedures with animals, sample collection, statistical evaluation of data and their interpretation, and supervised all stages of the experiment. AD was responsible for assistance in conduction all of the experimental procedures with animals and sample collection. JJ was responsible for the concept and experimental design of the study, conduction all of the experimental procedures with animals, supervision of all stages of the experiment and data interpretation. All authors participated in the preparation of, and have approved the final version of the manuscript.

Acknowledgements
The authors wish to thank HUVEPHARMA NV (Antwerp/Belgium) for providing Optiphos phytase and financial support for this project.

Author details
[1]Department of Animal Physiology, University of Life Sciences in Lublin, ul. Akademicka 12, 20-950 Lublin, Poland. [2]II Department of Radiology, Medical University of Lublin, ul. Staszica 16, 20-081 Lublin, Poland. [3]Department of Poultry Science, University of Warmia and Mazury in Olsztyn, ul. Oczapowskiego 5, 10-719 Olsztyn, Poland.

References
1. Nelson TS. The hydrolysis of phytate phosphorus by chicks and laying hens. Poult Sci. 1976;55:2262–4.
2. Ahmadi H, Rodehutscord M. A meta-analysis of responses to dietary nonphytate phosphorus and phytase in laying hens. Poult Sci. 2012;91:2072–8.
3. Selle PH, Ravindran V. Microbial phytase in poultry nutrition. Anim Feed Sci Technol. 2007;135:1–41.
4. Shaw AL, Macklin KS, Blake JP. Phytase supplementation in a reduced calcium and phosphorus diet fed to broilers undergoing an *Eimeria* challenge. J Poult Sci. 2012;49:178–82.
5. Pirgozliev V, Bedford MR, Acamovic T, Allimehr M. The effects of supplementary bacterial phytase on dietary true metabolisable energy, nutrient digestibility and endogenous losses in precision fed turkeys. Br Poult Sci. 2011;52:214–20.
6. Tykałowski B, Stenzel T, Koncicki A. Selected problems related to ossification processes and their disorders in birds. Med Weter. 2010;66:464–9.
7. Riddell C. Non-infectious skeletal disorders of poultry: an overview. In: Whitehead CC, editor. Bone Biology and Skeletal Disorders in Poultry, Poultry Science Symposium No. 23. Abingdon, UK: Carfax Publishing Co; 1992. p. 119–45.
8. Turner KA, Lilburn MS. The effect of early protein restriction zero to eight weeks on skeletal development in turkey toms from two to eighteen weeks. Poult Sci. 1992;71:1680–6.
9. Walser MM, Cherns FL, Dziuk HE. Osseus development tibial dyschondroplasia in five lines of turkeys. Avian Dis. 1982;26:265–70.

10. Nestor KE, Bacon WL, Moorhead PD, Saif YM, Havenstein GB, Renner PA. Comparison of bone and muscle growth in turkey lines selected for increased body weight and increased shank width. Poult Sci. 1987;66:1421–8.

11. Nelson TS, Kirby LK, Johnson ZB. Effect of calcium, phosphorus, and energy on the incidence of weak legs in heavy male broilers. J App Poult Res. 1992;1:11–8.

12. Dinev I. Leg weakness pathology in broiler chickens. J Poult Sci. 2012;49:63–7.

13. Hester PY, Krueger KK, Jackson M. The effect of restrictive and compensatory growth on the incidence of leg abnormalities and performance of commercial male turkeys. Poult Sci. 1990;69:1731–42.

14. Hester PY, Krueger KK, Jackson M. The effect of compensatory growth on carcass characteristics of male turkeys. Poult Sci. 1990;69:1743–8.

15. Naumann C, Bassler R. Methodenbuch Band III. Die chemische Untersuchung von Futtermitteln. Darmstadt, Germany: VDLUFA-Press; 1993.

16. Barreiro FR, Baraldi-Artoni SM, do Amaral LA, Barbosa JC, Girardi AM, Pacheco MR, et al. Determination of broiler femur parameters at different growth phases. Int J Poult Sci. 2011;10:849–53.

17. Simsa S, Ornan EM. Endochondral ossification process of the turkey (*Meleagris gallopavo*) during embryonic and juvenile development. Poult Sci. 2007;86:565–71.

18. Crespo R, Stover SM, Shivaprasad HL, Chin RP. Microstructure and mineral content of femora in male turkeys with and without fractures. Poult Sci. 2002;81:1184–90.

19. Charuta A, Majchrzak T, Czerwiński E, Cooper RG. Spongious matrix of the tibio-tarsal bone of ostriches (*Struthio camelus*) – a digital analysis. Bull Vet Inst Pulawy. 2008;52:285–9.

20. Shim MY, Karnuah AB, Mitchell AD, Anthony NB, Pesti GM, Aggrey SE. The effects of growth rate on leg morphology and tibia breaking strength, mineral density, mineral content, and bone ash in broilers. Poult Sci. 2012;91:1790–5.

21. Tatara MR. Current methods for *in vivo* assessment of the skeletal system in poultry. Med Weter. 2006;62:266–9.

22. Tatara MR, Sierant-Rozmiej N, Krupski W, Majcher P, Śliwa E, Kowalik S, et al. Quantitative computed tomography for the assessment of mineralization of the femur and tibia in turkeys. Med Weter. 2005;61:225–8.

23. Charuta A, Cooper RG, Pierzchała M, Horbańczuk JO. Computed tomographic analysis of tibiotarsal bone mineral density and content in turkeys as influenced by age and sex. Czech J Anim Sci. 2012;57:573–80.

24. Charuta A, Dzierzęcka M, Biesiada-Drzazga B. Evaluation of densitometric and geometric parameters of tibiotarsal bones in turkeys. Bull Vet Inst Pulawy. 2012;56:379–84.

25. Poulos Jr PW. Tibial dyschondroplasia (osteochondrosis) in the turkey. A morphologic investigation. Acta Radiol. 1978;358:197–227.

26. Wyers M, Chekel Y, Plassiart G. Late clinical expression of lameness related to associated osteomyelitis and tibial dyschondroplasia in male breeding turkeys. Avian Dis. 1991;35:408–41.

27. Lynch MM, Thorp BH, Withehead CC. Avian tibial dyschondroplasia as a cause of bone deformity. Avian Pathol. 1992;21:275–85.

28. Rath NC, Bayyari GR, Beasley JN, Huff WE, Balog JM. Age-related changes in the incidence of tibial dyschondroplasia in turkeys. Poult Sci. 1994;73:1254–9.

29. Crespo R, Stover SM, Droual R, Chin RP, Shivaprasad HL. Femoral fractures in a young male turkey breeder flock. Avian Dis. 1999;43:150–4.

30. Crespo R, Stover SM, Taylor KT, Chin RP, Shivaprasad HL. Morphometric and mechanical properties of femora in young adult male turkeys with and without femoral fractures. Poult Sci. 2000;79:602–8.

31. Charuta A, Dzierzecka M, Majchrzak T, Czerwinski E, Cooper RG. Computer-generated radiological imagery of the structure of the spongious substance in the postnatal development of the tibiotarsal bones of the Peking domestic duck (*Anas platyrhynchos var. domestica*). Poult Sci. 2011;90:830–5.

32. Charuta A, Cooper RG. Computed tomographic and densitometric analysis of tibiotarsal bone mineral density and content in postnatal Peking ducks (*Anas platyrhynchos var. domestica*) as influenced by age and sex. Pol J Vet Sci. 2012;15:537–45.

33. Olkowski AA, Laarveld B, Wojnarowicz C, Chirino-Trejo M, Chapman D, Wysokinski TW. Biochemical and physiological weaknesses associated with the pathogenesis of femoral bone degeneration in broiler chickens. Avian Pathol. 2011;40:639–50.

34. Charuta A, Dzierzecka M, Komosa M, Kalinowski Ł, Pierzchała M. Age- and sex-related differences of morphometric, densitometric and geometric parameters of tibiotarsal bone in Ross broiler chickens. Folia Biol (Krakow). 2013;61:211–20.

35. Charuta A, Dzierzecka M, Czerwiński E, Cooper RG, Horbańczuk JO. Sex- and age-related changes of trabecular bone of tibia in growing domestic geese (*Anser domesticus*). Folia Biol (Krakow). 2012;60:205–12.

36. Tatara MR, Majcher P, Krupski W, Studziński T. Volumetric bone density, morphological and mechanical properties of femur and tibia in farm turkeys with leg deformities. Bull Vet Inst Pulawy. 2004;48:169–72.

37. Tatara MR, Pierzynowski SG, Majcher P, Krupski W, Brodzki A, Studziński T. Effect of Alpha-Ketoglutarate (AKG) on mineralisation, morphology and mechanical endurance of femur and tibia in turkey. Bull Vet Inst Pulawy. 2004;48:305–9.

38. Kozłowski K, Jankowski J, Jeroch H. Efficacy of *Escherichia coli*-derived phytase on performance, bone mineralization and nutrient digestibility in meat-type turkeys. Vet Med Zoot. 2010;52:59–66.

39. Applegate TJ, Webel DM, Lei XG. Efficacy of a phytase derived from Escherichia coli and expressed in yeast on phosphorus utilization and bone mineralization in turkey poults. Poult Sci. 2003;82:1726–32.

40. Angel R, Saylor WW, Mitchell AD, Powers W, Applegate TJ. Effect of dietary phosphorus, phytase, and 25-hydroxycholecalciferol on broiler chicken bone mineralization, litter phosphorus, and processing yields. Poult Sci. 2006;85:1200–11.

41. Pirgozliev V, Acamovic T, Bedford MR. The effects of previous exposure to dietary microbial phytase on the endogenous excretions of energy, nitrogen and minerals from turkeys. Br Poult Sci. 2011;52:66–71.

15

Two cases of meningocele and meningoencephalocele in Jeju native pigs

In-Cheol Cho[1†], Yong-Sang Park[2†], Jae-Gyu Yoo[1], Sang-Hyun Han[3], Sang-Rae Cho[1], Hee-Bok Park[4], Kyong-Leek Jeon[2], Kyoung-Ha Moon[2], Han-Seong Cho[2] and Tae-Young Kang[2*]

Abstract

Background: Meningocele and meningoencephalocele of the skull are congenital deformities. Various species, such as pigs, dogs, and cats, are susceptible to congenital meningocele and meningoencephalocele and the incidence is higher in large white and landrace pigs.

Case presentation: In this study, swelling was observed in the fontanel areas of the median planes of the skull cap in two female piglets of the same litter. Gross clinical examination, neurological examination, computed tomography (CT), and magnetic resonance imaging (MRI) were conducted on the symptomatic piglets. The gross clinical and neurological examinations revealed no specific findings, except for the swellings. According to the CT results, the length of the defect on the sagittal section of the skull was 4.7 mm in case 1 and 20.62 mm in case 2. Connected flow between the skull swellings and the cerebrospinal fluid (CSF) of the lateral ventricles was observed, and partial herniation was identified in case 2. On MRI, CSF with high T2 signals was identified in the arachnoid spaces between the cerebrum and the cerebellum in the two cases, which is consistent with intracranial hypertension. The size of the swelling formed in the parietal bones was $1.6 \times 1.1 \times 1.8$ cm^3 (case 1) and $1.2 \times 1.38 \times 1.7$ cm^3 (case 2). The increase in intracranial pressure was more obvious in case 2 than in case 1, and was accompanied by posterior displacements of the mesencephalon and cerebellum.

Conclusions: Case 1 was diagnosed as meningocele resulting from meningeal herniation and case 2 was diagnosed as meningoencephalocele caused by brain tissue herniation.

Background

Meningocele and meningoencephalocele of the skull are congenital deformities. These deformities, which are observed as cyst-like swellings in the median part of the skull cap, occur very rarely. The intracranial material protrudes through a spontaneous cavity, such as the anterior fontanelle [1], and they are classified as encephalocele, meningocele, or meningoencephalocele according to the cranial bifida [2]. The condition is called meningocele when only cerebrospinal fluid (CSF) exists in the meningeal swelling, and it is called meningoencephalocele when brain tissues coexist in the swelling [3]. Dysraphism or a defect of the anterior fontanelle area triggers meningoencephalocele and meningocele. These defects take place in relation to agenesis of the surface ectoderm and neuroectoderm [2,4,5]. Congenital meningocele and meningoencephalocele occur in various animals, including horses, pigs, dogs, cats, and goats [1,4-10]. Their incidence is higher in large white and landrace pigs [1,5,11,12]. Experimentally, the incidence of meningoencephalocele upon crossing with a group with meningoencephalocele is between 0.95% and 1.37% [2,3]. Encephalocele and meningocele mostly occur in the suture line of the frontal region, and sometimes in the occipital region and the posterior occipital crest, whereas meningoencephalocele largely occurs in the occipital region [2,13]. Meningocele and meningoencephalocele have been diagnosed in humans and various animals by using computed tomography (CT) and magnetic resonance imaging (MRI). The occurrence of meningocele and meningoencephalocele in the indigenous pigs of Jeju Island has not been previously reported. In this study, we examined the brains

* Correspondence: tykang87@jejunu.ac.kr
†Equal contributors
2College of Veterinary Medicine, Jeju National University, Jeju 690-756, Republic of Korea
Full list of author information is available at the end of the article

of two Jeju Island indigenous pigs by using CT and MRI to diagnose meningocele and meningoencephalocele.

Materials and methods

We obtained two female piglets (age, 2 days; weight, ~1.4 kg) from a single Jeju native pig litter from a farm in Korea. The physical examination revealed a sac-like protrusion with fluctuant swelling in the frontoparietal region of the skull vault and a palpable skull defect on the top of the piglets' heads. A vault swelling may protrude through a normal opening, such as the anterior fontanelle. An ultrasound scanner (ProSoundAlpha 6, Hitachi Aloka, Japan) was used to examine the fluctuant swelling. The swelling appeared to be filled with anechoic fluid, which was likely CSF. The presence of brain tissue in the swelling could not be confirmed by the use of ultrasound examination and radiograph. Therefore, it was difficult to differentiate between meningocele and meningoencephalocele by using these methods. CT imaging (Asteion Super 4, Toshiba, Japan) and MRI (Vet-MR, Esaote, Italy) were performed to evaluate the swelling in the skull while the animals were under sedation with azaperone (Stresnil, Janssen Pharmaceutica, Belgium). The Animal Care Committee at the National Institute of Animal Science approved all experimental procedures (Approved No. 2014-095).

Case presentation

Case 1: In a 2-day old female piglet weighing approximately 1.4 kg, lesions connected with the swelling in the brain parenchyma of the prefrontal level were observed on MRI. The subarachnoid space between the cerebrum and cerebellum was filled with fluid, and the CSF was open and flowing. In addition, the corpus callosum was open, and the CSF flow measured by the MRI showed that the space was connected to the lateral ventricle (Figure 1D,E,F). On CT, the fissure lines of the skull and bone discontinuity were disappeared, and the regions in which the fissure lines met was identified (Figure 1C,D). A swelling containing matter of liquid density at the dorsolateral parietal bone was identified, and it was connected to the cerebral ventricle. The length of the defect in the cross-section of the skull was measured at 4.78 mm (Figure 1D). On MRI, a swelling with high T2/low T1 signals was identified in the dorsolateral parietal bone in the transverse cross-section. The size of the swelling was 10.67 × 16.31 (L × H, mm) (Figure 1G). Furthermore, the CSF flow of the lateral ventricle was connected with the defect of the skull. A swelling with high T2/low T1 signals was identified on the dorsolateral parietal bone from the median sagittal plane (Figure 1E,F), and bone discontinuity disappearance of the skull was also observed. The swelling on the median sagittal plane was 18.49 × 10.59 (L × H, mm). With CSF leakage through

the defective parietal bone, the mass observed in the parietal region formed a swelling with high T2/low T1 signals on MRI. The size of the swelling was 1.6 × 1.1 × 1.8 (L × H × W, cm). Case 1 was diagnosed as meningocele by meningeal herniation based on crania bifida of the skull in the anterior fontanelle region of the parietal bone. Morphologically, the case was diagnosed as extracranial (transcalvarial) herniation.

Case 2: Case 2, which was from the same litter as case 1, had two swellings in the frontal lobe region. As in case 1, both MRI and CT were used to examine case 2. The fluid of the case 1 swelling was an ahemorrhagic-serous exudate, but the fluid in case 2 was a hemorrhagic exudate. We observed characteristic changes in the brain structure, such as findings of ventrical herniation resulting from the exchange of CSF and posterior displacement of the cerebellum region due to increased brain pressure in the prosencephalic cavity. The length of the defective area of the transverse cross-section on CT of the skull was 20.62 mm (Figure 1K). The size of the protruding swelling was 12.02 × 10.62 (L × H, mm), and the matter of the swelling was connected with the cerebral ventricle.

On MRI, a swelling with high T2/low T1 signals in the transverse cross-section was identified, and the size of the protruding cyst was 11.66 × 11.38 (L × H, mm) (Figure 1M). Herniation of the brain tissue from the median sagittal plane to the defective area of the skull and posterior displacement of the cerebellum resulting from increased intracranial pressure were observed (Figure 1I). The size of the swelling on the median sagittal plane was measured at 17.24 × 12.92 (L × H, mm) (Figure 1L). As in case 1, case 2 had crania bifida of the skull in the anterior fontanelle region of the parietal bone. However, case 2 was diagnosed as meningoencephalocele because it was accompanied by herniation of the brain and the meninges encephali due to increased intracranial pressure. Morphologically, this case was diagnosed as extracranial (transcalvarial) herniation.

Discussion

Encephalocele is a deformity resulting from the herniation of brain tissue through a skull defect. Encephalocele and meningoencephalocele reflect imperfect osteogenesis of the skull and largely accompany protrusions of the brain structure [2,13]. The classification of encephalocele depends on the degree of brain tissue herniation. The defect is classified as cranium bifidum when only a skull defect is present. Herniation of the cranial dura mater through the defect is classified as meningocele, and herniation of the cranial dura mater and brain parenchyma are classified as meningoencephalocele. In humans, cranium bifidum occurs in one to four out of 10,000 live births [13]. Meningoencephalocele that caused the herniation of the cerebral tissue and meninges was found to occur in the

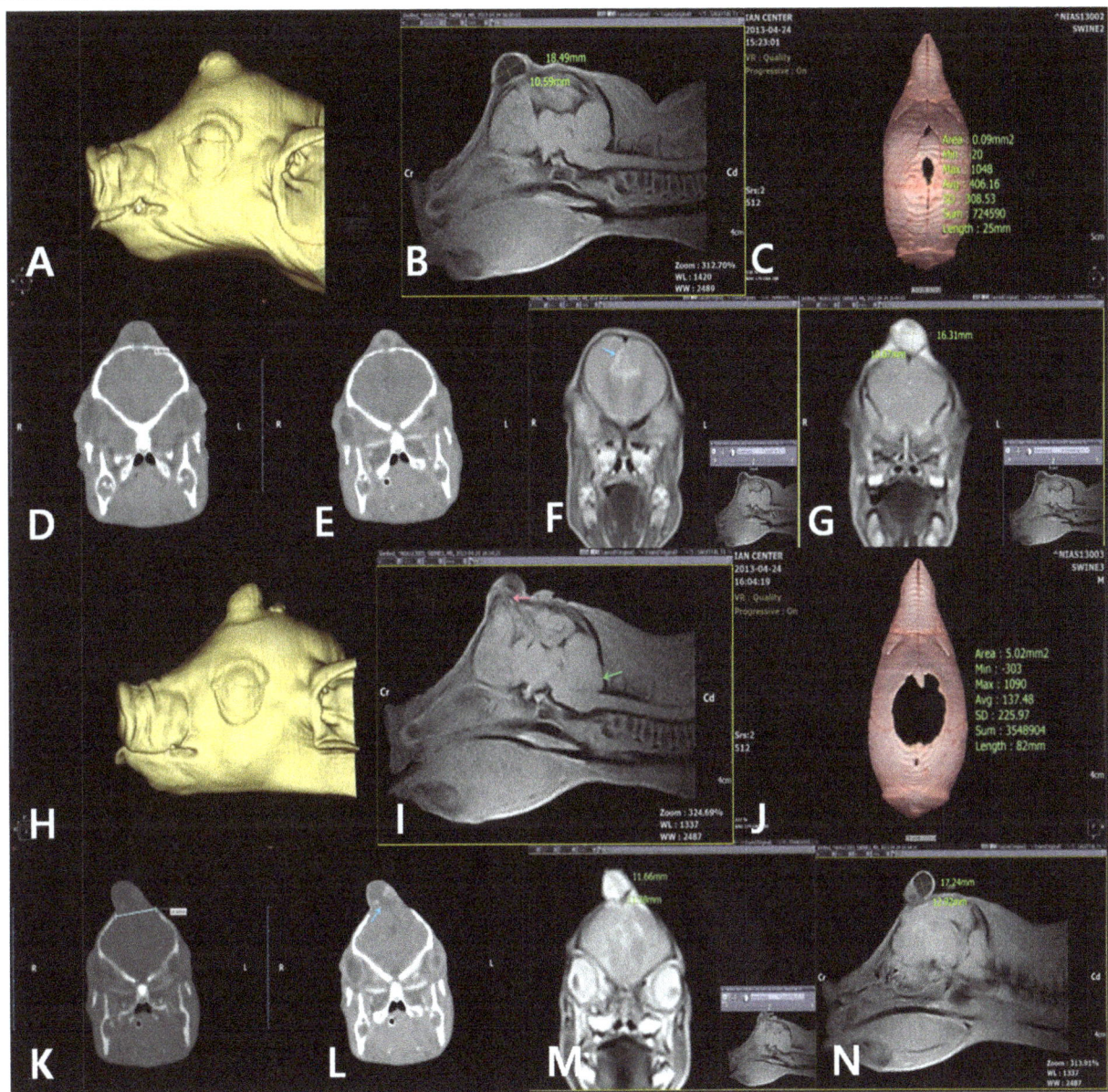

Figure 1 CT and MRI findings of the pig skull in case 1 (A–G) and case 2 (H–N). Three-dimensional volume reconstruction is shown in **A** (case 1) and **H** (case 2). The MRI of the pig's skull is shown in **B**, **F**, **G**, **I**, **M**, **L** and **N**. The imaging of the pig skull is shown in **C**, **D**, **E**, **K**, **L**, and **M**. **B**, The size of the swelling on the median sagittal plane on MRI was 18.49 × 10.59 (L × H, mm). **C** and **J**, Imaging of three-dimensional volume reconstruction of the pig skull defect, specifically a canal with irregular edges. **D**, Transverse-plane section through the skull showing the bone defect in case 1. The length of the defect was 4.78 mm, and a cyst containing matter of fluid density was apparent. **E** and **F**, The matter in the swelling was related to the cerebral ventricle. **G**, The size of the swelling on the cross-section was 10.67 × 16.31 (L × H, mm). **I** and **L**, Transverse-plane section through the skull showing the bone defect in case 2. The herniation of the brain tissues from the median sagittal plane to the skull defect was apparent. Posterior displacement of the cerebellum due to increased intracranial pressure was evident. The size of the swelling was 17.24 × 12.92 (L × H, mm). The transverse cross-section of case 2. The length of the defect was 20.62 mm. A swelling with matter of liquid density was apparent. Transverse cross-section of case 2 on MRI. A swelling with T2 high/T1 low signals was apparent. The size of the protruding swelling was 11.66 × 11.38 (L × H, mm).

occipital region, the frontal region, and the temporal region in 75%, 12%, and 13% of cases, respectively. Rare sites for protrusions are through the base of the skull, orbits, nose, or mouth [13]. Meningocele and meningoencephalocele are the result of a focal failure of the neuroectoderm and surface ectoderm to separate during fetal development, and these deformities have many potential causes, including genetic factors, nutritional deficiencies, and exposure to teratogenic agents during gestation [1,14,15]. Hereditary meningocele and meningoencephalocele cases have been reported in pigs and cats, and both of these hereditary diseases showed incomplete penetrance [3,5]. Cranium bifidum can be diagnosed by radiography, but differentiating between meningoencephalocele and meningocele with radiography and ultrasonography is difficult. However, meningoencephalocele and meningoceleare easily recognized by CT. CT scans enable differentiate between a meningocele and meningoencephalocele and measurement of the diameter of the defect. CT scans are a simple and valuable non-invasive diagnostic technique in animals. Nonetheless, when describing structural changes of the brain, CT scans should be combined with findings of changes in the brain parenchyma via MRI. An increase in intracranial pressure is commonly discovered in CT and MRI findings. CSF leakage is considered to occur in relation to the neural canal defect, and such neural canal defects are also associated with the size of the skull cap defect into meningoencephalocele and meningocele.

Conclusion

In this study, CT and MRI were used to make a diagnosis of encephalocele cases in pigs. The length of the defect on the sagittal section of two piglets' skull was estimated by using CT. Case 1 had a defect 4.7 mm in length and connected flow between the skull swellings and CSF. Case 2 had longer defect length (20.62 mm) than case 1 and partial herniation. On MRI imaging, both cases showed high T2 signals of CSF in the arachnoid spaces between the cerebrum and the cerebellum. The increase in intracranial pressure was more obvious in case 2 than in case 1, and accompanied posterior displacements of the mesencephalon and cerebellum. Case 1 was diagnosed as meningocele resulting from meningeal herniation, and case 2 was diagnosed as meningoencephalocele caused by brain tissue herniation.

Competing interests
The authors declare that they have no competing interests.

Authors' contributions
I-CC, Y-SP, J-GY, S-HH, S-RC, K-LJ, K-HM, and H-SC performed experiments; Y-SP, K-LJ, K-HM, H-SC, H-BP, and T-YK interpreted results of experiments; I-CC, Y-SP, and T-YK prepared figures; I-CC, Y-SP, H-BP, and T-YK drafted, edited and revised manuscript. I-CC, Y-SP, and T-YK conceived and designed the research. All authors read and approved the final manuscript.

Acknowledgements
This work was carried out with the support of "Cooperative Research Program for Agriculture Science & Technology Development (Project Numbers PJ01012301 and PJ0084972014)", Rural Development Administration, Republic of Korea.

Author details
[1]National Institute of Animal Science, Rural Development Administration, Jeju 690-150, Republic of Korea. [2]College of Veterinary Medicine, Jeju National University, Jeju 690-756, Republic of Korea. [3]Educational Science Research Institute, Jeju National University, Jeju 690-756, Republic of Korea. [4]Division of Animal and Dairy Science (Brain Korea 21 plus Program), Chungnam National University, Daejeon 305-764, Republic of Korea.

References

1. Lahunta A, Glass E, Lahunta A, Glass E. Development of the Nervous System: Malformation. In: Veterinary Neuroanatomy and Clinical Neurology. edn. St. Louis: Saunders; 2009. p. 23–53.
2. Sullivan ND. The nervous system. In: Jubb KVF, Kennedy PC, Palmer N, editors. Pathology of Domestic Animal, vol. 1. Orlando: Academic Press; 1985. p. 201–338.
3. Vogt DW, Ellersieck MR, Deutsch WE, Akremi B, Islam MN. Congenital meningocele-encephalocele in an experimental swine herd. Am J Vet Res. 1986;47(1):188–91.
4. Ohba Y, Iguchi T, Hirose Y, Takasu M, Nishii N, Maeda S, et al. Computer tomography diagnosis of meningoencephalocele in a calf. J Vet Med Sci. 2008;70(8):829–31.
5. Wijeratne WV, Beaten D, Cuthbertson JC. A field occurrence of congenital meningo-encephalocoele in pigs. Vet Rec. 1974;95(4):81–4.
6. Back W, van den Belt AJ, Lagerweij E, van Overbeeke JJ, van der Velden MA. Surgical repair of a cranial meningocele in a calf. Vet Rec. 1991;128(24):569–71.
7. MacKillop E. Magnetic resonance imaging of intracranial malformations in dogs and cats. Vet Radiol Ultrasound. 2011;52(1 Suppl 1):S42–51.
8. Parker AJ, Cusick PK. Meningoencephalocele in a dog (a case history). Vet Med Small Anim Clin. 1974;69(2):206–7.
9. Philip LM, Mohan MR, Bastin F, Sajesh MG. Surgical repair of frontal meningocele in a kid. J Indian Vet Assoc. 2012;10(2):50–2.
10. Sponenberg DP, Graf-Webster E. Hereditary meningoencephalocele in Burmese cats. J Hered. 1986;77(1):60.
11. Gilman JP. Congenital hydrocephalus in domestic animals. Cornell Vet. 1956;46(4):487–99.
12. Jackson P, Cockcroft P, Jackson P, Cockcroft P. Disease of the Nervous System. In: Handbook of Pig Medicine. edn. London: Saunders Elevier; 2007. p. 128–42.
13. Sandler MA, Beute GH, Madrazo BL, Hudak SF, Walter R, Haggar AH, et al. Ultrasound case of the day: Occipital meningoencephalocele. RadioGraphics. 1986;6(6):1096–9.
14. Dewey CW, Brewer DM, Cautela MA, Talarico LR, Silver GM. Surgical treatment of a meningoencephalocele in a cat. Vet Surg. 2011;40(4):473–6.
15. Braund KG. Degenerative and developmental diseases. In: Oliver JE, Hoerlein BF, Mayhew ZG, editors. Veterinary Neurology. Philadelphia: WB Saunders Co; 1987. p. 199.

16

Isolation of *Leptospira interrogans* serovar Hardjoprajitno from a calf with clinical leptospirosis in Chile

Miguel Salgado[1*], Barbara Otto[1], Manuel Moroni[2], Errol Sandoval[1], German Reinhardt[1], Sofia Boqvist[3], Carolina Encina[1] and Claudia Muñoz-Zanzi[4]

Abstract

Background: Although *Leptospira* isolation has been reported in Chilean cattle, only serological evidence of serovar Hardjo bovis infection has been routinely reported. The present report provides characterization of the pathological presentation and etiology of a clinical case of leptospirosis in a calf from the Los Rios Region in Chile.

Case presentation: In a dairy herd in southern Chile, 11 of 130 calves died after presenting signs such as depression and red-tinged urine. One of these calves, a female of eight months, was necropsied, and all the pathological findings were consistent with *Leptospira* infection. A urine sample was submitted to conventional bacteriological analysis together with highly specific molecular biology typing tools, in order to unravel the specific *Leptospira* specie and serovar associated with this clinical case.
A significant finding of this study was that the obtained isolate was confirmed by PCR as *L. interrogans*, its VNTR profile properly matching with *L. interrogans* Hardjoprajitno as well as its specific genomic identity revealed by *secY* gen.

Conclusion: *Leptospira interrogans* serovar Hardjoprajitno was associated with the investigated calf clinical case. This information adds to the value of serologic results commonly reported, which encourage vaccination improvements to match circulating strains. In addition, this finding represents the first case report of this serovar in Chilean cattle.

Keywords: *Leptospira*, Cattle, Clinical, Hardjoprajitno

Background

Leptospirosis is a zoonotic infectious disease caused by bacteria of the genus *Leptospira* that affects domestic and wild animals. The disease is distributed worldwide and of great public health importance, especially in warm and humid climates. The bacterium is shed in the urine of infected animals and this is the main transmission route for human infection [1]. The disease has also been recognized as one of the most important diseases in livestock, particularly in cattle, due to negative impacts on reproduction [2,3].

It is well established that *Leptospira* infection in Chile is present both in domestic and wild animals [4,5]. The apparent seroprevalences in different domestic animal species are high, ranging from 59 to 91% in cattle, 24% in goats, 7.1% sheep, 49% in equine, 70% in swine and 47% in wild mice [5]. In a study from Southern Chile 162/361 (45%) serum samples from apparently healthy cattle were seropositive for *Leptospira* using the Microscopic Agglutination Test. The proportion of seropositive samples was highest for *Leptospira* serovar Hardjo (68%), followed by serovars Pomona (11%), Tarassovi (8.6%), Bratislava (1.9%), Canicola (1.9%), Icterohaemorrhagiae (1.9%) and Ballum (1.2%) [4]. Recently, a study was carried out to determine *Leptospira* seroprevalence and to evaluate risk factors associated with seropositivity at herd level in smallholder bovine dairy herds in southern Chile, and 75% of the included herds (52/69) showed serological titers against one or more *Leptospira* serovar, where *Leptospira borgpetersenii* serovar Hardjo was the serovar

* Correspondence: miguelsalgado@uach.cl
[1]Department of Biochemistry and Microbiology, Faculty of Sciences, Universidad Austral de Chile, Edificio Instapanel, Campus Isla Teja, CC 567 Valdivia, Chile
Full list of author information is available at the end of the article

most frequently (81%) reported from animals with positive results [6].

Infection by *L. interrogans* serovar Hardjo (type Hardjoprajitno) in cattle has not been investigated previously in Chile. The importance of serovar Hardjoprajitno infection on the rate of abortion has been estimated to be 30% as opposed to what happens with *Leptospira borgpetersenii* Hardjo bovis where the rate reaches only a 3 to 10%. Additionally, acute infection of dairy cows with Leptospira *interrogans* Hardjoprajitno is associated with a drop in milk production [7]. Therefore, the aim of the present study was to present both pathological and microbiological evidence of the *Leptospira interrogans* Hardjoprajitno virulence from its isolation and characterization from a calf that died of clinical leptospirosis.

Case presentation
Study animal
In a dairy herd in southern Chile, eleven out of 130 calves died after presenting clinical signs such as depression and haematuria. One of these calves, a female of eight months, was submitted to the Department of Animal Pathology at the Faculty of Veterinary Science, Universidad Austral de Chile, Valdivia, Chile for necropsy.

Pathological findings
Necropsy showed a marked yellowing pigmentation in all mucosal body openings and in the subcutaneous tissue, fat and muscles. There were also isolated petechia in the kidneys and the bladder contained approximately two liters of red-tinged urine (Figure 1).

A urine sample was collected by puncturing the bladder and sent to the Leptospirosis and Paratuberculosis Laboratory, Department of Biochemistry and Microbiology, at the Faculty of Sciences, Universidad Austral de Chile, Valdivia, Chile. All the procedures were in strict accordance with the recommendations in the Guide of Use of Animals for Research of Universidad Austral de Chile, approved by the Committee on the Ethics of Animals for Research (www.uach.cl/direccion/ investigacion/uso_animales.htm).

Bacteriological analysis
The urine sample was investigated using dark field microscopy and bacterial structures consistent with *Leptospira* were found. Thereafter, 200 μl of urine sample with four replicates was cultured in EMJH medium at 29°C [8]. After a month of incubation, a positive result was reported with a typical Dinger ring growth.

Leptospira DNA was extracted from positive cultures and in order to identify *Leptospira* species, primers covering the most common pathogenic *Leptospira* species were used (664–665 *L. kirschneri* fla gene; 1280–1281 *L. interrogans* IS1500; 1805–1809 *L. borgpetersenii* IS1533) [9]. The total PCR reaction was 50 μl, of which 5 μl was 10× Taq polymerase buffer (Promega, Madison, WI), 2 μl dNTPs (2.5 mM stock containing all four dNTPs) (Promega, Madison, WI), 0.5 U Taq Polymerase (Promega, Madison, WI), 1 μl (each) primer (stock concentration = 100 pmol/μl; final concentration 2 pmol/μl), 35.5 μl dH$_2$O and 5 μl template. The PCR reactions considered 40 cycles of 94°C for 15 sec; 60°C for 30 sec and 68°C for 2 min. then 10°C hold. Negative and positive PCR controls were included as well as DNA extraction negative and positive controls.

To refine our understanding of the *Leptospira* specie and serovar associated with this clinical case, a Variable Number Tandem Repeat (VNTR) analysis was done. The VNTR primers were designed exclusively for use with *L. interrogans* [10-12]. PCR products for VNTR loci 4, 7, 10, 23, 27, 29, 30, 31, and 36 were assessed using the same PCR reaction as described above and the primers used were as previously reported [12]. PCR products were

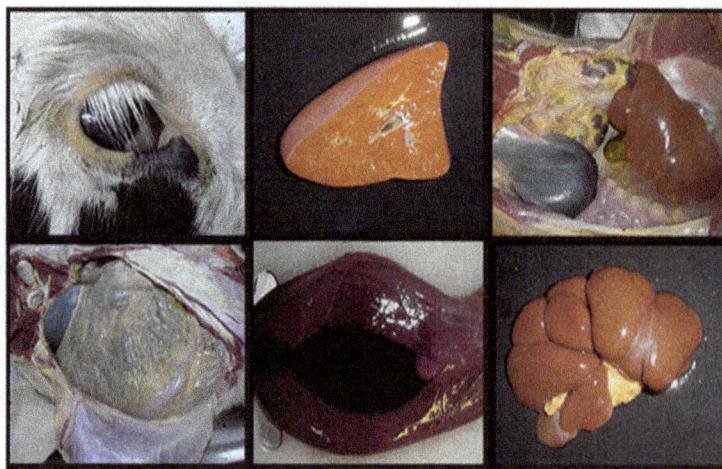

Figure 1 Calf with clinical sign and pathological findings consistent with *Leptospira* infection.

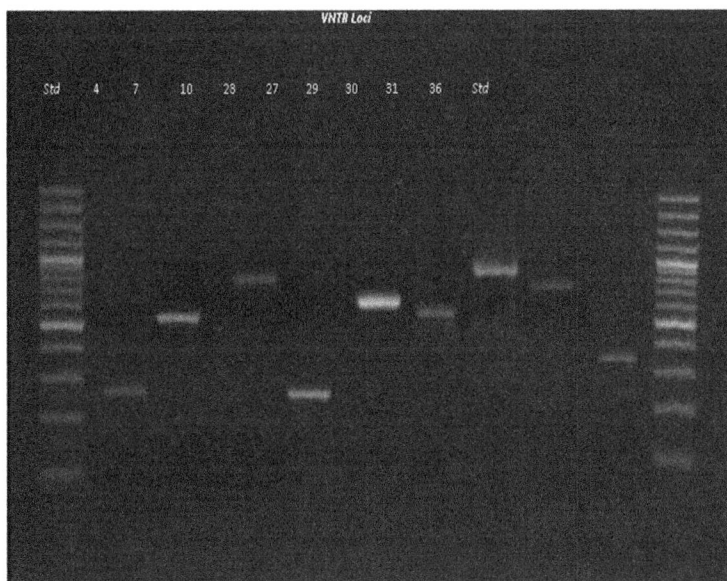

Figure 2 PCR analysis of the polymorphism of nine representative VNTR loci. Amplification was performed on the VNTR 4, 7, 10, 23, 27, 29, 30, 31, 36 loci of *L. interrogans* strains.

separated by agarose gel electrophoresis and visualized, and their sizes were calculated by comparing with reference standards (100-bp ladder; Invitrogen, Carlsbad, CA) and with the literature [10,11]. As a complement, we also amplified the gene *secY*, which is a house keeping gene that consists of alternating conserved and variable regions, making it suitable to deduce primers that generate amplicons with sufficient sequence heterogeneity to enable phylogenetic interpretation for *Leptospira* [13]. A 202 bp product was amplified by conventional PCR in 25 μl mixture containing 5 μl diluted template (1:100), 0.2 μM each primers SecYIVF (5'-GCGATTCAGTTTAATCCTGC-3') and SecYIV (5'-GAGTTAGAGCTCAAATCTA-AG-3'),

0.625 U GoTaq Flexi DNA Polymerase in 1X Green Buffer GoTaq (Promega, Madison, WI), 3.0 mM MgCl2, 0.3 mM dNTPs (Promega, Madison, WI), and 400 ng mL-1 bovine serum albumin (BSA; BioLabs, Ipswich, England). Cycle conditions included an initial denaturation step at 95°C for 5 min followed by 40 cycles at 94°C for 1 min, 57°C for 1 min and 72°C for 1 minute and a final elongation step at 72°C for 10 minutes. The PCR products obtained were separated on 1.5% agarose gel, stained with Gel Red (GelRed, Biotium Inc, Hayward, U.S), excised and purified using a commercial kit (E.Z.N.A® Gel Extraction Kit, Omega Bio-Tek, Norcross, U.S). Amplicons were sequenced by Macrogen Inc (Seoul, Korea). The consensus nucleotide

```
          CLUSTAL 2.1 multiple sequence alignment


L.int.Hardjo      GCGATTCAGTTTAATCCTGCAGAATTGGCTGAGAATTTGAAAAAATACGGTGGATTCATT 60
Ternero           GCGATTCAGTTTAATCCTGCAGAATTGGCTGAGAATTTGAAAAAATACGGTGGATTCATT 60
                  ************************************************************


L.int.Hardjo      CCAGGAATTCGTCCGGGTTCTCACACAAAAGAATACATTGAAAAAGTGTTAAATAGAATC 120
Ternero           CCAGGAATTCGTCCGGGTTCTCACACAAAAGAATACATTGAAAAAGTGTTAAATAGAATC 120
                  ************************************************************


L.int.Hardjo      ACTCTTCCCGGAGCTATGTTTCTTGCAGGTTTGGCATTAGCACCTTATATTATTATAAAA 180
Ternero           ACTCTTCCCGGAGCTATGTTTCTTGCAGGTTTGGCATTAGCACCTTATATTATTATAAAA 180
                  ************************************************************


L.int.Hardjo      TTCTTAGATTTGAGCTCTAACTC 203
Ternero           TTCTTAGATTTGAGCTCTAACTC 203
                  ***********************
```

Figure 3 ClustalW aligment for 202 bp fragment, *SecY* gen.

sequence obtained in this study was compared with *secY* gene of *Leptospira interrogans* serovar Hardjo prajitno (GenBank accession number EU357983.1). DNA alignments were done using clustalW tools (http://www.ebi.ac. uk/Tools/msa/clustalw2).

Results and discussion

The isolate obtained in this study was confirmed by PCR as *L. interrogans* and its VNTR profile properly matched with *L. interrogans* type Hardjo prajitno (Figure 2). The *secY* gene alignment done by clustalW did reveal sequence identity strain belonging to the species *L. interrogans* serovar Hardjo prajitno (Figure 3). This confirms that *L. interrogans* type Hardjo prajitno is associated with acute infection of cattle in Chile. Previous studies have shown that the abortion rate after *Leptospira borgpetersenii* serovar Hardjo bovis infection is 3 to 10% whereas the rate increases up to 30% for *L.* Hardjo prajitno infection [3-7], which underscores the importance of this serovar. The clinical information in the presented study was conveniently complemented with bacteriological findings to describe the isolated strain affecting the clinical case presented.

The typing method used based on VNTR polymorphism provided a rapid characterization together with the highly discriminatory power reported [10,11] to identify *L. interrogans* serovars using clinical specimens. Furthermore, the use of *secY* gene in combination with the latter allowed a more robust result due to its great phylogenetic potential [13].

Conclusions

The present finding represents the first isolation confirmed as *L. interrogans* serovar Hardjo prajitno from cattle with clinical disease in Chile. The importance of this serovar in Chilean cattle needs to be investigated further. This information add to the value of serologic results commonly reported, which encourage vaccination improvements to match circulating strains. The latter is based on a previous published study on serological cross-reactivity between Hardjo bovis and Hardjoprajitno serovars, which implies similar antigenic determinants; although with substantial genomic differences as well as in their pathogenicity in the bovine specie [14].

Due to above mentioned, we emphasize the need to isolate, preserve and characterized strains of *Leptospira* in order to improve and standardize currently available diagnostic techniques. This will help to improve our understanding of the epidemiology and impact of this infection as well as to identify optimal option for surveillance and control.

Competing interests
The authors declare that they have no competing interests.

Authors' contributions
MS: lab work and draft writing; BO lab work and draft writing; MM: pathological study and draft writing; ES: lab work and draft writing; GR: draft writing; SB: draft writing, CE: molecular analysis; CMZ: draft writing. All authors read and approved the final manuscript.

Acknowledgments
This work was supported by DID GRANT S-2012-19. We also wanted to acknowledge Dr Richard Zuerner for provide technical help, writing assistance, and lab support at the Department of Biomedical Sciences and Veterinary Public Health, Swedish University of Agricultural Sciences.

Author details
[1]Department of Biochemistry and Microbiology, Faculty of Sciences, Universidad Austral de Chile, Edificio Instapanel, Campus Isla Teja, CC 567 Valdivia, Chile. [2]Department of Animal Pathology, Faculty of Veterinary Sciences, Universidad Austral de Chile, Valdivia, Chile. [3]Department of Biomedical Sciences and Veterinary Public Health, Swedish University of Agricultural Sciences, Box 7028, SE-750 07 Uppsala, Sweden. [4]Division of Epidemiology and Community Health, School of Public Health, University of Minnesota, Minneapolis, Minnesota, USA.

References
1. Levett PN. Leptospirosis. Clin Microbiol Rev. 2001;14:296–326.
2. Adler B, Moctezuma A. *Leptospira* and Leptospirosis. Vet Microbiol. 2010;27:287–96.
3. Ellis WA. Leptospirosis as a cause of reproductive failure. Vet Clin North America Food Animal Pract. 1994;10:463–78.
4. Zamora J, Riedemann S, Montecinos MI, Cabezas X. Isolation of *Leptospira* serovars Hardjo and Kennewicki from apparently normal cattle. Arch Med Vet. 1991;23:131–5.
5. Zamora J, Riedemann S. Animales silvestres como reservorios de Leptospirosis en Chile. Una revisión de los estudios efectuados en el país. Arch Med Vet. 1999;31:151–6.
6. Salgado M, Otto B, Sandoval E, Reinhardt G, Boqvist S. A cross sectional observational study to estimate herd level risk factors for Leptospira spp. serovars in small holder dairy cattle farms in southern Chile. BMC Vet Res. 2014;10:126.
7. Koizumi N, Yasutomi I. Prevalence of leptospirosis in farm animals. Jpn J Vet Res. 2012;60:55–8.
8. Faine S, Adler B, Bolin C, Perolat B. *Leptospira* and Leptospirosis. 2nd ed. Melbourne, Australia: Medisci Press; 1999. p. 169–84.
9. Zuerner RL, Bolin C. Differentiation of *Leptospira interrogans* isolates by IS1500 hybridization and PCR assays. J Clin Microbiol. 1997;35:2612–7.
10. Majed Z, Bellenger E, Postic D, Pourcel C, Baranton G, Picardeau M. Identification of variable-number tandem-repeat loci in *Leptospira interrogans* sensu stricto. J Clin Microbiol. 2005;43:539–45.
11. Slack AT, Dohnt MF, Symonds ML, Smythe LD. Development of a multiple-locus variable number of tandem repeat analysis (MLVA) for *Leptospira interrogans* and its application to *Leptospira interrogans* serovar Australis isolates from Far North Queensland, Australia. Ann Clin Microbiol Antimicrob. 2005;4:10.
12. Zuerner RL, Alt DP. Variable nucleotide tandem-repeat analysis revealing a unique group of leptospira interrogans serovar pomona isolates associated with California Sea Lions. J Clin Microbiol. 2009;47:1202–120.
13. Ahmed A, Engelberts MF, Boer KR, Ahmed N, Hartskeerl RA. Development and validation of a real-time PCR for detection of pathogenic Leptospira species in clinical materials. PLoS One. 2009;4:e7093.
14. De La Peña-Moctezuma A, Bulach DM, Adler B. Genetic differences among the LPS biosynthetic loci of serovars of *Leptospira interrogans* and *Leptospira borgpetersenii*. FEMS Immunol Med Mic. 2001;31:73–81.

17

In vitro antihelmintic effect of fifteen tropical plant extracts on excysted flukes of Fasciola hepatica

José Manuel Alvarez-Mercado[1], Froylán Ibarra-Velarde[1*], Miguel Ángel Alonso-Díaz[2], Yolanda Vera-Montenegro[1], José Guillermo Avila-Acevedo[3] and Ana María García-Bores[3]

Abstract

Background: Fasciolosis due to *Fasciola hepatica* is the most important hepatic disease in veterinary medicine. Its relevance is important because of the major economical losses to the cattle industry such as: reduction in milk, meat and wool production; miscarriages, anemia, liver condemnation and occasionally deaths, are estimated in billons of dollars.

The emergence of fluke resistance due to over or under dosing of fasciolides as well as environmental damage produced by the chemicals eliminated in field have stimulated the need for alternative methods to control *Fasciola hepatica*. The aim of this study was to evaluate the *in vitro* anthelmintic effect of fifteen tropical plant extracts used in tradicional Mexican medicine, on newly excysted flukes of *Fasciola hepatica*.

Results: The flukes were exposed in triplicate at 500, 250 and 125 mg/L to each extract. The efficacy was assessed as the mortality rate based on the number of live and dead flukes after 24, 48 and 72 h post-exposure. The plants with anthelmintic effect were evaluated once again with a concentration of 375 mg/L in order to confirm the results and to calculate lethal concentrations at 50%, 90% and 99% (LC_{50}, LC_{90}, and LC_{99}). Plant extracts of *Lantana camara*, *Bocconia frutescens*, *Piper auritum*, *Artemisia mexicana* and *Cajanus cajan* had an *in vitro* anthelmintic effect (P <0.05). The LC_{50}, LC_{90} and LC_{99} to *A. mexicana*, *C. cajan* and *B. frutescens* were 92.85, 210.44 and 410.04 mg/L, 382.73, 570.09 and 788.9 mg/L and 369.96, 529.94 and 710.34 mg/L, respectively.

Conclusion: It is concluded that five tropical plant extracts had promising anthelmintic effects against *F. hepatica*. Further studies on toxicity and *in vivo* biological evaluation in ruminant models might help to determine the anthelmintic potential of these plant extracts.

Keywords: Plant extracts, *Fasciola hepatica*, Anthelmintic activity, *In vitro*

Background

Fasciolosis caused by *Fasciola hepatica* has a worldwide distribution affecting cattle, sheep, goats, pigs, horses, rabbits and humans as well. It causes major economical losses to the cattle industry (estimated in billons of dollars) by decreasing milk and/or meat production, low reproductive efficiency, liver seizures in slaughterhouses, high costs to control parasitism and deaths [1,2].

The control of this disease has been based on the application of anthelmintics, but due to the development of resistance it seems that the efficacy of some chemical drugs has decreased [3,4]. The use of plants with anthelmintic activity may be an alternative to fluke control, given the great diversity of ecosystems. The opportunity of finding bioactive compounds with anti-fluke properties significantly increases because, secondary metabolites (SM) are the most important compounds as new alternatives for parasite control. Some SM such us alkaloids, saponins, skimmiarins A and C, tannins, flavonoids, terpenes (mono, di and sesquiterpenes) have been shown to be active against a wide range of parasites [5].

* Correspondence: ibarraf@unam.mx
[1]Departamento de Parasitología, Facultad de Medicina Veterinaria y Zootecnia, Universidad Nacional Autónoma de México. Cd. Universitaria, C.P. 04510 México, DF, Mexico
Full list of author information is available at the end of the article

Recent studies have reported the anthelmintic effect of plants such as *Artemisia mexicana*, *Mentha piperita*, *Achillea millefolium*, *Allium sativum*, *Piper nigrum*, and *Carica papaya* with parasiticidal effects against *F. hepatica* [6-8].

Veracruz is the Mexican state with the highest livestock production in the country [9] and parasitic illnesses are the main threat to grazing bovines in this region. Because of the great diversity of ecosystems, the native vegetation of Veracruz has a wide variety of plant species (containing variable levels of SM) which potentially could be used as a fascioliscide. However, studies to evaluate the effect of plants with possible anthelmintic properties against *F. hepatica* in the area have been not carried out. The aim of the present study was to evaluate the anthelmintic effect of fifteen plants extracts from Veracruz, Mexico.

Methods
Plant material
Fresh leaves (700 g) of *Acacia cornigera* (2147 IZTA), *Acacia farnesiana* (2164 IZTA), *Artemisia absinthium* (2155 IZTA), *Artemisia mexicana* (2156 IZTA), *Bocconia frutescens* (2153 IZTA), *Cajanus cajan* (2164 IZTA), *Cordia spp*, *Hibiscus rosa – sinensis* (2149 IZTA), *Lantana camara* (2160 IZTA), *Leucaena diversifolia* (2169 IZTA), *Melia azedarach* (2161 IZTA), *Mentha sp* (2163 IZTA), *Ocimum basilicum* (2154 IZTA), *Piper auritum*

(2165 IZTA) and *Teloxys ambrosioides* (2157 IZTA) were collected from villages in Veracruz, Mexico.

Prior to the beginning of this trial, samples of different plants were collected and identified by Dr. Edith López Villafranco of the IZTA Herbarium at the Facultad de Estudios Superiores Iztacala for the purpose of authenticating them. A voucher specimen was deposited in the IZTA herbarium for future reference (a reference number was assigned). The plants were chosen based on the traditional practices [10-12]; moreover reports of other authors [7,13-15] and interviews with local people have shown to be effective in finding remedies against other parasites.

Extraction procedure
Extraction procedures were undertaken in the phytochemistry laboratory of FES Iztacala and the evaluation of in vitro anthelmintic efficacy was carried out in the laboratory of experimental chemotherapy of the parasitology department, (FMVZ-UNAM).

The leaves of each plant (100 g) were dried in an oven for three days at 60°C, ground into powder and sequentially extracted with hexane, ethyl acetate and methanol. The extracts were filtered and successively concentrated. Each extract was concentrated under low pressure at low temperature and revolutions per minute (RPM) as follows: 1) hexane, at 60°C, 50 RPM, 2) ethyl acetate, at 78°C, 60 RPM and 3) methanol, at 65°C, 90 RPM using a

Table 1 In vitro anti-fluke effectiveness of fifteen plant extracts

Plant extract		Reference control (%)[d]		Untreated control (%)[e]	Efficacy (%)[c]		
		10 mg/L	50 mg/L	0 mg/L	125 mg/L	250 mg/L	500 mg/L
A. cornigera	n = 10	100[a]	100[b]	0[a]	0[a]	0[a]	0[a]
C. cajan		100[a]	100[b]	0[a]	0[a]	0[a]	100[b]
A. farnesiana		100[a]	100[b]	0[a]	0[a]	0[a]	0[a]
L. camara		100[a]	100[b]	0[a]	0[a]	0[a]	100[b]
H. rosa - sinensis		100[a]	100[b]	0[a]	0[a]	0[a]	0[a]
B. frutescens		100[a]	100[b]	0[a]	10 ± 0.1[a]	100[b]	100[b]
M. azedarach		100[a]	100[b]	0[a]	7 ± 0.11[a]	7 ± 0.11[a]	13 ± 0.11[a]
L. diversifolia		100[a]	100[b]	0[a]	0[a]	0[a]	0[a]
C. spp		100[a]	100[b]	0[a]	0[a]	0[a]	0[a]
C. ambrosioides		100[a]	100[b]	0[a]	0[a]	0[a]	0[a]
P. auritum		100[a]	100[b]	0[a]	0[a]	0[a]	100[b]
M. sativa		100[a]	100[b]	0[a]	0[a]	0[a]	0[a]
A. absinthium L.		100[a]	100[b]	0[a]	0[a]	0[a]	0[a]
O. basiliam		100[a]	100[b]	0[a]	0[a]	0[a]	0[a]
A. mexicana		100[a]	100[b]	0[a]	100[b]	100[b]	100[b]

[a,b]A different letter between columns indicates statistically significant differences. Significant at $p < 0.05$ level. Control—nil mortality.
[c]Average of three replicates ± standard deviation.
[d]Triclabendazole, average of three replicates ± standard deviation.
[e]Destilled water, average of three replicates ± standard deviation.

Table 2 Second assessment of anti-fluke effectiveness of five plant extracts

Plant extract		Reference control (%)[d]		Untreated control (%)[e]	Efficacy (%)[c]			
		10 mg/L	50 mg/L	0 mg/L	125 mg/l	250 mg/l	500 mg/l	500 mg/l
A. mexicana	n = 10	100[a]	100[b]	0[a]	93 ± 0.06[b]	100[a]	100[a]	100[a]
B. frutescens		100[a]	100[b]	0[a]	0[a]	100[b]	100[b]	100[b]
L. camara		100[a]	100[b]	0[a]	0[a]	0[a]	93 ± 0.06[b]	100[b]
P. auritum		100[a]	100[b]	0[a]	0[a]	0[a]	83 ± 0.06[b]	100[b]
C. cajan		100[a]	100[b]	0[a]	0[a]	0[a]	93 ± 0.06[b]	93 ± 0.06[b]

[a,b]A different letter between columns indicates statistically significant differences. Significant at p < 0.05 level. Control—nil mortality.
[c]Average of three replicates ± standard deviation.
[d]Triclabendazole, average of three replicates ± standard deviation.
[e]Distilled water, average of three replicates ± standard deviation.

rotaevaporator [16,17]. The plant extracts were kept in the dark at 4°C until tested.

Bioassays

To determine the antihelmintic effect of the 15 plant extracts on the mortality of excysted flukes a series of in vitro experiments were undertaken. Newly excysted flukes were obtained by the artificial excysment of *F. hepatica* metacercariae following the methodology described by Ibarra and Jenkins [18].

Formulation of plant extracts for screening

All compounds were formulated as follows: 500 mg of the compound were placed in a screw-capped 15 ml Eppendorf® tube to which 0.1 ml of methanol were added to dissolve the extract. Then two fold dilutions using distilled water were made to prepare concentrations of 500, 250 and 125 mg/L.

Plant extracts were placed in NUNC® culture dishes. Each well contained 1.6 mL of RPMI-1640® of the culture medium, 0.2 mL of solubilized extract and 0.2 ml containing 10 liver flukes. Four wells were used as untreated controls, three containing only a complete medium (RPMI-1640®), the last one containing a culture medium and 0.2 ml of methanol. In addition there were four more wells containing triclabendazole (SOFOREN®, Novartis) at a 10 and 50 mg/L, respectively. Each test remained incubated at 37°C for four days under a 5%

CO_2 atmosphere; each experiment was replicated three times.

The plant extracts with in vitro anthelmintic efficacy higher than 80% were re-evaluated twice in order to confirm the results, and a concentration of 375 mg/L was added to calculate the lethal concentration to kill 50%, 90% and 99% of the flukes (LC_{50}, LC_{90} and LC_{99}). All procedures were performed under aseptic conditions using a laminar flow hood.

Test interpretation

The flukes under study were examined at 24, 48 and 72 hours post-exposure. Activity was measured by comparing the survival of the treated flukes relative to those of the control group. At each evaluation time, these flukes without motility were considered as dead.

Efficacy measurement

The effectiveness of the plant extracts was assessed with the following formula [19]:

$$\text{Efficacy}(\%) = \frac{\text{No. of flukes alive in control group} - \text{No. of flukes alive in treated group}}{\text{No. of flukes alive in control group}} \times 100$$

When an extract showed an in vitro efficacy greater than 80%, it was considered to possess fascioliscide activity.

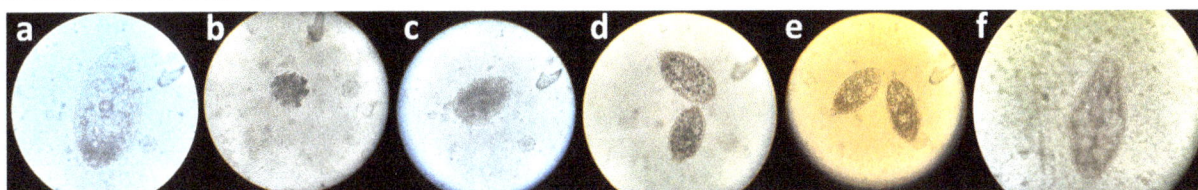

Figure 1 Flukicide activity of plant extracts. a. Untreated control flukes. **b**. Flukes treated with *L. camara* extract 72 hrs post exposition. Dead flukes being severely affected in the tegument and internal organs. **c**. Flukes treated with *A. mexicana* extract 72 hrs post exposition. Flukes showed no motility and internal changes. **d**. Flukes treated with *P. auritum* extract 72 hrs post exposition. Flukes showed no motility and no internal changes. **e**. Flukes treated with *C. cajan* extract 72 hrs post exposition. Flukes showed no motility and no internal changes. **f**. Flukes treated with *B. frutescens* extract 72 hrs post exposition. Flukes showed no motility, but presented internal changes and litghtly affected tegument.

Table 3 Lethal concentration estimates from plant extracts with anthelmintic efficacy in vitro

Plant extract	LC$_{50}$ (mg/L)	LCL-UCL	LC$_{90}$ (mg/L)	LCL-UCL	LC$_{99}$ (mg/L)	LCL-UCL	SD	x^2 (df = 10)
A. mexicana	92.85	42.16-124.50	210.44	166.78-306.78	410.04	288.46-1135.26	±2.197	5.893
C. cajan	382.73	327.13-444.12	570.09	479.89-908.48	788.9	603.92-1768.3	±3.653	15.258
B. frutescens	369.96	318.77-419.83	529.94	457.78-748.36	710.34	567.74-1298.47	±3.813	14.702

LC50 — lethal concentration that kills 50% of the exposed flukes, LC90 — lethal concentration that kills 90% of the exposed flukes, LC99 — lethal concentration that kills 99% of the exposed flukes, UCL: upper confidence limit; LCL: lower confidence limit, SD: standard deviation. x^2 — Chi-square; df: degree of freedom. Significant at p < 0.05 level.

Phytochemical screening

The active extracts were subjected to phytochemical analysis to determine the presence of SM groups following standard published protocols [20,21].

Statistical analyses

A Kruskal-Wallis test, P <0.05 was used to determine significant differences [22] and a PROBIT test was performed with POLO PLUS [23] to determine the LC$_{50}$, LC$_{90}$ and LC$_{99}$ of the extracts that showed in vitro fascioliscide efficacy.

Results

Efficacy of the extracts

The flukes placed in the control wells remained alive and healthy throughout all the tests. From 15 plants evaluated (Table 1), five plant extracts at different dose levels effectively killed *Fasciola hepatica* (P <0.05). At a dose of 500 mg/L, *C. cajan*, *L. camara* and *P. auritum* had an efficacy of 100%, while *B. frutescens* and *A. mexicana* had a 100% efficacy at a dose of 125 mg/L.

The five extracts showing *in vitro* anthelmintic activity greater than 80% are indicated in Table 2. These were evaluated for a second time including a concentration of 375 mg/L to determine LC$_{50}$, LC$_{90}$ and LC$_{99}$. The results were consistent with the previous one described above.

Figure 1 shows the flukicide activity before and after exposition with some plant extracts at 40×.

Lethal concentration estimates at 50%, 90% and 99% for exposed flukes to plant extracts

The slopes LC 50, LC 90 and LC 99% in *A. mexicana*, *C. cajan* and *B. frutescens* tested plant extracts are shown in Table 3. *A. mexicana* showed significantly lower LC$_{50}$, LC$_{90}$ and LC$_{99}$ than *C. cajan* and *B. frutescens*, but it was not possible to calculate LC for *P. auritum* and *L. camara* due to their high efficacy (100%), but it was possible to be done in the two higher doses.

Phytochemical screening

Table 4 shows that most crude extracts contain MS such as alkaloids, phenolic compounds as well as coumarins, flavanones and flavonoids. Furthermore, sesquiterpen lactones, steroids, triterpenes and glycosides were also detected.

Discussion

Plant extracts currently represent a potencial alternative for the effective control of fasciolosis in domestic ruminants. However, since this area has been explored only to a limited extent, there is a manifest need to carry out new research to determine their potential against *F. hepatica*.

Jeyathilakan et al. [24] evaluated on *Fasciola gigantica* adults the efficacy of ethno-medicinal plant aqueous extracts such as *Allium sativum*, *Lawsonia inermis*, and *Opuntia ficus indica* in vitro in comparison with Oxyclozanide with efficacies from 40 – 100%. Jeyathilakan et al.

Table 4 Results of phytochemical screening

Colorimetric reaction	Plant extract				
	L. camara	B. frutescens	P. auritum	C. cajan	A. mexicana
Phenolic compounds (FeCl3)	++	+	++	++	+
Coumarins (UV)	–	++	–	–	+
Flavanones (NH3)	+ Yellow	–	+ Yellow	+ Yellow	+ Yellow
Flavonoids (Shinoda)	–	–	+ Red	+ Orange	+ Red
Sesquiterpene lactones (Baljet)	+	–	+	+	+
Alkaloids (Meyer)	+++	+++	+++	+++	+++
Alkaloids (Dragendorff)	+++	+++	+++	+++	+++
Steroids and triterpenoids (Liberman, Burchard)	++	++	+	+	+
Glycosides (α-naphtol)	–	–	–	–	+

Symbology: –– negative; + weak positive; ++ positive; +++ strong positive.

[25] evaluated the essential oils of *Cymbopogan nardus* and *Azadirachta indica*. The results indicate that the essential oil of citronella showed a potential anthelmintic activity (100%) whereas neem oil did not show any significant effect. Their results indicated the potential for developing herbal-based anthelmintics to control *F. gigantica* in livestock.

In this study, five plant extracts showed fascioliscide activity: *A. mexicana*, *B. frutescens*, *L. camara*, *P. auritum* and *C. cajan* (P <0.05). Recent studies have reported that, at the same concentrations used in our study, *A. mexicana* extract had an anthelmintic of efficacy 100% [19,26]. The latter findings show that at the doses tested, *A. mexicana* has an intrinsic anti-fluke activity; it also indicates that this extract may be an alternative to the chemical control of *F. hepatica* only after evaluation and *in vivo* toxicity studies. In this regard, studies by Ibarra-Moreno et al. [27] in CD1 mice demonstrated that the *A. mexicana* extract had no toxicity in renal or liver tissue.

To our knowledge, this is the first report of the anthelmintic effect of *P. auritum*, *B. frutescens* and *C. cajan* against *F. hepatica*. Although these plants have not been evaluated against trematodes before, they are found to possess some interesting and additional positive characteristics which deserve to be considered for future *in vivo* studies. For example, Ghanem et al. [28] reported a protective and an antioxidant effect in the plants of the Piperaceae family as well in *P. auritum* with cultured hepatocytes of mice. In addition, Estrada et al. [29] mention that acute toxicity tests show that the intake of extracts of different polarities of *P. auritum* involves no health risks. Kundu et al. [30] have also found in the *C. cajan* extract a hepato protective effect on mice. Since there are no reported toxic effects of these plants, it is possible to obtain a similar *in vivo* effect by direct administration to ruminants.

Up to now there have been no reports of anti-fluke effectiveness for *L. camara* despite its well – known toxicity in cattle and sheep. This is the first report of *in vitro* anthelmintic activity in the *L. camara* extract. However, it is necessary to consider the undesirable effects such as photosensitivity and liver disorders that are caused in the animals that consume this plant. If this plant demonstrates great anthelmintic activity in continued studies, there will be sufficient reason for further study in order to identify the causal agents responsible for this toxicity. It is, therefore, convenient to find other species of *Lantana spp* that have no toxicity reports [31].

Secondary metabolites such as alkaloids, terpenes, tannins or flavonoids contained in crude plant extracts have been related to parasiticidal activity [32-35]. Nevertheless, since these are not the only compounds that these and other plant species possess, it would be wrong to discard the effect of other bioactive compounds. Hence, it is necessary to determine the chemical composition of the extracts that show anthelmintic efficacy. Interestingly, all extracts gave a positive reaction for alkaloids. The literature shows reports of the presence of these compounds in *L. camara* [36], *B. frutescens* [37], and *P. auritum* [38], but not in *C. cajan* and *A. mexicana*. It is likely that the positive reactions in the latter species are due to the presence of nitrogen compounds such as amino acids or other amines of a non-alkaloid origin. These alkaloids are probably responsible for the biological activity; however, there are reports of non-nitrogenous substances isolated from these plants with biocide activity as well as pentacyclic triterpenoids isolated from *L. camara* [39] and sterols and sesquiterpene lactones isolated from *C. cajanus* [40] and *A. mexicana* [41], respectively.

Consequently, the present study represents preliminary information for the continuing research to demonstrate whether the data obtained can be amplified or not in order to get their SM to determine finally whether it is one SMs or a combination of SM responsible for fascioliscide activity.

Conclusion

Of the fifteen extracts tested, five showed promising in vitro fascioliscide efficacy, thus indicating that they could possibly be strong candidates for further biological and toxicological analyses aimed at demonstrating their real potential for liver fluke control in ruminants.

Competing interests
The authors of this manuscript have no financial or personal relationships with other people or organizations that could inappropriately influence or bias the content of the paper.

Authors' contributions
FIV, MAAD, YVM and JGAA contributed to conception and design of the study. JMAM, AMGB were responsible for execution and data collection. JMAM and MAAD were primarily responsible for data analysis and interpretation and all authors were involved in drafting the manuscript critical reading, editing and final approval of the submitted version.

Acknowledgments
This research was supported by the Council of Science and Technology (CONACYT, Mexico) and Project UNAM-DGAPA-PAPIIT IN 220313. We are thankful to Dr. Estephanie Ibarra Moreno, for her kind technical assistance in the evaluation of extracts.

Author details
[1]Departamento de Parasitología, Facultad de Medicina Veterinaria y Zootecnia, Universidad Nacional Autónoma de México. Cd. Universitaria, C.P. 04510 México, DF, Mexico. [2]Centro de Enseñanza Investigación y Extensión en Ganadería Tropical, Facultad de Medicina Veterinaria y Zootecnia, Universidad Nacional Autónoma de México, Km. 5.5, Carretera Federal Tlapacoyan-Martínez de la Torre, C.P. 93600 Veracruz, Mexico. [3]Lab. de Fitoquímica, UBIPRO, Facultad de Estudios Superiores Iztacala, UNAM, Avenida de los Barrios 1, C.P. 54090 Edo. de México, Mexico.

References

1. OPS (Organización Panamericana de la Salud). Zoonosis y enfermedades transmisibles comunes al hombre y a los animales. USA: OPS; 2003.
2. FAO. (Food and Agriculture Organization of the United Nations). Resistencia a los antiparasitarios. Estado actual con énfasis en América Latina. Italy: FAO; 2003.
3. Ceballos L, Moreno L, Alvarez L, Shaw L, Fairweather I, Lanusse C. Unchanged triclabendazole kinetics after co-administration with ivermectin and methimazole: failure of its therapeutic activity against triclabendazole-resistant liver fluke. BMC Vet Res. 2010;6:1–8.
4. Olaechea F, Lovera V, Larroza M, Raffo F, Cabrera R. Resistance of *Fasciola hepatica* against triclabendazole in cattle in Patagonia (Argentina). Vet Parasitol. 2011;178:364–6.
5. Anthony JP, Fyfe L, Smith H. Plant active components – a resource for antiparasitic agents? Trends Parasitol. 2005;21:462–8.
6. Vera-Montenegro Y, Ibarra-Velarde F, Ramirez-Avila G, Munguia-Xochihua J. In vitro fasciolicide activity of some plant extracts against newly excysted flukes. Ann NY Acad Sci. 2008;1149:180–2.
7. Singh TU, Kumar D, Tandan SK, Mishra KS. Inhibitory effect of essential oils of Allium sativum and Piper longumon spontaneous muscular activity of liver fluke, Fasciola gigantica. Exp Parasitol. 2009;123:302–8.
8. Ferreira JFS, Peaden P, Keiser J. In vitro trematocidal effects of crude alcoholic extracts of *Artemisia annua, A. absinthium, Asimina triloba, and Fumaria officinalis*: trematocidal plant alcoholic extracts. Parasitol. 2011;109:585–1592.
9. INEGI (Instituto Nacional de Estadística, Geografía e Información). Boletín de información oportuna del sector agropecuario. Aguascalientes: Instituto Nacional de Estadística, Geografía e Informática; 2010.
10. Cano ALM. Flora Medicinal de Veracruz I. Inventario Etnobotánico. México: Universidad Veracruzana; 1997.
11. Columba M. Plantas medicinales utilizadas en el estado de Morelos. México: Universidad Autónoma del estado de Morelos; 2007.
12. Rodríguez A, Coombes J, Jimenez R. Plantas silvestres de Puebla: herbario y jardín botánico BUAP. México: Herbario BUAP; 2009.
13. Fernandes FF, Freitas SEP. Acaricidal activity of an oleoresinous extract of Copaifera reticulata (Leguminosae: Caesalpinioideae) against larvae of the southern cattle tick, Rhipicephalus (Boophilus) microplus (Acari: Ixodidae). Vet Parasitol. 2007;147:150–4.
14. Camurça-Vasconcelos ALF, Bevilaqua CML, Morais SM, Maciel MV, Costa CTC, Macedo ITF, et al. Anthelmintic activity of Lippia sidoides essential oil on sheep gastrointestinal nematodes. Vet Parasitol. 2008;154:167–70.
15. Alonso-Díaz MA, Torres-Acosta JFJ, Sandoval-Castro CA, Hoste H. Comparing the sensitivity of two in vitro assays to evaluate the anthelmintic activity of tannin rich plant extracts against Haemonchus contortus. Vet Parasitol. 2011;181:360–4.
16. Harnborne JB. Phytochemical phylogeny; proceedings of the Phytochemical Society Symposium. London: Academic; 1970.
17. Trease GE. Tratado de farmacognosis. México: Interamericana; 1987.
18. Ibarra OF, Jenkins DC. An in vitro screen for new fasciolicidal agents. Z Parasitenkd. 1984;70:655–61.
19. Ibarra-Moreno S, Ibarra-Velarde F, Ávila-Acevedo JG. In vitro evaluation of anthelmintic activity with hexane, methanol and ethyl acetate with extracts processed and obtained from some mexican plants used in traditional medicine based on ethno Botanical Studies. Am J Plant. 2012;3:506–11.
20. Evans WC. Trease and Evans' Pharmacognosy. 15th ed. Edinburgh, U.K: Saunders Ltd; 2002.
21. Sampietro DA, Sgariglia M, Soberón J, Quiroga E, Vattuone M. (2009) Colorimetric reactions. In: Sampietro D, Catalan C, Vattuone M, editors. Isolation, Identification and Characterization of Allelochemicals/Natural Products. U.S.A: CRC Press; 2009. p. 73–101.
22. Statgraphics Centurion XVI (Computer program) Statpoint Technologies, INC. version 16.1.17(64-bits) EUA, 2011.
23. LeOra Software In: ROBERTSON JL, PREISLER HK, RUSSELL RM. (Eds.) A user's guide to Probit or Logic Analysis. Berkley, USA; 2003.
24. Jeyathilakan N, Murali k, Anandaraj A, Latha BR, Abdul Basith S. Anthelmintic activity of essential oils of Cymbopogan nardus and Azadirachta indica on Fasciola gigantica. Tamilnadu J Vet Anim Sci. 2010;6(5):204–9.
25. Jeyathilakan N, Murali K, Anandaraj A, Abdul-Basith S. In vitro evaluation of anthelmintic property of ethno-veterinary plant extracts against the liver fluke Fasciola gigantica. J Parasit Dis. 2012;36(1):26–30.
26. Elango G, Rahuman AA. Evaluation of medicinal plant extracts against ticks and fluke. Parasitol Res. 2011;108(3):513–19.
27. Ibarra-Moreno S, Ibarra-Velarde F, Ávila-Acevedo JG. Obtaining the minimum lethal dose against Fasciola hepatica in vitro using plant extract hexanes with anthelmintic activity and toxicity evaluation on CD1 male mice. Am J Plant Sci. 2012;3:899–903.
28. Ghanem MTM, Radwan HMA, Mahdy ESM, Elkholy YM, Hassanein HD, Shahat AA. Phenolic compounds from Foeniculum vulgare (Subsp. Pipertum) (Apiaceae) herb and evaluation of hepatoprotective antioxidant activity. Phcog Res. 2012;4:104–8.
29. Estrada-Reyes R, Martínez-Laurrabaquio A, Ubaldo Suárez D, Araujo-Escalona AG. Neuropharmacological studies of Piper auritum Kunth (Piperaceae): antinociceptive and anxiolytic-like effects. J Med Plants Res. 2013;7 (23):1718–29.
30. Kundu R, Dasgupta S, Biswas A, Bhattacharya A, Pal BC, Bandyopadhyay D, et al. Cajanus cajan Linn. (Leguminosae) prevents alcohol-induced rat liver damage and augments cytoprotective function. J Ethnopharmacol. 2008;118:440–7.
31. Ghisalberti EL. Review Lantana camara L (Verbenaceae). Fitoterapia. 2000;71:467–86.
32. Hoste H, Jackson F, Athanasiadou S, Thamsborg SM, Hoskin SO. The effects of tannin-rich plants on parasitic nematodes in rumiants. Trends Parasitol. 2006;6:253–61.
33. Athanasiadou S, Githiori J, Kyriazakis I. Medicinal plants for helminth parasite control: facts and fiction. Animal. 2007;1:1392–400.
34. Calzada F, Yépez-Mulia L, Tapia-Contreras A. Effect of Mexican medicinal plant used to treat trichomoniasis on *Trichomonas vaginalis* trophozoites. J Ethnopharmacol. 2007;113:248–51.
35. Von son-de Fernex E, Alonso-Díaz MA, Valles-De la Mora B, Capetillo-Leal CM. In vitro anthelmintic activity of five tropical legumes on the exsheathment and motility of *Haemonchus contortus* infective larvae. Exp Parasitol. 2012;131:413–8.
36. Ntalli NG, Caboni P. Botanical Nematicides: A Review. J Agric Food Chem. 2012;60:9929–40.
37. Montgomery CT, Cassels B, Maurice S. The Rhoeadine Alkaloids. J Nat Prod. 1983;46:441–53.
38. Parmar VS, Jain SC, Bisht KS, Jain R, Taneja P, Jha A, et al. Phytochemistry of the genus piper. Phytochemistry. 1997;46:597–673.
39. Siddiqui BS, Raza SM, Begum S, Siddiqui S, Firdous S. Pentacyclic triterpenoids from *Lantana camara*. Phytochemistry. 1995;38:681–5.
40. Akihisa T, Nishimura Y, Nakamura N, Roy K, Ghosh P, Thakur S, et al. Sterols of *Cajanus cajan* and three other leguminosae seeds. Phytochemistry. 1992;31:1769–8.
41. Mata R, Delgado G, Romo DVA. Sesquiterpene lactones of *Artemisia mexicana* var. Angustifolia. Phytochemistry. 1984;23:1665–8.

18

Evaluation of the specificity of a commercial ELISA for detection of antibodies against porcine respiratory and reproductive syndrome virus in individual oral fluid of pigs collected in two different ways

Tatjana Sattler[1,2*], Eveline Wodak[2] and Friedrich Schmoll[2]

Abstract

Background: The monitoring of infectious diseases like the porcine reproductive and respiratory syndrome (PRRS) using pen-wise oral fluid samples becomes more and more established. The collection of individual oral fluid, which would be useful in the monitoring of PRRSV negative boar studs, is rather difficult. The aim of the study was to test two methods for individual oral fluid collection from pigs and to evaluate the specificity of a commercial ELISA for detection of PRRSV antibodies in these sample matrices. For this reason, 334 serum samples from PRRSV negative pigs (group 1) and 71 serum samples from PRRSV positive pigs (group 2) were tested for PRRSV antibodies with a commercial ELISA. Individual oral fluid was collected with a cotton gauze swab from 311 pigs from group 1 and 39 pigs from group 2. Furthermore, 312 oral fluid samples from group 1 and 67 oral fluid samples from group 2 were taken with a self-drying foam swab (GenoTube). The recollected oral fluid was then analysed twice with a commercial ELISA for detection of PRRSV antibodies in oral fluid.

Results: All serum samples from group 1 tested negative for PRRSV antibodies. The collection of oral fluid was sufficient in all samples. Sampling with GenoTubes was less time consuming than sampling with cotton gauze swabs. False positive results were obtained in 7 (measure 1) respectively 9 (measure 2) oral fluid samples recollected from cotton gauze swabs and in 9 and 8 samples from GenoTubes. The specificity of the oral fluid ELISA was 97.4% for cotton gauze swabs and 97.3% for GenoTubes. 70 out of 71 serum samples and all oral fluid samples from group 2 tested positive for PRRSV antibodies. The sensitivity of the oral fluid ELISA was 100%. According to the kappa coefficient, the results showed an almost perfect agreement between serum and oral fluid collected in both ways (kappa > 0.8).

Conclusions: Both methods used for individual oral fluid collection proved to be practical and efficient and can be used for PRRSV antibody detection. It has to be considered, however, that false positive results may occur more often than in serum samples.

Keywords: PRRSV, ELISA, Swine, Cotton gauze swabs, GenoTubes, Sensitivity

* Correspondence: tasat@vetmed.uni-leipzig.de
[1]Large Animal Clinic for Internal Medicine, University of Leipzig, An den Tierkliniken 11, 04103 Leipzig, Germany
[2]Institute for Veterinary Disease Control, AGES, Robert-Koch-Gasse 17, 2340 Mödling, Austria

Background

In recent years, the applicability of oral fluid samples for diagnostics of infectious disease like porcine reproductive and respiratory syndrome (PRRS), caused by the PRRS virus (PRRSV) has seen increased discussion in scientific literature. Several methods of detecting PRRSV RNA and PRRSV antibodies (Ab), using both different molecular diagnostic methods and serological techniques, were developed [1-3]. Sampling techniques were evaluated [4] and the effect of the stabilization of the oral fluid [5] and sample processing [6] was determined with the intention to improve the results. Different ropes for the oral fluid collection were tested [6,7]. Some ELISAs, specifically developed for PRRSV Ab detection in oral fluid, show results comparable to serum ELISAs [2,8]. The usage of cotton ropes as chewing material for oral fluid collection was found to be the method of choice [6,7]. This system is highly suitable for pen-wise oral fluid collection in weaning pigs and fatteners. For individual oral fluid collection, however, especially from sows and boars, the animals have to be trained to chew on the cotton rope [4,7]. This is a time consuming measure and is not widely accepted among European pig producers. On the other hand, the continuous testing of individual animals via oral fluid sampling would be a substantial improvement in the monitoring in PRRSV negative herds like boar studs. This presupposes an easy, rapid, animal friendly and efficient sampling method as well as the uncomplicated storage and transport of the samples. Self-drying foam swabs like GenoTubes Livestock (Prionics, Schlieren, Switzerland) that were developed for the detection of minimal DNA amounts in forensic medicine have a small sample volume and can be stored at room temperature for several weeks [9].

For the collected oral fluid samples, test systems with a high specificity and sensitivity are needed, as they are continuously developed and improved for serum samples [10,11]. A recently developed ELISA detecting IgG Ab against PRRSV in individual oral fluid collected with cotton ropes has according to Kittawornrat et al. [8] a specificity of 100% (95% confidence interval at 99%, 100%) and a sensitivity of 94.7% (92.4%, 96.5%). According to the manufacturer of the cited IDEXX PRRS OF ELISA (IDEXX, Ludwigsburg, Germany), the specificity is quoted at 98.7% (92.2%, 100%) in 77 tested individual oral fluid samples whereas the sensitivity is 100% (94.2%, 100%) in 78 tested samples. For the IDEXX PRRS X3 Ab test (IDEXX), which is generally considered to be the de facto gold standard ELISA in the detection of PRRSV Ab in serum, the manufacturer quotes a sensitivity of 98.8% and a specificity of 99.9%.

The objective of the study was to test the efficacy and practicability of oral fluid collection from individual pigs via cotton gauze swabs and a dry foam swab (GenoTube)

as well as the re-collection of oral fluid from these materials. Furthermore, the specificity of the IDEXX PRRSV OF ELISA for the detection of PRRSV Ab in oral fluid collected with these methods was evaluated in comparison to the IDEXX PRRS X3 in serum samples. To ensure the sensitivity of the oral fluid ELISA, a number of PRRSV positive pigs were tested as well.

Methods

Animals and serum samples

A total of 395 pigs (405 samples) were included in the study. The pigs consisted of 2 groups. Group 1 (n = 334) included 152 boars from four German boar studs, 67 boars from one Austrian boar stud, 35 fatteners from one German pig breeding farm and 57 sows and gilts as well as 23 nursery piglets from two Austrian pig breeding farms. All farms were classified as PRRSV negative (category IV according to Holtkamp et al. [12]). Group 2 included a total of 71 samples from the following pigs: a) 39 fatteners from one Austrian and one German PRRSV positive fattening farm, b) 12 nursery piglets injected with a PRRSV type 2 strain at pre-vaccine stage and c) 20 fatteners challenged with a highly pathogenic PRRSV type 2 strain. Ten of the pigs mentioned under c) were the same as in b) and used twice for sampling with a time lag of 28 days between both sampling times. A blood sample was taken from each pig. All blood samples, except of the pigs mentioned under b) and c) in group 2, were collected in the course of monitoring programs and not taken for the purpose of this study. Housing, animal care and experimental protocol of the pigs mentioned under b) and c) were approved by the local ethics committee (Agency of the Government in Lower Austria, Department of Agrarian Law). Blood samples were centrifuged for 10 minutes at 2400 g within 4 hours after sampling and serum was kept frozen at minus 20°C until analysis.

Collection and handling of oral fluid samples

Oral fluid was collected from the above mentioned pigs in two different ways while they were fixated for blood sampling or, in case of the boars, during semen collection:

1. Individual oral fluid samples were collected via cotton gauze swab. For this purpose, the swab was held into the mouth of the respective pig with a serrefine and the oral fluid was allowed to soak into the swab (Figure 1a). The swabs were stored in a 50-ml-falcon tube at minus 20°C until re-collection of the oral fluid and analysis. For the re-collection of the oral fluid, the swab was centrifuged for 10 minutes at 2500 g in a 50-ml-falcon tube with filter (Figure 1b).

2. Individual oral fluid samples were collected via GenoTubes (Figure 2a). The GenoTubes soaked with oral fluid

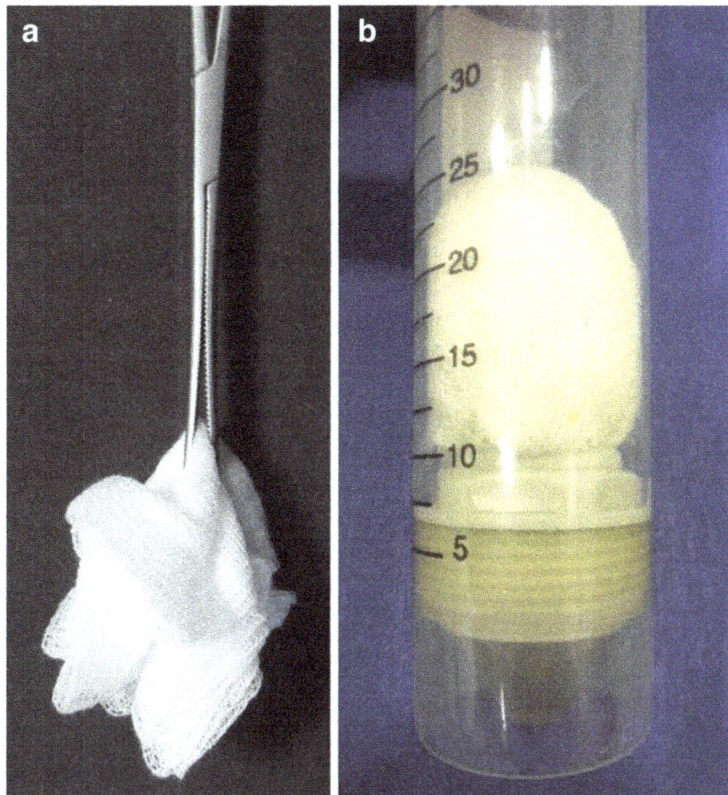

Figure 1 Oral fluid collection via cotton gauze swabs (a), centrifugation for re-collection of oral fluid (b).

were stored at room temperature up to four weeks until analysis.

Group 1: In 289 pigs oral fluid could be collected in both described ways. In 22 pigs (boars from Austria) only cotton gauze swabs were used and in another 23 pigs (nursery piglets from Austria) only GenoTubes were utilised. Group 2: Oral fluid samples were collected from 35 pigs both via cotton gauze swab and via GenoTube. In another 4 pigs only cotton gauze swabs and in 22 pigs (32 samples) only GenoTubes were collected.

Oral fluid collection was done on the same day that the blood samples were taken from the respective pigs.

Detection of PRRSV antibodies by ELISA

All serum samples were analysed with the IDEXX PRRS X3 Ab test for the presence of antibodies against PRRSV.

All oral fluid samples were analysed with the IDEXX PRRS OF ELISA, designed for detection of antibodies against PRRRSV in oral fluid. To test the reproducibility of results, samples of group 1 were tested in two different measures. The capacity of the foam swab of the GenoTube was measured experimentally. For this reason, 10 GenoTubes were dived into oral fluid for some seconds and the amount of fluid soaked into the swab was measured with weighing. The average was at approximate

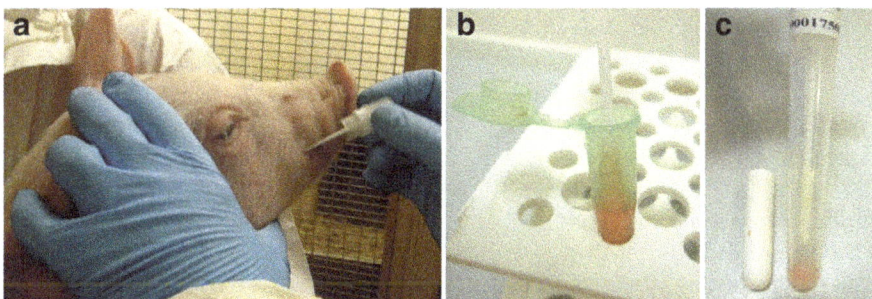

Figure 2 Oral fluid collection via GenoTubes (a), reconstitution of oral fluid by resuspension (b) and following centrifugation (c).

200 μl with no considerable deviation. To reconstitute the dried oral fluid, the foam swab of the GenoTube was re-suspended in a 1.5 ml microcentrifuge tube with 400 μl of the dilution buffer of the ELISA kit (Figure 2b) which means a 1:2 dilution of the contained oral fluid as is required in manufacturer's instructions. To remove the remaining oral fluid from the foam swab, the GenoTubes were centrifuged for 10 minutes at 2500 g after removing the SafeDry medium from the tube (Figure 2c). The gained fluid was added into the respective microcentrifuge tube.

All serum and oral fluid ELISAs were conducted according to the manufacturer's instructions. A brief description of the IDEXX PRRSV OF ELISA is given in [1]. In both ELISAs, samples with sample-to-positive (S/P) ratios ≥0.4 (cut-off value) were considered positive for PRRSV antibodies.

Statistical analysis

The specificity of the IDEXX PRRS OF ELISA in oral fluid from cotton gauze swabs and GenoTubes compared to the IDEXX PRRS X3 Ab test in serum was estimated using group 1. The sensitivity of the IDEXX PRRS OF ELISA in oral fluid from cotton gauze swabs and Geno-Tubes compared to the IDEXX PRRS X3 Ab test in serum was tested using the samples from group 2. The correlation of S/P values of the ELISAs were tested in group 2 with the correlation coefficient after Spearman. Over all samples, the accuracy of the IDEXX PRRS OF ELISA in oral fluid from cotton gauze swabs and GenoTubes was calculated. In measure one, the agreement of the IDEXX PRRS OF ELISA in oral fluid from cotton gauze swabs and GenoTubes with the IDEXX PRRS X3 Ab test in serum was determined with the kappa coefficient (κ) and interpreted according to Landis and Koch [13].

Results

Collection of oral fluid samples

From all cotton gauze swabs, a sufficient amount of oral fluid (between 0.5 and 5.0 ml) could be collected. The collection from each pig took between 30 seconds and three minutes. The limiting factor for the collection of oral fluid samples via cotton gauze swabs was the dryness of the mouth of the respective pig. This was more often the case in smaller pigs while the mouths of sows and especially breeding boars contained more oral fluid. The collection of oral fluid via cotton gauze swabs from boars during semen collection is possible without any fixation.

The collection of oral fluid with GenoTubes took only a few seconds and went therefore much faster than with cotton gauze swabs. The usage of GenoTubes in fatteners and adult pigs is mostly possible without fixation of the pig.

Detection of PRRSV antibodies by ELISA

The serum samples of all group 1 pigs tested negative for PRRSV antibodies. The calculated specificity of the serum ELISA was therefore 100%.

The results of the oral fluid ELISA from cotton gauze swabs and GenoTubes compared to the serum ELISA are shown in Table 1. The S/P values in the PRRSV antibody negative oral fluid samples ranged from 0.00 to 0.39 both in cotton gauze swabs and in GenoTubes. S/P values from false positive oral fluid samples from cotton gauze swabs ranged from 0.40 to 0.95, those from Geno-Tubes ranged from 0.41 to 0.84. In cotton gauze swabs as well as in GenoTubes, respectively, five false positive samples agreed between measure 1 and 2. No agreement of false positive samples was found between cotton gauze swabs and GenoTubes.

The S/P values of the PRRSV antibody ELISAs in group 2 can be seen in Figure 3. 70 of the 71 serum samples, all cotton gauze samples and all GenoTubes were tested positive for PRRSV antibodies. The S/P values of the positive samples in serum ranged from 0.48 to 2.60, in cotton gauze swabs from 0.89 to 8.93 and in GenoTubes from 0.44 to 8.60. The negative serum sample had a S/P value of 0.39, the S/P value of the corresponding Genotube was at 3.94. There was a positive correlation of S/P values between serum and GenoTubes ($r = 0.40$) and between cotton gauze swabs and Geno-Tubes ($r = 0.82$) in the samples of group 2.

Descriptive test parameters and measurements of agreement for all three samplings are shown in Table 2.

Discussion

In this study, two different ways of individual oral fluid sampling were evaluated for their effectiveness and

Table 1 Two-by-two contingency table comparing results of ELISA for detection of PRRSV antibodies in serum and oral fluid collected via cotton gauze swabs and GenoTubes

IDEXX PRRS OF - oral fluid			IDEXX PRRS X3 Ab - Serum	
			Negative	Positive
Cotton gauze swabs	Measure 1	Negative	304	0
		Positive	7	39
	Measure 2	Negative	302	-
		Positive	9	-
		Total	311	39
GenoTubes	Measure 1	Negative	303	0
		Positive	9	67
	Measure 2	Negative	304	-
		Positive	8	-
		Total	312	67

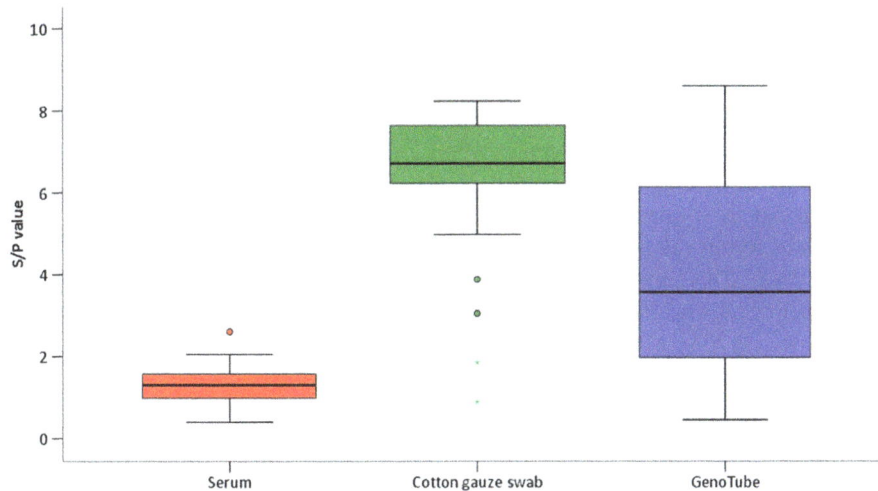

Figure 3 PRRSV antibodies in serum and oral fluid collected via cotton gauze swab and GenoTubes in PRRSV positive pigs.

practicability. Using these oral fluid samples, the descriptive test parameters of the IDEXX PRRSV OF ELISA for detection of PRRSV antibodies in oral fluid were calculated in comparison to the IDEXX PRRSV X3 ELISA in serum samples.

Until now, besides the usage of GenoTubes Livestock for DNA analysis of the tested individuals, only a few studies described the use of GenoTubes for detection of infectious agents in animals [14,15]. In the mentioned studies, *Brachyspira* DNA in rectal swabs of pigs, respectively classical and African swine fever virus DNA in wild boars were detected by PCR. One study is published that describes the usage of GenoTubes for sampling and detection of antibodies against African swine fever virus [16]. However, no study referring to the usage of GenoTubes for PRRSV antibody detection by ELISA was available until now.

Both of the sampling techniques used, cotton gauze swabs as well as GenoTubes, proved to be efficient for oral fluid collection from individual pigs. The collection by both sampling methods was successful in all pigs. Individual oral fluid collection by cotton or polyester ropes is not always that successful even in trained pigs (success between 37.5 and 87.5% of the cases) [17]. The

Table 2 Descriptive test parameters and measures of agreement of the IDEXX PRRSV OF using oral fluid collected via cotton gauze swabs and GenoTubes

	Cotton gauze swabs	GenoTubes
Specificity (%)	97.4	97.3
Sensitivity (%)	100.0	100.0
Accuracy (%)	97.7	97.6
Kappa coefficient (κ)	0.91	0.91

IDEXX PRRS X3 Ab in serum was used as reference test.

collection via cotton gauze swabs, however, was time consuming and more difficult in smaller pigs than in fatteners or adult pigs. Sampling adult boars without fixation is possible for instance during semen collection. It has to be considered, however, that the swab must be taken from within the mouth. Collection of frothy saliva around the mouth was proven to be insufficient in other studies [4]. The collection of oral fluid with GenoTubes was easier and less time consuming than with cotton gauze swabs and can be done in larger and adult pigs mostly without the fixation of the animal. The re-collection of oral fluid from GenoTubes was efficient and can be standardised. The GenoTube contains a Safe-Dry medium that causes a rapid active drying of the sample. The absence of fluid makes the samples very stable. Samples collected with a GenoTube can therefore be stored for several weeks and transported at room temperature [9].

According to the kappa coefficient, almost perfect agreement (κ > 0.80) [13] was found between ELISA results in serum and oral fluid from cotton gauze swabs and GenoTubes. The sensitivity of the ELISA was 100% in both oral fluid sample species. This number agrees with the sensitivity given by the manufacturer of the ELISA for oral fluid collected with cotton ropes. The one serum sample of group 2 that was PRRSV Ab negative in serum had a S/P value slightly beneath the cutoff, whereas the corresponding GenoTube sample was found clearly positive. It has to be considered, however, that for an accurate analysis of sensitivity a larger number of samples must be analysed. Other studies defined the sensitivity of the ELISA with 94.7%, tested in PRRSV type 2 antibody positive samples exclusively [8], and with 94.7% (n = 19) in cotton ropes and 93.3% (n = 15) in polyester ropes, tested in PRRSV type 1 inoculated pigs

[17], and were thereby lower than calculated in this study. Some false positive results can occur by analysing PRRSV antibodies in oral fluid by ELISA. The specificity of the ELISA in this study is with 97.4% for cotton gauze swabs and 97.3% for GenoTubes within the confidence interval given by the manufacturer but lower than calculated in other studies for oral fluid samples collected with cotton ropes [8]. In group 2, a correlation was found between the S/P values of serum samples and oral fluid collected with GenoTubes. This underlines the good agreement between serum and oral fluid samples found in other studies as well [17,18]. There was a strong correlation between S/P values of PRRSV ab positive oral fluid samples collected with GenoTubes and with cotton gauze swabs, confirming the reproducibility of the results of the oral fluid ELISA in samples collected with different sampling methods. The sampling techniques used in this study are therefore equally suitable for oral fluid collection and subsequent testing with the IDEXX PRRS OF ELISA as cotton ropes.

Conclusions
This study shows that oral fluid samples can be used for the PRRSV antibody detection on individual pig level. The use of GenoTubes proved to be an especially practical method both for oral fluid collection and for storage and transport of the samples. The ELISA detecting PRRSV Ab in oral fluid collected by cotton gauze swabs and GenoTubes proved to be highly sensitive. It has to be considered, however, that false positive samples needing re-testing may occur. This can cause irritations, especially in PRRSV negative farms like boar studs.

Competing interests
The authors declare that they have no competing interests.

Authors' contributions
TS: Study coordination and design, performance of ELISAs, statistical analysis, drafting of the manuscript. EW: Acquisition of data, participating in study design FS: Conceived of the study, study design. All authors read and approved the final manuscript.

Acknowledgements
The authors want to thank the teams of the department of Virology/Electron Microscopy of the Institute of Veterinary Disease Control, AGES Mödling, especially Jutta Pikalo and Manfred Berger, for excellent technical assistance. Further thanks go to Dr. Bettina Fasching, Dr. Doris Verhovsek and Dr. Oliver Habeck for organization of and help with sample taking. Financial support to this study was provided by the Verein der Freunde und Förderer der Schweinemedizin, Austria and by Sanphar Asia. We acknowledge support from the German Research Foundation (DFG) and Universität Leipzig within the program of Open Access Publishing.

References
1. Kittawornrat A, Panyasing Y, Goodell C, Wang C, Gauger P, Harmon K, et al. Porcine reproductive and respiratory syndrome virus (PRRSV) surveillance using pre-weaning oral fluid samples detects circulation of wild-type PRRSV. Vet Microbiol. 2014;168:331–9.
2. Gerber PF, Giménez-Lirola L, Halbur PG, Zhou L, Meng XJ, Opriessnig T. Comparison of commercial enzyme-linked immunosorbent assays and fluorescent microbead immunoassays for detection of antibodies against porcine reproductive and respiratory syndrome virus in boars. J Virol Methods. 2014;197:63–6.
3. Ouyang K, Binjawadagi B, Kittawornrat A, Olsen C, Hiremath J, Elkalifa N, et al. Development and Validation of an Assay To Detect Porcine Reproductive and Respiratory Syndrome Virus-Specific Neutralizing Antibody Titers in Pig Oral Fluid Samples. Clin Vaccine Immunol. 2013;20:1305–13.
4. Pepin BJ, Kittawornrat A, Liu F, Gauger PC, Harmon K, Abate S, et al. Comparison of specimens for detection of Porcine Reproductive and Respiratory Syndrome Virus infection in boar studs. Transbound Emerg Dis 2013, doi:10.1111/tbed.12135 [Epub ahead of print].
5. Decorte I, Van der Stede Y, Nauwynck H, De Regge N, Cay AB. Effect of saliva stabilisers on detection of porcine reproductive and respiratory syndrome virus in oral fluid by quantitative reverse transcriptase real-time PCR. Vet J. 2013;197:224–8.
6. Olsen C, Karriker L, Wang C, Binjawadagi B, Renukaradhya G, Kittawornrat A, et al. Effect of collection material and sample processing on pig oral fluid testing results. Vet J. 2013;198:158–63.
7. Decorte I, Van Breedam W, Van der Steede Y, Nauwynck H, De Regge N, Cay AB. Detection of total and PRRSV-specific antibodies in oral fluids collected with different rope types from PRRSV-vaccinated and experimentally infected pigs. BMC Vet Res. 2014;10:134.
8. Kittawornrat A, Prickett J, Wang C, Olsen C, Irwin C, Panyasing Y, et al. Detection of Porcine reproductive and respiratory syndrome virus (PRRSV) antibodies in oral fluid specimens using a commercial PRRSV serum antibody enzyme-linked immunosorbent assay. J Vet Diagn Invest. 2012;24:262–9.
9. Garvin AM, Holzinger R, Berner F, Krebs W, Hostettler B, Lardi E, et al. The forensiX Evidence Collection Tube and Its Impact on DNA Preservation and Recovery. Biomed Res Int. 2013;2013:105797.
10. Sattler T, Wodak E, Revilla-Fernández S, Schmoll F. Comparison of different commercial ELISAs for detection of antibodies against porcine respiratory and reproductive syndrome virus in serum. BMC Vet Res. 2014;10:300.
11. Cong Y, Huang Z, Sun Y, Ran W, Zhu L, Yang G, et al. Development and application of a blocking enzyme-linked immunosorbent assay (ELISA) to differentiate antibodies against live and inactivated porcine reproductive and respiratory syndrome virus. Virology. 2013;444:310–6.
12. Holtkamp DJ, Polson DD, Torremorell M, Morrison B, Classen DM, Becton L, et al. Terminology for classifying swine herds by porcine reproductive and respiratory syndrome virus status. J Swine Health Prod. 2011;19:44–56.
13. Landis JR, Koch GG. An application of hierarchical kappa-type statistics in the assessment of majority agreement among multiple observers. Biometrics. 1977;33:363–74.
14. Costa MO, Hill JE, Fernando C, Lemieux HD, Detmer SE, Rubin JE, et al. Confirmation that "Brachyspira hampsonii" clade I (Canadian strain 30599) causes mucohemorrhagic diarrhea and colitis in experimentally infected pigs. BMC Vet Res. 2014;10:129.
15. Petrov A, Schotte U, Pietschmann J, Dräger C, Beer M, Anheyer-Behmenburg H, et al. Alternative sampling strategies for passive classical and African swine fever surveillance in wild boar. Vet Microbiol. 2014;173:360–5.
16. Blome S, Goller KV, Petrov A, Dräger C, Pietschmann J, Beer M. Alternative sampling strategies for passive classical and African swine fever surveillance in wild boar–extension towards African swine fever virus antibody detection. Vet Microbiol. 2014;174:607–8.
17. Decorte I, Van Campe W, Mostin L, Cay AB, De Regge N. Diagnosis of the Lelystad strain of Porcine reproductive and respiratory syndrome virus infection in individually housed pigs: comparison between serum and oral fluid samples for viral nucleic acid and antibody detection. J Vet Diagn Invest. 2015;27:47–54.
18. Kittawornrat A, Engle M, Panyasing Y, Olsen C, Schwartz K, Rice A, et al. Kinetics of the porcine reproductive and respiratory syndrome virus (PRRSV) humoral immune response in swine serum and oral fluids collected from individual boars. BMC Vet Res. 2013;9:61.

19

Characterization of a caprine model for the subclinical initial phase of *Mycobacterium avium* subsp. *paratuberculosis* infection

Heike Köhler[1*], Anneka Soschinka[1,2], Michaela Meyer[1,3], Angela Kather[1,4], Petra Reinhold[1] and Elisabeth Liebler-Tenorio[1]

Abstract

Background: Paratuberculosis caused by *Mycobacterium avium* subsp. *paratuberculosis* (MAP) is difficult to control due to a long phase of clinically non-apparent (latent) infection for which sensitive diagnostics are lacking. A defined animal model for this phase of the infection can help to investigate host-MAP interactions in apparently healthy animals and identify surrogate markers for disease progress and might also serve as challenge model for vaccines. To establish such a model in goats, different age at inoculation and doses of oral inoculum of MAP were compared. Clinical signs, faecal shedding as well as MAP-specific antibody, IFN-γ and IL-10 responses were used for in vivo monitoring. At necropsy, about one year after inoculation (pi), pathomorphological findings and bacterial organ burden (BOB) were scored.

Results: MAP infection manifested in 26/27 inoculated animals irrespective of age at inoculation and dose. Clinical signs developed in three goats. Faecal shedding, IFN-γ and antibody responses emerged 6, 10–14 and 14 wpi, respectively, and continued with large inter-individual variation. One year pi, lesions were detected in 26 and MAP was cultured from tissues of 23 goats. Positive animals subdivided in those with high and low overall BOB. Intestinal findings resembled paucibacillary lesions in 23 and multibacillary in 4 goats. Caseous and calcified granulomas predominated in intestinal LNN. BOB and lesion score corresponded well in intestinal mucosa and oGALT but not in intestinal LNN.

Conclusions: A defined experimental infection model for the clinically non-apparent phase of paratuberculosis was established in goats as suitable basis for future studies.

Keywords: Experimental animal model, MAP, Goat, Faecal shedding, Antibody, IFN-γ, Culture, Pathology

Background

Paratuberculosis is a chronic granulomatous enteritis caused by *Mycobacterium avium* subsp. *paratuberculosis* (MAP) and affects domestic and wild ruminants worldwide, causing considerable economic losses for the livestock industry [1,2]. Research to improve diagnostic methods and prophylactic measures has been performed for many years, but still many questions remain unanswered. One reason is the extended clinically non-apparent initial phase of the infection and the still insufficient knowledge about the interactions between the host organism and the pathogen during this time period.

Despite large numbers of naturally MAP infected animals, elucidation of host-pathogen interactions in the early phase of the disease is only possible using the defined conditions and variables of experimental animal models. This is due to a diagnostic gap that allows in vivo identification of infected animals only after seroconversion or after the onset of faecal shedding, which become detectable late in the course of the disease with large inter-individual variation [3]. Experimental animal infection models allow the investigation of relevant numbers of animals with defined infection status and under identical conditions during the clinically non-apparent phase of disease.

* Correspondence: heike.koehler@fli.bund.de
[1]Institute of Molecular Pathogenesis, Friedrich-Loeffler-Institut, Federal Research Institute for Animal Health, Jena, Germany
Full list of author information is available at the end of the article

Experimental infections have been performed in diverse domestic species, and furthermore, in small laboratory animals [4]. Study conditions were not standardized among the experiments making comparisons difficult. Generally, age at infection, dose and frequency of inoculation, and duration of the experiment are decisive for disease development [4,5]. International guidelines for standardization of animal models for paratuberculosis have been proposed only recently [5]. While cattle, sheep and deer have been used extensively studies in goats are rare and only small numbers of animals were included [6-12]. Since marked individual variations of host immune response and lesions were observed even in the same experiment, the conclusions vary widely.

Performing experimental infections in goats has several advantages in comparison to cattle and sheep. Goats are susceptible to the three main groups of MAP, Type I, II and III [13-15]. They are considered the least naturally MAP resistant species due to a rather fast disease progress [16]. This allows a shorter duration of experiments. In a study using Angora goats, specific IFN-γ responses were observed already one month after challenge with MAP positive gut mucosa and sero-conversion as early as four months post infection (mpi). Clinical signs occurred between 22 and 29 mpi [17]. In addition, the feeding and housing requirements of goats are easier to fulfil compared to cattle.

The aim of the present study was to establish a well characterized experimental animal model for the clinically non-apparent phase of paratuberculosis in goats as a basis for future studies of the early pathogenesis of MAP infection.

Results
Clinical signs
Severe clinical signs of paratuberculosis were observed in three of the MAP-inoculated animals (3/27). One animal each of group V2 and V4 developed non-treatable diarrhea at 37 and 35 wpi, respectively, and had to be necropsied, while the third goat of group V1 was cachectic at 48 wpi. At 37, 38 and 39 wpi, 3 other goats of group V2 died or had to be euthanized because of neurologic signs. Post mortem examination revealed cerebrocortical necrosis.

Shedding of MAP
MAP was detected repeatedly in the faeces of most of the animals during the inoculation period (not shown). Shedding stopped at 1 wpi in 13 of the 14 early inoculated goats and in eight of the 13 late inoculated goats and re-emerged about 6 wpi in all animals except one goat of group V2. A large inter-individual variability of shedding in terms of intensity (not shown) and time course was observed independent from inoculation time

and dose. Essentially, three different shedding patterns occurred: animals that stopped shedding before 34 wpi (1), animals that shed MAP intermittently until necropsy (2) and animals that shed MAP continuously during the entire course of the experiment (3). Animals which had to be necropsied before the end of the observation period were not defined (Table 1).

Antibody response
The specific antibody response against MAP started at 14 wpi in the MAP-inoculated animals. The proportion of antibody positive animals as well as antibody levels increased until 22–26 wpi. S/P% varied largely between individuals with no significant differences between inoculation groups in general (Figure 1A). No seroconversion was observed in three MAP-inoculated goats from different groups (V1, V2 and V4) and in all control animals.

IFN-γ response
A specific IFN-γ response of the MAP-inoculated animals against jPPD was first detected at 10–14 wpi. IFN-γ release of the PBMC reached peak values at 22–26 wpi and decreased afterwards. At 14 and 18 wpi, the IFN-γ response of group V4 (late inoculated animals that received 20 mg bwm per dose) exceeded that of the other inoculated groups. Because of the large variation of the response within the groups, statistically significant differences between inoculation groups occurred only incidentally. In the control groups no jPPD-specific IFN-γ release was induced (Figure 1B).

IL-10 response
A marked release of IL-10 was induced by in vitro stimulation of PBMC from MAP-inoculated and control animals with jPPD at 6–14 wpi (K1, V1 and V2, Figure 2A) or 6–10 wpi (K2, V3 and V4, Figure 2B). Time course and magnitude of the response differed between early and late inoculated groups including the respective controls with peak responses at 14 wpi in group K1, V1 and V2 and at 10 wpi in groups K2, V3 and V4. The control groups tended to have a lower IL-10 response than the two age matched MAP-inoculated groups. This was more pronounced in the younger animals (K1, V1 and V2). At later sampling dates the IL-10 response of all groups decreased considerably (Figure 2A and B).

Bacterial organ burden (BOB)
MAP was culturally isolated after necropsy from at least one tissue sample of 23 of the 27 MAP-inoculated goats. The four MAP negative goats belonged to the groups V1 (n = 2), V2 (n = 1) and V4 (n = 1). These animals were allocated to BOB category I. MAP positive animals could be sub-divided into two categories (Table 2):

Table 1 Faecal shedding of MAP before and after oral inoculation and shedding category of animal

Group	Animal No.	Week p. i. -3	1	6	10	14	18	22	26	30	34	38	42	44	46	Shedding category[a]
K1	1	-	-	-	-	-	-	-	-	-	-	-	-	-	-	-
	2	-	-	co.	-	-	-	-	-	-	-	-	#			-
	3	-	n.a.	-	-	-	-	-	-	-	-	-	-	-	-	-
	4	-	-	co.	-	-	-	-	-	-	-	-	-	-	-	-
	5	-	-	co.	-	-	-	-	-	-	-	-	-	-	-	-
	6	-	-	-	-	-	-	-	-	-	-	-	-	-	-	-
V1	7	-	-	X	X	X	X	X	X	-	-	-	-	-	-	1
	8	-	-	X	X	X	X	X	X	X	X	X	X	X	X	3
	9	-	-	X	X	X	X	X	X	X	X	X	X	X	X	3
	10	-	-	X	X	X	X	X	X	X	X	X	X	X	X	3
	11	-	-	X	X	X	X	X	X	X	-	-	-	-	-	1
	12	-	-	X	X	X	X	X	X	X	-	-	-	-	-	1
	13	-	-	X	X	X	-	-	-	-	-	X	X	X	X	2
V2	14	-	-	X	X	X	X	X	X	-	X	-	#			nd
	15	-	-	X	X	-	-	X	-	-	-	-	X	-	-	2
	16	-	-	X	X	X	X	X	X	X	-	#				nd
	17	-	X	X	X	X	X	X	-	-	-	-	#			nd
	18	-	-	X	X	X	X	X	X	-	-	-	-	-	-	1
	19	-	-	-	X	X	X	X	X	X	X	X	X	X	X	3
	20	-	-	X	X	-	-	-	n.a.	-	-	-	#			nd
K2	21	-	-	-	-	-	-	-	-	-	-	-	-	-	-	-
	22	-	-	-	-	-	-	-	-	-	-	-	-	-	-	-
	23	-	-	-	-	-	-	-	-	-	-	-	-	-	-	-
	24	-	-	-	-	-	-	-	-	-	-	-	-	-	-	-
	25	-	-	-	-	-	-	-	-	-	-	-	-	-	-	-
	26	-	-	-	-	-	-	-	-	-	-	-	-	-	-	-
V3	27	-	X	X	X	X	X	-	-	X	X	X	X	X	X	2
	28	-	-	X	X	X	X	X	X	X	-	-	-	-	-	1
	29	-	X	X	X	X	X	X	-	-	-	-	-	#		nd
	30	-	-	X	X	X	X	X	-	-	-	-	-	X	-	2
	31	-	-	X	X	X	-	-	-	-	-	-	-	-	-	1
	32	-	X	X	X	X	-	X	-	-	-	-	-	-	-	1
V4	33	-	-	X	X	X	X	X	X	-	-	X	-	X	-	2
	34	-	-	X	X	-	-	-	-	-	-	-	X	-	-	2
	35	-	X	X	X	X	X	X	X	X	X	X	X	X	X	3
	36	-	-	X	X	X	-	-	-	-	X	#				nd
	37	-	-	X	X	X	X	X	X	X	X	X	X	X	X	3
	38	-	-	X	X	X	X	-	-	-	-	-	-	-	-	1
	39	-	X	X	X	-	-	-	-	-	-	-	-	-	-	1

[a]Shedding category: 1 – stopping before 34 wpi; 2 – intermittent; 3 – continuously; **X**, positive faecal culture; n.a., not available; co., contaminated; #, animal no longer available (necropsy); nd, not defined.

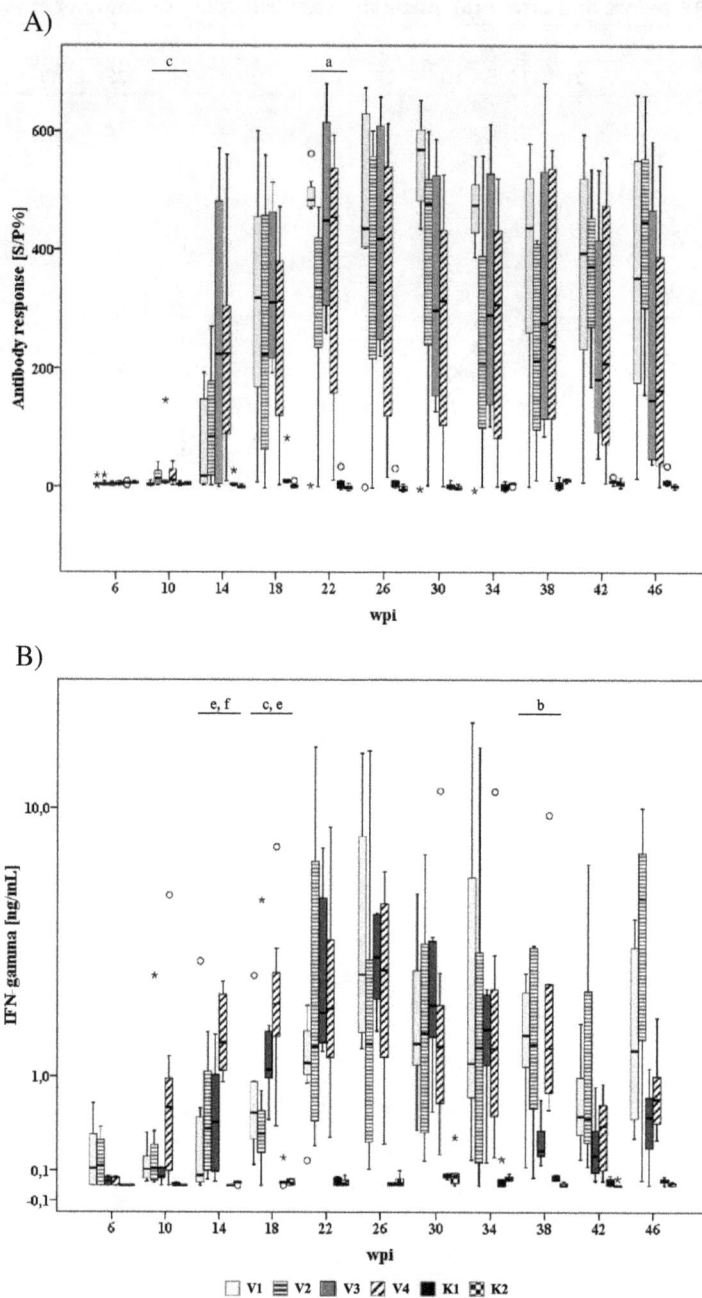

Figure 1 Time course and intensity of MAP-specific antibody response (A) and antigen-induced (Johnin, 4 µg/mL) IFN-γ response (B) of **inoculated and control goats.** Box and Whisker Plot represents median value, 25% and 75% percentiles (box), range, outlier values (o), and extreme values (*). Different letters indicate significant differences between groups (Mann–Whitney-U test, P ≤ 0.05): a – V1 vs. V2, b – V1 vs. V3, c – V1 vs. V4, d – V2 vs. V3, e – V2 vs. V4, f – V3 vs. V4.

BOB category II: Animals that harbored only low to moderate amounts of MAP in intestinal tissues and associated lymph nodes. The proportion of MAP positive organs varied largely between these animals. MAP could be recovered most often from the ICV-LN, followed by the M-LN and ICVPP. The IPP and the mucosa of the duodenum were positive only in a few cases.

BOB category III: Animals that had moderate to very high amounts of MAP in most of the samples from intestinal tissues and associated lymph nodes. High amounts of MAP were most frequently recovered from the ICV-LN, the proximal and median jejunal LN and the mucosa of the mid jejunum.

MAP was also isolated from extra-intestinal tissue of nine animals, three from group V1, two each from groups

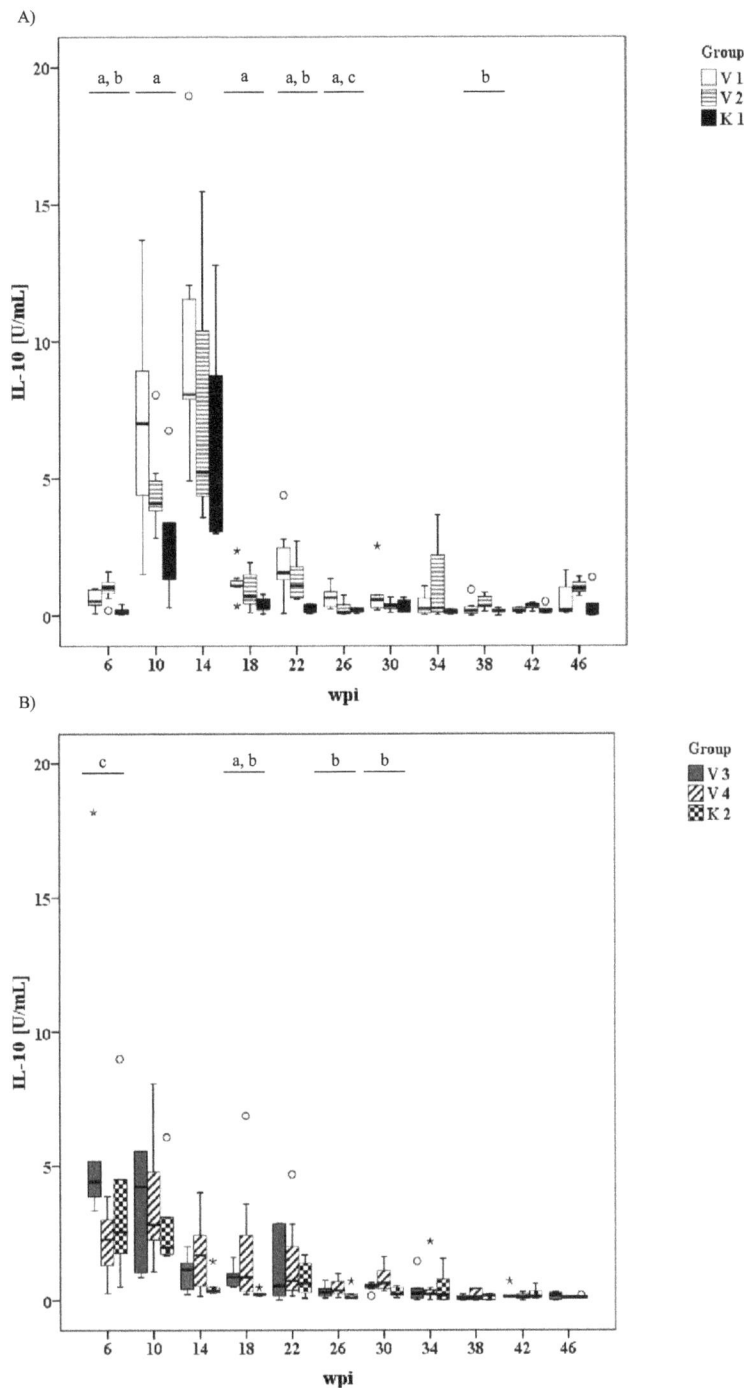

Figure 2 Time course and intensity of the antigen-induced (Johnin, 4 μg/mL) IL-10 response of early inoculated goats (A) and late inoculated goats (B) and the corresponding control animals. Box and Whisker Plot: see Figure 1. Different letters indicate significant differences between groups (Mann-Whitney-U test, P ≤ 0.05): Figure 2A: a – K1 vs. V1, b – K1 vs. V2, c – V1 vs. V2; Figure 2B: a – K2 vs. V3, b – K2 vs. V4, c – V3 vs. V4.

V2 and V4 and one from group V3. Regarding lymphatic tissue, the hepatic LN was most often positive (n = 8), followed by the retropharyngeal LN (n = 5) and the tonsils (n = 2). MAP was isolated from liver of five and spleen of two animals (Table 3). Notably, most tissue samples of the

cachectic goat were MAP positive, including superficial cervical LN, kidney, diaphragm and gluteal muscle (not shown).

On the individual animal level, no marked differences in the BOB of intestinal lymph nodes, oGALT and

Table 2 Cultural detection of MAP in intestinal mucosa, oGALT and intestinal lymph nodes of the MAP-inoculated goats at necropsy

Group	Animal No.	Jejunal LNN prox.	Jejunal LNN median	Jejunal LNN distal	Ileocol LN	LNN BOB	LNN BOB cat.	JPP	IPP prox.	IPP distal	ICVPP	PCPP	oGALT BOB	oGALT BOB cat.	Duoden	Jejunum 1	Jejunum 2	Jejunum 3	Intestine BOB	Intestine BOB cat.	Summary BOB cat.
V1	7	0[a]				0	I[b]				0	0	0	I	0	0	0	0	0	I	I
	8[c]	3.85	25.00	25.00	37.50	22.84	III	25.00	0	20.14	21.53	21.53	17.64	III	25.00	8.42	8.33	20.14	15.47	III	III
	9	22.63	50.00	40.00	40.00	38.16	III	40.00	35.00	40.00	62.50	co.	44.38	III	co.	23.57	40.00	40.00	34.52	III	III
	10	15.00	32.50	25.00	40.00	28.13	III	38.75	33.33	26.25	co.	co.	32.78	III	7.50	40.00	38.75	37.50	30.94	III	III
	11	0	4.96	6.75	6.25	4.49	II	0	0	0	3.13	0	0.63	II	co.	0	16.52	0	5.51	II	II
	12	0	0	0	0	0	I	0	0	0	co.	0	0	I	0	0	0	0	0	I	I
	13	17.80	11.11	0	22.22	12.78	II	0	0	0	22.22	5.56	5.55	II	0	16.67	16.67	25.00	14.58	II	II
V2	14[d]	0	0	7.29	0	1.82	II	0	0	co.	8.33	0	2.08	II	0	0	co.	0	0	I	II
	15	16.67	8.33	8.33	8.33	10.42	II	16.67	0	4.17	0	8.33	5.83	II	0	8.33	0	0	2.08	II	II
	16[e]	12.46	8.33	10.06	0	7.71	II	14.38	16.67	12.79	12.11	0	11.19	II	0	12.84	0	5.55	4.60	II	II
	17[f]	0	0	0	7.50	1.88	II	n.a.	0	0	0	1.85	0.46	II	0	0	0	0	0	I	II
	18	0	0	0	0	0	I	0	0	0	0	0	0	I	0	0	0	0	0	I	I
	19	6.25	20.83	25.00	31.89	20.97	III	20.83	11.11	26.39	16.67	co.	18.75	III	0	16.67	20.83	20.83	14.58	II	III
	20[g]	0	0	0	0	0	I	0	0	0	0	0	0	I	0	16.67	0	0	0.42	II	I
V3	27	17.14	12.33	15.48	36.61	20.39	III	4.17	9.72	15.47	16.67	8.33	10.87	II	0	15.08	32.14	20.24	16.87	III	III
	28	13.26	14.44	4.17	9.33	10.30	II	8.33	2.17	0	9.33	co.	4.96	II	5.00	8.33	11.11	10.00	8.61	II	III
	29	0	4.80	5.88	0	2.67	II	co.	0	0	5.00	co.	1.67	II	co.	0	0	0	0	I	II
	30	0	3.75	0	8.69	3.11	II	16.67	0	2.50	10.00	33.33	12.50	II	0	10.00	0	0	2.50	II	II
	31	0	0	0	8.63	2.16	II	co.	0	0	0	co.	0	I	co.	0	0	0	0	I	II
	32	0	0	0	2.00	0.5	I	0	0	0	0	0	0	I	0	0	0	0	0	I	I
V4	33	10.24	12.54	9.42	20.51	13.18	II	4.76	0	0	0	18.89	4.73	II	0	8.33	25.00	0	8.33	II	II
	34	9.40	16.91	0	11.11	9.35	II	co.	0	0	0	0	0	I	0	0	19.09	8.33	6.86	II	II
	35	33.33	33.33	1.85	41.67	27.55	III	37.37	0	25.00	16.67	20.21	19.85	III	4.17	16.67	25.00	16.67	15.62	III	III
	36[h]	8.89	13.29	16.67	0	9.71	II	0	10.00	8.33	14.34	13.33	9.20	II	3.33	0	co.	0	1.11	II	II
	37	35.00	30.00	35.00	40.00	35.00	III	33.33	23.81	8.33	co.	4.76	17.56	III	0	33.33	35.71	10.00	19.76	III	III
	38	6.67	0	18.75	15.86	10.31	II	co.	0	co.	0	0	0	I	0	co.	co.	0	0	I	II
	39	0	0	0	0	0	I	0	0	0	0	0	0	I	0	co.	co.	0	0	I	I

[a]Growth Index [b]BOB category: I, no growth; II, BOB ≤ 15; III, BOB > 15; [c]cachectic; [d]died 39 wpi; [e]necropsied 37 wpi, diarrhea; [f]died 37 wpi; [g]necropsied 35 wpi, diarrhea; [h]necropsied 38 wpi; diarrhea; prox. proximal; Ileocol Ileocolic; Duoden Duodenum; n.a. not available.

Table 3 Cultural isolation of MAP and lesions in extra-intestinal sites

Group	Animal No.	Liver Culture	Liver glnf	Liver MAP-IHC	Hepatic LN Culture	Hepatic LN glnf	Hepatic LN MAP-IHC	Spleen Culture	Spleen glnf	Spleen MAP-IHC	Retropharyngeal LN Culture	Retropharyngeal LN glnf	Retropharyngeal LN MAP-IHC	Tonsil Culture	Tonsil glnf	Tonsil MAP-IHC
V1	7	0[a]	0	0	0	0	0	0	0	0	0	0	0	0	0	0
	8	33.33	+++[b]	0	25.00	++	0	12.50	0	0	10.42	0	0	26.04	++	0
	9	0	0	0	13.93	0	0	0	0	0	0	0	0	0	0	0
	10	21.78	++	0	14.16	0	0	11.46	0	0	0	0	0	0	0	0
	11	0	0	0	0	0	0	0	0	0	0	0	0	0	0	0
	12	0	+	0	0	0	0	0	0	0	0	0	0	0	0	0
	13	0	0	0	0	0	0	0	0	0	0	0	0	0	0	0
V2	14[c]	co.	0	0	0	++	0	0	0	0	0	0	0	0	0	0
	15	0	0	0	0	0	0	0	0	0	0	0	0	0	0	0
	16[c]	0	0	0	1.9	+	0	0	0	0	5.26	0	0	0	0	0
	17[c]	0	0	0	0	++	0	0	0	0	0	0	0	0	0	0
	18	0	0	0	0	0	0	0	0	0	0	0	0	0	0	0
	19	0	+++	0	6.6	++	0	0	0	0	4.16	+	0	3.57	0	0
	20[c]	0	0	0	0	0	0	0	0	0	0	0	0	0	0	0
V3	27	12.50	0	0	8.33	0	0	0	0	0	0	0	0	0	0	0
	28	co.	0	0	0	0	0	0	0	0	0	0	0	0	0	0
	29	0	0	0	0	0	0	0	0	0	0	0	0	0	0	0
	30	0	0	0	0	0	0	0	0	0	0	0	0	0	0	0
	31	0	0	0	0	0	0	0	0	0	0	0	0	0	0	0
	32	0	0	0	0	0	0	0	0	0	0	0	0	0	0	0
V4	33	0	0	0	0	0	0	0	0	0	0	0	0	0	0	0
	34	0	0	0	0	0	0	0	0	0	0	0	0	0	0	0
	35	16.78	0	0	8.33	0	0	0	0	0	8.33	0	0	0	0	0
	36[d]	0	0	0	0	0	0	0	0	0	0	0	0	0	0	0
	37	4.29	0	0	22.50	0	0	0	0	0	7.94	0	0	0	0	0
	38	co.	0	0	0	0	0	0	0	0	0	0	0	0	0	0
	39	co.	0	0	0	0	0	0	0	0	0	0	0	0	0	0

[a]Growth Index [b]granulomatous infiltrate: 0, none; +, mild, focal; ++, moderate, multifocal; +++, severe, diffuse; [c]necropsy at 37–39 wpi; [d]necropsy at 35 wpi; co. contaminated; na. not available; glnf, granulomatous infiltrate; MAP IHC, MAP antigen detected by IHC.

intestinal mucosa could be detected in animals with BOB category III, while variability was higher in category II animals. Culturally negative and the two categories of culturally positive animals were distributed over all inoculation groups.

Gross pathology

Macroscopic lesions were most frequently (21 out of 27 goats) seen in mesenteric and ileocolic lymph nodes and oGALT, especially JPPs. Affected lymph nodes were enlarged and had areas of necrosis and calcification varying from 1 mm to extensive throughout the entire lymph node (Figure 3A). JPPs had reduced thickness and were indented in most of the goats (Figure 4A), in a few goats they were thickened and firm (Table 4). The surface was occasionally ulcerated. Chronic villous serositis was regularly seen at the serosal aspect of altered JPPs (Figure 4B). Lesions were inconsistently seen in the IPP, ICVPP and PCPP. Both intestinal lymph nodes as well as oGALT were altered in most goats. Intestinal wall outside oGALT was affected less frequently (12 out of 27 goats, Table 4). Multiple small (0.5–2 cm) foci of thickened intestinal mucosa were seen in the small intestine of seven, thickening of segments in three and of the entire length in another three goats. The latter was associated with corrugated intestinal mucosa. Thickened and nodular lymphatics were frequent in the altered segments of intestine. Intestinal lesions were restricted to the small intestine and were seen only in goats which had also lesions in JPPs and intestinal lymph nodes. All goats from the control groups and one goat of groups V3 and V4 each were without paratuberculous lesions. A few helminths were seen in a few goats of all groups.

Histopathology and immunohistochemistry for MAP

Histopathology confirmed the macroscopic lesions in intestinal lymph nodes (Table 4). Granulomas with extensive central necrosis and calcification surrounded by a variable amount of granulomatous infiltrate, fibrocytes and lymphocytes predominated (Figure 3B). Small amounts of mycobacterial material (paucibacillary) were regularly seen by IHC in the necrotic centers (Figure 3C). Multibacillary lesions were seen in four of the early inoculated goats (Figure 3D). Multifocal granulomatous infiltrates of epitheloid cells and multinucleated giant cells (MGCs) were seen in subcapsular sinuses, along trabeculae and adjacent to granulomas in 18 goats additionally to granulomas and in 2 goats as only lesions. Single mycobacteria were detected occasionally in these infiltrates.

To allow better comparison with immunologic and bacterial culture data, lesions in intestinal lymph nodes were scored as no lesions (category I), mild lesions (category II) or severe lesions (category III). Animals with category III lesions predominated. Goats with mild lesions were particularly frequent in V3. One goat of V2 and three of V4 had no lesions in intestinal lymph nodes (category I).

Macroscopic lesions in JPPs were confirmed in all affected goats by histology. In the majority of goats (16 out of 20), the architecture of the organized lymphoid tissue was markedly altered with few and small lymphoid follicles and severe and sometimes complete loss of interfollicular lymphoid tissue (Figure 5A). Lesions were characterized by small focal to multifocal groups of epitheloid cells and few MGCs and extensive infiltration with lymphocytes and plasma cells (lesion type C, Figure 5B). The mucosal surface was irregular with occasional ulcers. A mild to severe chronic fibro-proliferative serositis was seen regularly. Lesions were paucibacillary in one goat, multibacillary in one goat and without mycobacteria by IHC in 14 goats (Figure 5C). In three goats, small granulomatous infiltrates without changes of the tissue architecture were seen in addition (lesion type A). Two goats from the early inoculated groups had more extensive

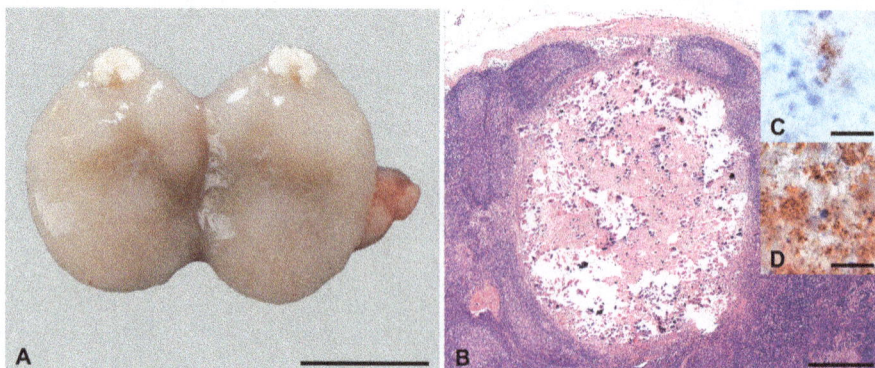

Figure 3 Lesions in mesenteric lymph nodes. Enlarged lymph node with focal necrosis and calcification (**A**, goat 9, bar = 1 cm), granuloma with extensive necrosis and calcification (**B**, goat 38, HE, bar = 500 μm). Small foci of granular staining for mycobacteria possibly associated with a degenerated cell were seen in granulomas of most goats (**C**, goat 11, immunohistochemistry MAP, bar = 10 μm), numerous mycobacteria throughout granulomas in 4 goats (**D**, goat 19, immunohistochemistry MAP, bar = 10 μm).

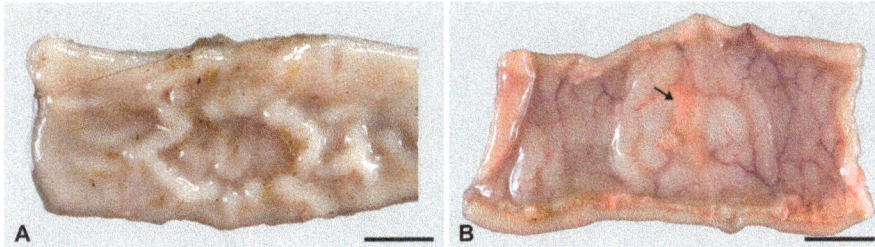

Figure 4 Lesions at Peyer's patches. Indented Peyer's patch in jejunum. (**A**, goat 13). Circumscribed villous serositis (arrow) is frequent in altered Peyer's patches (**B**, goat 31). Bar = 1 cm.

infiltrates of epitheloid cells and MGCs admixed with lymphocytes predominantly in the interfollicular areas (lesion type B). Mycobacteria were not detected in type A and B lesions by IHC. Multifocal, moderate to severe infiltrates of predominantly epitheloid cells (lesion type D) occurred in one goat of group V1 and one goat of group V4 (Figure 6A, B). Numerous mycobacteria were present in the epitheloid cells of these lesions (Figure 6C). Comparable lesions were detected in other sites with oGALT, e.g. IPP, ICVPP, PCPP and in the rectum, but less frequently.

Lesions in the intestine outside oGALT were characterized by multifocal infiltrates of epitheloid cells and few MGCs. MGCs predominated in small and focal lesions which were often missed by the macroscopic examination. Mycobacteria were detected in 3 of the 15 goats with intestinal lesions.

Lesions in oGALT and small intestine were also classified as lesions category I to III. Besides the extent of lesions and number of mycobacteria detected by IHC, the number of oGALT (n = 7) and intestinal sites (n = 5) collected for histology with lesions was included. A mix of goats with all lesions categories were seen in all groups. Goats with lesions category II in oGALT and without lesions (category I) in small intestine were more frequent in group V2.

Association between lesion category and BOB category

A clear association between lesion and BOB category was noted in oGALT and small intestinal tissue (Table 5, A and B). No to mild lesions predominated in those tissues where no bacterial growth had been detected. Tissues with bacterial organ burden were characterized by mild to severe lesions, the strongest association between severe lesions and high BOB was noted in the oGALT. In contrast, no association between lesion and BOB category could be established in the intestinal lymph nodes. Severe lesions predominated in LNN with low and even without BOB (Table 5, C).

Discussion

A well characterized experimental model for the clinically non-apparent phase of paratuberculosis was established which fulfils the following requirements for the experimental design [18]: (1) defined host, (2) standardized infection, (3) standardized stage of disease, (4) appropriate controls.

Goats of the breed Thüringer Wald Ziege were selected as host species. This is an independent native German breed of dairy goats which has been maintained without cross-breeding since 1935 [19]. All kids came from one pedigree herd with no history of clinical paratuberculosis. Freedom from disease had been verified by the negative outcome of faecal culture of all adult goats prior to purchase of the kids and was confirmed by lack of lesions as well as negative results of faecal and tissue culture of all control animals.

For standardization of the infection special attention was paid to the strain selection and preparation of the inoculum. The isolate used for inoculation (JII-1961) is a Type II (C-) strain of MAP genetically highly similar to K10 (P. Möbius, personal communication). It was isolated from the ICV-LN of a dairy cow with paratuberculosis [20]. The inoculum was prepared from a bacterial stock which had been established after a few passages of the isolate. Aliquots of this stock are available for further experiments. The MAP dose was standardized as recommended [5] by adjusting the bacterial wet mass used for preparation of the inoculum.

Four different inoculation regimens were compared in order to optimize the model to be representative for the clinically non-apparent phase of the disease. Three animals of the group inoculated with the high dose at early age developed neurological signs which could not be attributed to MAP infection. An association between cerebrocortical necrosis and paratuberculosis has not been reported in the literature.

In addition to clinical signs, the course of the disease was monitored in vivo by four parameters (faecal shedding, specific serum antibodies against MAP, antigen-induced IFN-γ and IL-10 response), which have also been used by other investigators (reviewed by [5]), thus allowing comparison between studies. The blood parameters in particular were seen as surrogates of host-pathogen interactions in clinically healthy animals.

Table 4 Lesions in intestinal lymph nodes, oGALT and small intestine of the MAP-inoculated goats at necropsy: macroscopic and histological lesions and MAP detection by IHC

Group	Anim. No.	Mesenteric and ileocolic LNN				oGALT (e.g. JPP, #of sites examined = 7)					Small intestine (#of sites examined = 5)					Lesion cat. summary
		Macro	Histo	MAP IHC	Lesion cat. LNN	Macro	Histo	MAP IHC	#of sites affected	Lesion cat. oGALT	Macro	Histo	MAP IHC	#of sites affected	Lesion cat. intestine	
V1	7	✓,e	G	2	III	–	–	0	0	I	–	–	0	0	I	II
	8	✓,e	G, glnf	2	III	✓	mf, D	2	7	III	✓,E	mf +++	2	4	III	III
	9	✓,e	G, glnf	1	II	✓	mf, C	2	5	III	✓,S	mf ++	0	4	III	III
	10	✓,f	G, glnf	1	III	✓	mf, C	1	4	III	✓,S	mf +	2	4	III	III
	11	✓,e	G, glnf	1	III	✓	f/mf, C/A	0	2	II	–	f +	0	1	I	II
	12	✓,e	G	1	III	–	–	0	0	I	–	–	0	0	I	II
	13	–	glnf	1	II	✓	f/mf, B	0	1	II	✓,MF	mf +	0	2	II	II
V2	14[a]	✓,e	G, glnf	1	III	✓	f, C	0	3	II	–	–	0	0	I	II
	15	–	–	0	I	✓	mf, C	0	1	II	✓,MF	–	0	0	I	II
	16[a]	✓,e	G, glnf	1	III	✓	mf, B	0	3	II	✓,E	mf ++	0	4	III	II
	17[a]	✓,e	G, glnf	1	III	✓	mf, C	0	1	II	–	–	0	0	I	II
	18	✓,e	G, glnf	2	II	✓	mf, C	0	3	II	–	–	0	0	I	II
	19	✓,e	G, glnf	2	III	✓	mf/d, C	0	6	III	✓,S	mf ++	0	4	III	III
	20[a]	✓,f	G, glnf	1	II	–	–	0	0	I	–	–	0	0	I	II
V3	27	✓,f	G	0	II	✓	mf, C/A	0	5	III	✓,S, MF	f +	0	1	II	II
	28	✓,e	G, glnf	1	II	✓	mf, C	0	1	II	✓,MF	f ++	0	3	II	II
	29	✓,f	G, glnf	1	II	✓	f, C	0	2	II	–	–	0	0	I	II
	30	✓,f	G, glnf	1	II	✓	mf, C	0	4	III	–	–	0	0	I	II
	31	–	glnf	0	II	–	–	0	0	I	–	–	0	0	I	II
	32	✓,e	G, glnf	1	III	✓	f, C	0	2	II	–	f ++	0	1	II	II
V4	33	✓,e	G, glnf	1	III	✓	f/mf, C/A	0	2	II	✓,MF	mf +	0	1	II	II
	34	–	–	0	I	✓	mf, C	0	1	II	–	f +	0	2	II	II
	35	✓,e	G, glnf	1	III	✓	mf, C	0	7	III	✓,MF	mf ++	0	4	III	III
	36[b]	–	–	0	I	✓	mf, C	0	4	III	–	f +	0	1	I	II
	37	✓,e	G, glnf	1	III	✓	mf, D	2	4	III	✓,MF	mf +/++	1	4	III	III
	38	✓,e	G, glnf	1	III	–	–	0	0	I	–	–	0	0	I	II
	39	–	–	0	I	–	–	0	0	I	–	–	0	0	I	I

✓ paratuberculous lesion; – no paratuberculous lesion; G granuloma; glnf granulomatous infiltrate; LNN lymph nodes; MAP IHC MAP detected by IHC; nd not done; [a] necropsy at 37–39 wpi; [b] necropsy at 35 wpi; 0 no MAP; 1 paucibacillary; 2 multibacillary; f focal; mf multifocal; e extensive; A–D type of histological lesion (see text); +, ++, +++ mild, moderate, severe granulomatous infiltrates; E entire small intestine with thickened intestinal wall and corrugated mucosa; S segments of small intestine with thickened intestinal wall and corrugated mucosa; MF 0.5 – 2 cm thickening of the intestinal mucosa with central depression; lesion categories: I – no lesions; II – mild lesions; III – severe lesions.

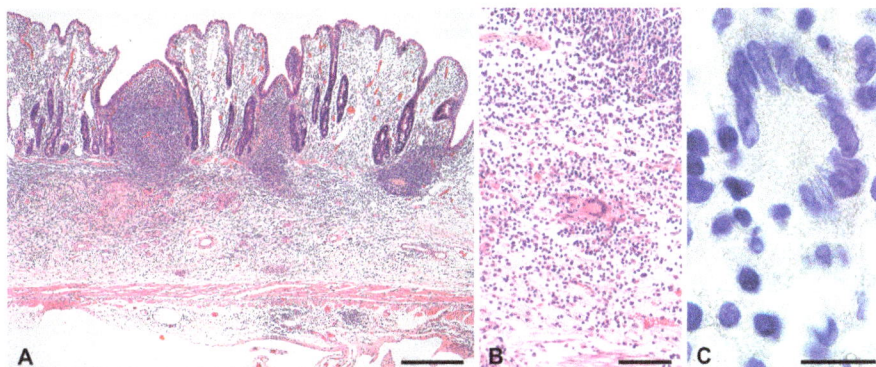

Figure 5 Severely atrophic Peyer's patch in jejunum lacking lymphoid follicles and interfollicular areas, but with marked villous serositis. (**A**, goat 28). The organized lymphoid tissue is replaced by multiple small foci of epitheloid cells and MGCs and an extensive infiltrate of lymphocytes and plasma cells (**A**, **B** higher magnification of **A**, HE). There are no mycobacteria in the granulomatous infiltrate (**C**, immunohistochemistry MAP). Bar in A = 500 μm, bar in B = 100 μm, bar in C = 10 μm.

The experiment was terminated about one year after inoculation independent of the appearance of clinical signs. At that time, the proportion of animals that developed clinical signs characteristic of paratuberculosis was rather low and independent from group allocation. Tissue lesions and level of tissue colonization with MAP were quantified as measure for the manifestation and dissemination of the infection. The results confirmed that the majority of the inoculated goats were in the clinically non-apparent phase of paratuberculosis. The results of the in vivo parameters indicate that even the animal without signs of infection at necropsy (goat no. 39) had undergone transient infection.

Appropriate numbers of age-matched control animals of the same origin were included in the study and examined in the same manner as the inoculated goats. The animals were kept in a separate room of the same animal facility as the inoculated groups to assure similar environmental, feeding and housing conditions. They were neither exposed to nor infected by MAP as proven by the results of the examinations conducted in vivo and after necropsy. This confirms that the applied sanitary and management measures were sufficient to prevent unwanted carry-over of MAP.

Onset and time course of faecal shedding, antibody response, and antigen-specific IFN-γ response was similar to one [10] and completely different from another study in goats [6], further supporting the need for standardization of the model. In both studies the total inoculation doses were considerably higher than in the present one, and the goats were challenged with a MAP strain of caprine origin whereas our goats received an isolate of bovine origin. Differences in virulence or host adaptation of the MAP strains used for inoculation have to be taken into account. However, direct comparison of the virulence of bovine and caprine MAP isolates for goats has not been performed yet. Higher responsiveness and/or a quicker onset of the host response to C-strains of MAP in comparison to S-strains has been demonstrated in sheep, goats, cattle [16,17,21] and deer [22]. Another explanation might be a different susceptibility of different goat breeds to MAP although scientific evidence is lacking [23].

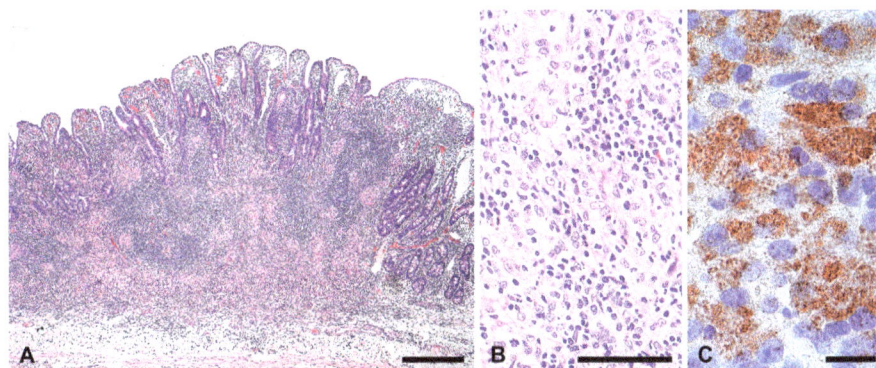

Figure 6 Jejunum Peyer's patch with severe granulomatous infiltrate. (goat 37, **A**, **B** higher magnification of A, HE). Many mycobacteria in the granulomatous infiltrate (**C**, immunohistochemistry MAP). Bar in A = 500 μm, bar in B = 100 μm, bar in C = 10 μm.

Table 5 Relation between histological score and bacterial organ burden of selected organs

		Bacterial organ burden category (n)				p χ²-test (Pearson)
	A) Intestinal mucosa	I	II	III	Total	
Lesion category (n)	I	9	3	0	12	0.002
	II	1	5	1	7	
	III	0	4	4	8	
	Total	10	12	5	27	
	B) oGALT	I	II	III	Total	
	I	6	0	0	6	≤ 0.001
	II	3	9	0	12	
	III	0	3	6	9	
	Total	9	12	6	27	
	C) Intestinal LNN	I	II	III	Total	
	I	1	3	0	4	0.703
	II	1	5	2	8	
	III	3	7	5	15	
	Total	5	15	7	27	

In the present experiment, IFN-γ response and antibody response started almost at the same time. This matches with findings in naturally infected goats where the onset of the IFN-γ response usually preceded the humoral response, but positive antibody titers could sometimes be seen simultaneously with, or even prior to the IFN-γ response [24]. The paradigm of a Th1 over Th2 dominancy in the early stages of MAP infection, that has been postulated for many years, is challenged by these data, which are further confirmed by the results of experimental MAP infections of sheep [25]. Considerable variation of the individual host responses was seen in the further course of the experiment which is in agreement with findings in naturally infected goats [24,26] as well as experimentally infected sheep [21,25] and cattle [16].

Transient elevation of antigen-induced IL-10 release by PBMC was observed in MAP-inoculated and control goats up to 14 wpi depending on the age at inoculation, with significantly higher levels in MAP-inoculated animals compared to age–matched controls (K1) in the early inoculated groups (V1, V2). Similar findings were reported from calves after experimental oral inoculation of mucosal scrapings from a cow with clinical paratuberculosis [27]. It can be speculated that a transient anti-inflammatory response is induced in very young goats shortly after MAP infection which is subsequently down-regulated by a strong IFN-γ response indicative of pro-inflammatory mechanisms. In a leprosy model, IFN-γ differentially modulated IL-12 and IL-10 production resulting in up-regulation of IL-12 and down-regulation of IL-10 release in response to *Mycobacterium leprae* stimulation [28].

Morphological investigation and cultivation of MAP from tissues collected at necropsy one year after inoculation were used to confirm the infection. Lesions and/or MAP were detected in 26 of the 27 goats inoculated indicating a very high infection rate. This has been reported in several other studies in goats and confirms the good reproducibility of MAP-infection using this model [10,17,29,30]. Lesions induced by the experimental infection were comparable to those in natural infection [31,32]. There were minor differences: (1) Naturally infected goats had a higher frequency of diffuse lesions in the small intestine indicating a more advanced stage of infection in the goats sampled at slaughter [31,32]. (2) JPP and ICVPP were most consistently affected in the present and other experimental studies [30,33], whereas lesions predominated in IPP, terminal ileum and ICVPP in naturally infected goats and also some experimental studies [29,31,32,34]. Lesions were seen in intestinal lymph nodes in similar frequency as in oGALT, whereas other studies report a predominance of lesions in intestinal lymph nodes [29]. These differences might be related to the sampling procedures. (4) The number of intestinal lymph nodes with caseous and calcified granulomas was markedly higher compared to naturally infected goats [31]. It remains unresolved whether virulence of the MAP strain, stage of infection or susceptibility of the breed have contributed to this. Caseous and calcified granulomas are characteristic of MAP infection in goats and not common in other ruminant species. They may allow comparative studies for other mycobacterial infections even beyond the scope of paratuberculosis.

Isolation of MAP from tissues was not possible in four of the inoculated goats, confirming findings in other experimental studies [6,7,9]. Obviously, the organism was cleared to a large extent or changed to a viable-but-non-culturable state after manifestation of infection, since all four goats shed MAP until at least 10 wpi, all mounted a specific IFN-γ response, and tissue lesions were found in three of them. Culture results were assessed semi-quantitatively, an approach utilized only in a few other published studies in goats and sheep [10,29,35]. This allowed allocation of the animals to BOB categories as a prerequisite for additional comparative analyses. In agreement with another experimental study [6] viable MAP was most often recovered from lymph nodes and to a lesser extent from intestinal mucosa and oGALT. In contrast, no difference in the proportion of positive lymph nodes and intestinal samples was obvious in naturally infected adult goats [26]. This seems to be due to the more advanced stage of the disease in these animals in comparison to the experimental studies. Viable MAP was also recovered from extra-intestinal sites, pointing to dissemination of the organisms already in the clinically non-apparent phase of the disease and confirming findings in experimentally [10] and naturally infected goats [26].

Two different doses of MAP and two different age periods for inoculation were compared in order to identify the optimal infection regimen. There was considerable inter-individual variation in faecal shedding, the in vivo-host responses, BOB and lesions at necropsy, but no significant differences between the treatment groups except for an earlier onset of the IFN-γ response and a reduced IL-10 response in the animals that received high MAP doses starting at 42 days after birth (group V4). This is not unexpected, since the modifications of the inoculation dose and the age at inoculation were only minimal in the present experiment in comparison to other studies performed in sheep and deer [22,35-37].

The readout parameters, lesion scores and BOB, used at the end of the experiment were closely matching in the intestinal tract, but markedly different in the intestinal LN. Differences between lesion scores and BOB were more frequent in goats with milder lesions where oGALT and intestinal mucosa were not uniformly affected. In the intestinal LN, histological classification did not allow conclusions about BOB. In particular, low BOB was associated with no, mild and severe lesions. These differences are not unexpected, since the lesions reflect tissue damage caused by MAP and the reaction of the host to MAP, and cultural results the ability of MAP to survive, replicate and spread. It can be speculated that MAP is more efficiently cleared from intestinal LN than from mucosa or oGALT because of tissue-specific control mechanisms. The granulomas that predominated in the intestinal LN may either allow the host to control the mycobacterial infection or MAP to persist [38].

Overall lesion and BOB categories showed agreement in the majority of goats. Only in three goats, MAP was not cultivated, but caseous and calcifying granulomas were present in intestinal lymph nodes and in three goats, lesions were considered severe, but BOB was low. Two factors might have contributed to these discrepancies: (1) the massive host immune response – seen as severe lesions - may have reduced the amount of viable MAP in the tissue and (2) organization and removal of lesions after the clearance of the pathogen take an extended period of time. Lesions and BOB categories will allow subgrouping of animals for retrospective analyses of in vivo data.

Conclusions

A well characterized experimental animal model of paratuberculosis was established in goats. The lack of clinical signs and the finding of paucibacillary lesions in the majority of goats indicate that this experimental model targets as intended the clinically non-apparent phase of infection. Monitoring of host-pathogen interaction in vivo and post mortem findings confirmed inter-individual differences in the progress of disease and will allow subgrouping for comparative investigations. This animal model provides the basis for future studies of pathogenesis and early diagnosis of MAP infection.

Methods
Legislation and ethical approval
This study was carried out in strict accordance with European and National Law for the Care and Use of Animals. The protocol was approved by the Committee on the Ethics of Animal Experiments and the Protection of Animals of the State of Thuringia, Germany (Permit Number: 04-002/08). All experiments were done in containment of biosafety level 2 under supervision of the authorized institutional Agent for Animal Protection. During the entire study, every effort was made to minimize suffering.

Animals
Thirty nine male goats kids (breed: 'Thüringer Wald Ziege') were included. Animals originated from a conventionally raised herd of dairy goats with no history of clinical paratuberculosis. Before purchase, all adult goats of the herd were tested once for the presence of MAP by faecal culture and were proved to be negative. Clinically healthy goat kids aged 3 to 5 days and weighing between 2.6 and 6.0 kg (4.01 ± 0.76 kg; mean

± SD) were transferred to the animal facility of the Friedrich-Loeffler-Institut in Jena.

The goats were allocated to six different groups (n = 6-7) considering weight at birth, age, sire and dam in order to prevent full siblings in the same group, get an equal distribution of the offspring of one sire over the groups and adjust the mean body weight and the mean age of the groups. Throughout the entire study, animals of the different groups were kept in separate rooms but under equal housing and feeding conditions, and in accordance with international guidelines for animal welfare [39,40].

Feeding was adjusted to the age-dependent nutritional needs of the animals. The kids received goat milk from the herd of origin up to day 8 after birth, then commercial milk replacer for goat kids (Denkamilk capritop, Denkavit, Warendorf, Germany) up to the age of 10 weeks. Water, mineral blocks without copper, containing 37 % sodium, 1.1 % calcium, 0.6 % magnesium and trace elements (Mineralleckstein ohne Kupfer, esco – european salt company, Hannover, Germany) and hay were supplied *ad libitum* during the whole course of the experiment. Small amounts of pelleted concentrates were offered already during milk feeding. After weaning protein rich pelleted concentrates for goats (Alleinfuttermittel für Ziegenmastlämmer and Milchleistungsfutter II, both LHG Landhandelsgesellschaft, Schmölln, Germany) containing vitamin A, D3 and E were fed. The ration of concentrates was gradually increased up to 500 grams per day. None of the given feed contained antibiotics. The animals were castrated at the age of 12 weeks. During the whole course of the experiment the animals were neither treated with systemic antibiotics nor immunosuppressive drugs.

Study design

Four of the six groups were challenged with MAP (V1 – V4; n = 6-7), two groups served as controls (K1, K2; n = 6, Table 6). With respect to the suggested guidelines [5,23], four different inoculation regimens were compared. Treatment of the groups differed as follows: Oral inoculation with MAP started 3–5 days post natum

(dpn) for two early inoculated groups (V1, V2) and at 42 dpn for two late inoculated groups (V3, V4). Inoculation was performed ten times every two to three days. One group each of the early and the late inoculated goats received 10 mg bacterial wet mass (bwm, V1, V3) per dose, the others received 20 mg bwm of MAP per dose (V2, V4). The age matched controls were sham-inoculated at the same time (K1 starting at 3–5 dpn, K2 starting at 42 dpn, Table 6).

Each goat underwent daily clinical examination from the beginning of the experiment until necropsy. Parameters to follow the course of infection were faecal shedding of MAP, antibody response in serum and specific IFN-γ and IL-10 responses of peripheral blood mononuclear cells (PBMC). Individual blood and faecal samples were collected to examine humoral immune response and faecal shedding of MAP before the first inoculation and in regular intervals after inoculation. The amount of blood that could be collected from very young goat kids was limited because of animal welfare reasons, therefore, testing of the cellular immune response started only 5–6 weeks post inoculation (wpi) and continued until necropsy (Figure 7).

As scheduled, goats were euthanized and necropsied about 12 months after the last inoculation. A few animals died or had to be necropsied earlier for animal welfare reasons (Table 6). Gross and histologic lesions, amount of MAP in lesions detected by immunohistochemistry, and bacterial organ burden were recorded. Emphasis was laid on elaboration of detailed qualitative and semi-quantitative scoring systems for bacteriological and pathomorphological parameters.

Preparation of bacteria used for inoculation

A low passage MAP field isolate from the ICV-LN of a cow (JII-1961) was propagated in Middlebrook 7H9 broth (MB, Becton Dickinson, Heidelberg, Germany) containing glycerine (Merck, Darmstadt, Germany), OADC (Becton Dickinson, Heidelberg, Germany) and Mycobactin J (Allied Monitor, Fayette, MO, US) at 37 ± 2 °C. No antibiotics were added. After centrifugation,

Table 6 Study design: group allocation, time point and dose of inoculation and time point of necropsy

Start of inoculation period	3-5 dpn			41-43 dpn		
Group	K1	V1	V2	K2	V3	V4
Number of animals (n)	6	7	7	6	6	7
Inoculation dose per day (mg bwm)	-	10	20	-	10	20
Average bacterial counts/mL	-	$2.08 \pm 0.57 \times 10^7$		-	$1.62 \pm 0.73 \times 10^7$	
Average bacterial counts/inoculum	-	2.08×10^8	4.16×10^8	-	1.62×10^8	3.24×10^8
Total inoculation dose	-	2.08×10^9	4.16×10^9	-	1.62×10^9	3.24×10^9
Time of necropsy (wpi)	48[a]	48	49[b]	46	47	48[c]

dpn, days post natum; bwm, bacterial wet mass; wpi, weeks post infection; [a]one animal was necropsied at 39 wpi; [b]one animal each died at 37 and 39 wpi, one animal each was necropsied at 37 and 38 wpi; [c]one animal was necropsied at 35 wpi.

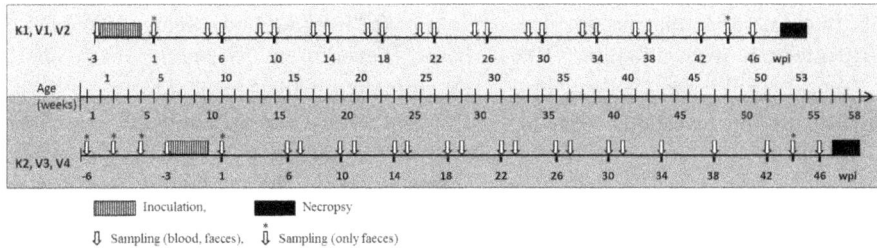

Figure 7 Schematic representation of the time course of the experiment. Challenge time and dose, animal number: V1 – 3–5 dpn, 10 mg bwm, n = 7; V2 – 3–5 dpn, 20 mg bwm, n = 7; V3 – 42 dpn, 10 mg bwm, n = 6; V4 – 42 dpn, 20 mg bwm, n = 7. Controls: K1 – 3–5 dpn, n = 6; K2 – 42 dpn, n = 6.

the bacterial pellet was recovered. The pellets from different parallel culture batches originating from the same pre-culture were re-suspended in small volumes of culture medium, pooled, and dispensed to form the bacterial inoculum stocks. After centrifugation of the stocks, the bacterial wet mass (bwm) of each pellet was determined. The stocks were stored at 5 ± 3 °C for a maximum of 9 weeks. One stock was used per inoculation day. Two to three days before inoculation the pellet was re-suspended to a concentration of 1 mg bwm/mL using PBS. This batch suspension was incubated at 37 ± 2 °C until the day of inoculation. Then, either 10 mL (groups V1 and V3) or 20 mL (groups V2 and V4) of the suspension were dispensed into separate tubes to form the inoculum for each individual animal. Bacterial counts of the respective batch suspension were determined on plates of Middlebrook 7H10 agar (Becton Dickinson, Heidelberg, Germany) containing OADC, Mycobactin J and Amphotericin B (AppliChem, Darmstadt, Germany). Serial dilutions from 10^{-1} to 10^{-9} were performed in MB and 100 µl of each dilution was plated on the agar plates. Plates were incubated at 37 °C for six weeks. Colony numbers were counted from the three highest dilutions showing visible colonies. Bacterial counts were expressed as the mean of the colony numbers corrected for the dilution. The bacterial inoculum amounted to $1.62 - 4.16 \times 10^8$ cfu/dose (Table 6). For further characterization of the batch suspensions, acid-fast bacilli (AFB) were confirmed by Ziehl-Neelsen staining, MAP was confirmed by IS900 PCR using primers according to Englund et al. [41]. Freedom from contaminating bacteria was proved by inoculation on blood agar plates.

Oral administration

Each individual MAP dose was suspended in 50 mL of pre-warmed milk replacer in a baby bottle. The goats were bottle-fed with the inoculum prior to regular morning feeding. Control animals received the same amount of pure milk replacer.

Faecal culture

Three gram of faeces were placed into 30 mL of 0.75% HPC. The solution was mixed vigorously, allowed to settle for five min and the supernatant transferred to a fresh vial. The samples were agitated on a shaker for 30 min and then incubated in upright position for 48 hours at room temperature (RT) in the dark. The supernatants were discarded and 200 µL of the pellet were transferred on each of four slopes of Herrold's Egg Yolk Medium with Mycobactin J and Amphotericin, Nalidixic acid and Vancomycin (ANV, HEYM, Becton Dickinson, Heidelberg, Germany). The cultures were incubated up to 6 months at 37 ± 2 °C and checked every 2 weeks for contamination and occurrence of visible colonies. As soon as colonies became visible, colony counts were estimated semi-quantitatively by a colony score (CS) from 1 to 5, with $1 = 0 - 10$; $2 = 11 - 20$; $3 = 21 - 50$; $4 = 51 - 100$ individual colonies per slope; $5 =$ bacterial lawn, and the week of appearance (WA) was recorded. To correct for the time until colonies became visible, a growth index (GI) allowing a numerical estimation of the MAP concentration in the samples was calculated by the formula: $GI = CS \times 100/WA$. The mean GI of the four corresponding slopes was determined.

Serum preparation and antibody detection

Blood without anti-coagulants was kept for 2–3 hours at RT, centrifuged at $2000 \times g$ for 20 min, the serum recovered, aliquoted and stored at –20 °C until use. MAP specific antibodies were detected with the ID Screen Paratuberculosis Indirect ELISA (ID Vet, Montpellier, France) according to the instructions of the manufacturer. The antibody response is demonstrated by the sample-to-positive ratio (S/P%) as recommended by the manufacturer.

Preparation of PBMC

Twenty mL blood containing 75 units per mL sodium-heparin (SIGMA Taufkirchen, Germany) was layered over 20 mL lymphocyte separation medium (PAA, Pasching, Austria) and centrifuged at $1500 \times g$ for 30 min at RT.

The PBMC were removed, washed three times with Hank's buffer without calcium and magnesium, resuspended in RPMI 1640 medium with glutamine, 10% foetal calf serum (FCS), 10 mM HEPES and 1% Penicillin/Streptomycin (all Biochrom, Berlin, Germany) and adjusted to 2×10^6 PBMC per mL.

Stimulation assay

PBMC were transferred to 96-well round bottom culture plates (NUNC, Roskilde, Denmark) to a final cell number of 2×10^5 PBMC per well. Cells were stimulated in triplicate with Concanavalin A (Con A, 20 µg/mL, SIGMA, Taufkirchen, Germany) or Johnin purified protein derivative (jPPD, 4 µg/mL, kindly provided by D. Bakker, CVI-WUR, Lelystad, The Netherlands) at $37 \pm 2\,°C$, 5% CO_2. Non-stimulated cells served as controls. Cell supernatants were collected after 24 hours of stimulation for measurement of IFN-γ and after 64 hours for IL-10.

IFN-γ ELISA

IFN-γ was measured with an in-house capture ELISA using monoclonal antibodies against bovine IFN-γ (capture antibody: clone CC330, AbD Serotec, Kidlington, UK; detection antibody: clone CC302-Biotin, AbD Serotec), HRP-labelled biotin as conjugate (AbD Serotec) and 3,3′,5,5′-tetramethylbenzidine (TMB) as substrate (SIGMA, Taufkirchen, Germany). IFN-γ concentration was determined relative to a dilution series of recombinant bovine IFN-γ (AbD Serotec) from 9.167-0.013 ng/mL.

IL-10 ELISA

IL-10 was measured with an in-house capture ELISA using monoclonal antibodies against bovine IL-10 (capture antibody: clone CC318, AbD Serotec; detection antibody: clone CC320-Biotin, AbD Serotec), HRP-labelled biotin and TMB as described for the IFN-γ ELISA. IL-10 concentration was determined relative to a dilution series of recombinant bovine IL-10 (kindly provided by G. Entrican and S. Wattegedera, Moredun Research Institute, Penicuik, Scotland, UK) from 30–0.041 U/mL.

The validity of both, the IFN-γ and the IL-10 ELISA for caprine samples was determined in preceding stimulation experiments using PBMC of healthy adult goats (data not shown).

Necropsy and collection of tissue samples

Goats inoculated with MAP were necropsied between 47 and 49 wpi and controls 46 and 48 wpi. Special sampling was done to obtain intestinal samples of high quality. At necropsy, the sites of intestine to be collected for histology were selected while the animals were under deep anesthesia. For this, they were sedated with Xylazin at a dose of 0.25 mg/kg body weight (BW) IM (Rompun® 2%, Bayer, Leverkusen, Germany) and anesthetized with Ketamin hydrochloride at 2.5 mg/kg BW IV (Ketamin 10%, Intervet, Unterschleißheim, Germany) and Diazepam at 0.5 mg/kg BW IV (Faustan®, AWD, Radebeul, Germany) [42]. The intestine was exposed, segments of about 5 cm were ligated and filled with 4% neutral buffered formalin (NBF) in the duodenum, four sites of jejunum (3 m apart), one jejunal Peyer's patch (JPP) from the proximal and from the distal jejunum and three sites (terminal ileum, 50 cm and 150 cm proximal to the ileocaecal valve (ICV)) of ileal Peyer's patch (IPP). Then, goats were euthanized with 20 mL of pentobarbital IV (Release®, WDT, Garbsen, Germany), the intestine removed *in toto*, detached from the mesentery and spread full length on a table. In addition to the sites mentioned above, samples were collected from caecum, organized lymphoid tissue in the colon next to the ileocaecal valve (ICVPP), at the end of the proximal colon (PCPP) and in the rectum, central flexure of the colon and descending colon. JPP, IPP, ICVPP and PCPP are referred to as organized lymphoid tissue in the intestinal wall (oGALT). Samples for histology were opened, pinned flat on styrofoam and fixed in NBF. Samples were also collected at the respective sites for bacterial organ culture. The remaining intestine was opened, ingesta and mucosa examined and macroscopic lesions documented.

All intestinal lymph nodes were examined and samples collected from proximal, mid (only bacterial organ culture) and distal mesenteric lymph nodes (M-LN), ileocolic lymph nodes (ICV-LN) and colonic lymph nodes (Co-LN, only histology). Then a complete necropsy was performed and representative tissue samples were collected from tonsils, retropharyngeal LN, spleen, kidney, liver, hepatic LN for cultural isolation and histology, diaphragm, gluteal muscle, and superficial cervical LN (only for cultural isolation), and from thymus, lung, heart, aorta, pancreas, adrenal, rumen, abomasum, bone marrow, and superficial inguinal LN (only for histology).

Histology and immunohistochemistry (IHC)

Tissue samples were embedded in paraffin and lesions examined in hematoxylin and eosin (HE)-stained paraffin sections. Severity of lesions was graded from + to +++, with + (mild), ++ (moderate) and +++ (severe), distribution of lesions as focal (f) – up to 3 distinct granulomatous infiltrates per section; multifocal (mf) – more than 3 distinct granulomatous infiltrates per section and diffuse (d) – infiltrates throughout the section. In the intestinal lymph nodes, granulomatous infiltrates and distinct granulomas with central necrosis and calcification were seen. In oGALT the following types of lesions were distinguished: A – small foci of epitheloid cells and multinucleated giant cells without changes of the tissue architecture; B – extensive granulomatous infiltrates with many lymphocytes; C – small foci of granulomatous infiltrate embedded in numerous lymphocytes and plasma cells and atrophy of the organized lymphoid tissue; D – multifocal to diffuse granulomatous infiltrates with numerous epitheloid cells.

Paraffin sections of all intestinal sites, intestinal lymph nodes, liver, tonsil, hepatic LN, superficial inguinal LN and tissues with granulomatous lesions were examined for MAP by the indirect immunoperoxidase method. Polyclonal rabbit anti-MAP serum (Dako, Glostrup, Denmark) was used as primary antibody and peroxidase-conjugated goat anti-rabbit IgG as secondary antibody (Dianova, Hamburg, Germany). Sections were pretreated with trypsin (0.1%, 37 °C, 20 min) for antigen retrieval. 3-amino-9-ethyl carbazole (AEC) was used as chromogen. Sections were counter stained with hematoxylin. As positive control, a slide from an experimentally inoculated goat in which mycobacteria had been detected by Ziehl-Neelsen staining and from which MAP had been isolated by culture was included. As negative control, a consecutive section of the positive control was incubated with a polyclonal antiserum directed against non-related bacteria (*Brachyspira hyodysenteriae*) instead of the polyclonal rabbit anti-MAP serum. For each section which had areas of necrosis, a consecutive section was incubated with the antiserum against non-related bacteria as negative control. The number of mycobacteria per section was graded using a scoring system adapted from previous studies as none (less than two labeled bacteria per section), paucibacillary (up to 50% of macrophages contain MAP, on average 1–10 MAP per macrophage, few areas in necrotic centers of granulomas) and multibacillary (most macrophages contain MAP, on average >10 MAP per macrophage or uncountable, extensive areas in necrotic centers of granulomas) [43].

Macroscopic lesions, histological findings and immunohistochemical detection of MAP were summarized as lesion categories for the intestinal lymph nodes, oGALT, small intestine and as overall lesions for the individual animal to be able to correlate the morphological findings with cultural isolation of MAP from organs, faecal shedding and immune reactions. The different sites were discriminated, because severity of lesions varied within individual goats. The criteria are listed in Table 7.

Tissue culture

Fat and connecting tissue was removed from lymph nodes and other tissue. Intestine was opened and ingesta removed. One gram of sample was cut from different locations, minced with scissors and transferred into a plastic bag containing 7 mL 0.9% HPC. The samples were homogenized in a stomacher for 6 min, transferred to a 50 mL tube and agitated on a shaker at 200 rpm for 10 min at RT. Afterwards they were incubated in upright position for 24 hours at RT in the dark. After centrifugation at $1880 \times g$ for 20 min at RT, supernatants were discarded and the pellet re-suspended with 1 mL of sterile phosphate buffered saline (pH 7.2). 200 μL of the pellet were transferred on each of four slopes of HEYM (Becton Dickinson, Heidelberg, Germany). The cultures were further treated and GI was calculated as described above.

The bacterial organ burden (BOB) was calculated for the samples from intestine, oGALT and intestinal lymph nodes separately and in summary by dividing the sum of the GI's of the respective tissues by the number of tissues involved. BOB categories were designated as follows: category I – no growth, category II - BOB ≤ 15, category III - BOB > 15.

Statistics

Response intensities of inoculation groups were analysed with the Mann–Whitney U-test, frequencies of categories of parameters were compared using Pearson's χ^2-test. The level of significance for all statistical methods applied was P ≤ 0.05. Results were displayed as 'Box and Whisker' plots. Outlier values are 1.5-3 times of the length of a box away from the median and extreme values are further away than three times of the length of the box.

Table 7 Assignment of lesion categories for mesenteric and ileocecal LNN, oGALT and small intestine and in summary

Lesion category	mesenteric and ileocecal LNN	oGALT	small intestine	summary
I	no lesions (macroscopic, histological), no MAP	no lesions (macroscopic, histological), no MAP	no lesions (macroscopic, histological), no MAP	all 3 sites (LNN, oGALT and small intestine) are category I
II	predominantly small circumscribed lesions, lesions in 1–2 out of the 3 LNN examined, paucibacillary	lesions in up to 3 sites of oGALT, f/mf, paucibacillary	lesions in up to 2 sites of small intestine, f/mf, paucibacillary	at least 2 of the 3 sites (LNN, oGALT, small intestine) are category II **or** 1 site is category II, 2 are category I **or** 1 site each is category I, category II and category III
III	predominantly extensive lesions, lesions in all 3 LN, pauci-/multibacillary	lesions in >3 sites of oGALT, mf, pauci-/multibacillary	lesions in >2 sites of intestine, mf, pauci-/multibacillary	at least 2 of the 3 sites (LNN, oGALT, small intestine) are category III **or** 1 site is category III and the others are category I

LNN lymph nodes, oGALT gut-associated lymphoid tissue, f focal, mf multifocal.

Abbreviations
AFB: Acid fast bacilli; BOB: Bacterial organ burden; bwm: Bacterial wet mass; dpn: Days post natum; oGALT: Organized lymphoid tissue in the intestinal wall; GI: Growth index; ICV: Ileocaecal valve; IFN-γ: Interferon-γ; IL-10: Interleukin-10; IPP: Ileal Peyer's patch; JPP: Jejunal Peyer's patch; jPPD: Johnin purified protein derivative; LN: Lymph node; MAP: Mycobacterium avium subsp. paratuberculosis; mpi: Months post infection; PBMC: Peripheral blood mononuclear cells; wpi: Weeks post infection.

Competing interests
The authors declare that they have no competing interests.

Authors' contributions
HK conceived of the study, HK, ELT and PR participated in its design and coordination and in the in vivo sampling. AK established and AS performed the IFN-γ and IL-10 assays. HK, ELT and MM performed the necropsies, MM and ELT did the histological and immunohistochemical investigations. AS, MM, ELT and HK contributed to the analysis and interpretation of the data. HK, ELT, AS and PR contributed to drafting and revision of this article. All authors have read and approved the final article.

Acknowledgements
We thank Uta Brommer, Danny Michel, Monica Godat and Sabine Lied for excellent technical assistance. The support from the goat breeder and from the staff of the animal facilities at the Friedrich-Loeffler-Institut in Jena is kindly acknowledged. The study was partially supported by the animal disease compensation funds of Thuringia, Hesse, Mecklenburg-Western Pomerania, Lower Saxony, Rhineland-Palatinate, and Baden-Wuerttemberg.

Author details
[1]Institute of Molecular Pathogenesis, Friedrich-Loeffler-Institut, Federal Research Institute for Animal Health, Jena, Germany. [2]Present address: Tierärztliche GmbH Hagenow, Hagenow, Germany. [3]Present address: Tierarztpraxis Dr. Peitzmeier, Hille, Germany. [4]Present address: Institute of Immunology, Jena University Hospital, Jena, Germany.

References
1. Bhattarai B, Fosgate GT, Osterstock JB, Fossler CP, Park SC, Roussel AJ. Comparison of calf weaning weight and associated economic variables between beef cows with and without serum antibodies against or isolation from feces of Mycobacterium avium subsp paratuberculosis. Javma-J Am Vet Med A. 2013;243:1609–15.
2. Chi J, VanLeeuwen JA, Weersink A, Keefe GP. Direct production losses and treatment costs from bovine viral diarrhoea virus, bovine leukosis virus, Mycobacterium avium subspecies paratuberculosis, and Neospora caninum. Prev Vet Med. 2002;55:137–53.
3. Whitlock RH, Buergelt C. Preclinical and clinical manifestations of paratuberculosis (including pathology). Vet Clin N Am-Food A. 1996;12:345.
4. Begg DJ, Whittington RJ. Experimental animal infection models for Johne's disease, an infectious enteropathy caused by Mycobacterium avium subsp paratuberculosis. Vet J. 2008;176:129–45.
5. Hines ME, Stabel JR, Sweeney RW, Griffin F, Talaat AM, Bakker D, et al. Experimental challenge models for Johne's disease: a review and proposed international guidelines. Vet Microbiol. 2007;122:197–222.
6. Storset AK, Hasvold HJ, Valheim M, Brun-Hansen H, Berntsen G, Whist SK, et al. Subclinical paratuberculosis in goats following experimental infection - an immunological and microbiological study. Vet Immunol Immunop. 2001;80:271–87.
7. Sigurdardottir OG, Press CM, Saxegaard F, Evensen O. Bacterial isolation, immunological response, and histopathological lesions during the early subclinical phase of experimental infection of goat kids with Mycobacterium avium subsp paratuberculosis. Vet Pathol. 1999;36:542–50.
8. Munjal SK, Tripathi BN, Paliwal OP, Boehmer J, Homuth M. Application of different methods for the diagnosis of experimental paratuberculosis in goats. Zoonoses Public Hlth. 2007;54:140–6.
9. Munjal SK, Tripathi BN, Paliwal OP. Progressive immunopathological changes during early stages of experimental infection of goats with Mycobacterium avium subspecies paratuberculosis. Vet Pathol. 2005;42:427–36.
10. Hines ME, Stiver S, Giri D, Whittington L, Watson C, Johnson J, et al. Efficacy of spheroplastic and cell-wall competent vaccines for Mycobacterium avium subsp paratuberculosis in experimentally-challenged baby goats. Vet Microbiol. 2007;120:261–83.
11. Malone AN, Fletcher DM, Vogt MB, Meyer SK, Hess AM, Eckstein TM. Early weight development of goats experimentally infected with Mycobacterium avium subsp paratuberculosis. PLoS ONE. 2013;8:e84049. doi:10.1371/journal.pone.0084049.
12. Singh PK, Singh SV, Saxena VK, Singh MK, Singh AV, Sohal JS. Expression profiles of different cytokine genes in peripheral blood mononuclear cells of goats infected experimentally with native strain of Mycobacterium avium subsp paratuberculosis. Anim Biotechnol. 2013;24:187–97.
13. Biet F, Sevilla IA, Cochard T, Lefrancois LH, Garrido JM, Heron I, et al. Inter- and intra-subtype genotypic differences that differentiate Mycobacterium avium subspecies paratuberculosis strains. BMC Microbiol. 2012;12:264.
14. de Juan L, Mateos A, Dominguez L, Sharp JM, Stevenson K. Genetic diversity of Mycobacterium avium subspecies paratuberculosis isolates from goats detected by pulsed-field gel electrophoresis. Vet Microbiol. 2005;106:249–57.
15. Liapi M, Botsaris G, Slana I, Moravkova M, Babak V, Avraam M, et al. Mycobacterium avium subsp. paratuberculosis sheep strains isolated from Cyprus sheep and goats. Transboundary and Emerging Diseases. 2013. doi: 10.1111/tbed.12107.
16. Stewart DJ, Vaughan JA, Stiles PL, Noske PJ, Tizard MLV, Prowse SJ, et al. A long-term bacteriological and immunological study in Holstein-Friesian cattle experimentally infected with Mycobacterium avium subsp paratuberculosis and necropsy culture results for Holstein-Friesian cattle, Merino sheep and Angora goats. Vet Microbiol. 2007;122:83–96.
17. Stewart DJ, Vaughan JA, Stiles PL, Noske PJ, Tizard MLV, Prowse SJ, et al. A long-term study in Angora goats experimentally infected with Mycobacterium avium subsp paratuberculosis: Clinical disease, faecal culture and immunological studies. Vet Microbiol. 2006;113:13–24.
18. Whittington RJ, Begg DJ, de Silva K, Plain KM, Purdie AC. Comparative immunological and microbiological aspects of paratuberculosis as a model mycobacterial infection. Vet Immunol Immunop. 2012;148:29–47.
19. Thüringer Wald Ziege. [http://www.thueringerwaldziege.de/]
20. Borrmann E, Mobius P, Diller R, Kohler H. Divergent cytokine responses of macrophages to Mycobacterium avium subsp. paratuberculosis strains of Types II and III in a standardized in vitro model. Vet Microbiol. 2011;152:101–11.
21. Stewart DJ, Vaughan JA, Stiles PL, Noske PJ, Tizard ML, Prowse SJ, et al. A long-term study in Merino sheep experimentally infected with Mycobacterium avium subsp. paratuberculosis: clinical disease, faecal culture and immunological studies. Vet Microbiol. 2004;104:165–78.
22. O'Brien R, Mackintosh CG, Bakker D, Kopecna M, Pavlik I, Griffin JFT. Immunological and molecular characterization of susceptibility in relationship to bacterial strain differences in Mycobacterium avium subsp paratuberculosis infection in the red deer (Cervus elaphus). Infect Immun. 2006;74:3530–7.
23. Hines II ME. Experimental Ruminant Models of Paratuberculosis. In: Behr MA, Collins DM, editors. Paratuberculosis: Organism, Disease, Control. Wallingford, Cambridge: CAB International; 2010. p. 201–22.
24. Lybeck KR, Storset AK, Djonne B, Valheim M, Olsen I. Faecal shedding detected earlier than immune responses in goats naturally infected with Mycobacterium avium subsp paratuberculosis. Res Vet Sci. 2011;91:32–9.
25. Begg DJ, de Silva K, Carter N, Plain KM, Purdie A, Whittington RJ. Does a Th1 over Th2 dominancy really exist in the early stages of Mycobacterium avium subspecies paratuberculosis infections? Immunobiology. 2011;216:840–6.
26. Manning EJB, Steinberg H, Krebs V, Collins MT. Diagnostic testing patterns of natural Mycobacterium paratuberculosis infection in pygmy goats. Can J Vet Res. 2003;67:213–8.
27. Stabel JR, Robbe-Austerman S. Early immune markers associated with Mycobacterium avium subsp paratuberculosis infection in a neonatal calf model. Clin Vaccine Immunol. 2011;18:393–405.
28. Libraty DH, Airan LE, Uyemura K, Jullien D, Spellberg B, Rea TH, et al. Interferon-gamma differentially regulates interleukin-12 and interleukin-10 production in leprosy. J Clin Invest. 1997;99:336–41.
29. Hines ME, Turnquist SE, Ilha MRS, Rajeev S, Jones AL, Whittington L, et al. Evaluation of novel oral vaccine candidates and validation of a caprine model of Johne's disease. Front Cell Infect Mi. 2014;4. doi: 10.3389/fcimb.2014.00026.
30. Valheim M, Sigurdardottir OG, Storset AK, Aune LG, Press CM. Characterization of macrophages and occurrence of T cells in intestinal lesions of subclinical paratuberculosis in goats. J Comp Pathol. 2004;131:221–32.

31. Corpa JM, Garrido J, Marin JFG, Perez V. Classification of lesions observed in natural cases of paratuberculosis in goats. J Comp Pathol. 2000;122:255–65.

32. Tafti AK, Rashidi K. The pathology of goat paratuberculosis: Gross and histopathological lesions in the intestines and mesenteric lymph nodes. J Vet Med B. 2000;47:487–95.

33. Kruger C, Kohler H, Liebler-Tenorio EM. Sequential development of lesions 3, 6, 9, and 12 months after experimental infection of goat kids with *Mycobacterium avium* subsp *paratuberculosis*. Vet Pathol. 2014, doi: 10.1177/0300985814533804.

34. Thomas GW. Paratuberculosis in a large goat herd. Vet Rec. 1983;113:464–6.

35. Reddacliff LA, Whittington RJ. Experimental infection of weaner sheep with S strain *Mycobacterium avium* subsp *paratuberculosis*. Vet Microbiol. 2003;96:247–58.

36. Mackintosh CG, Clark RG, Thompson B, Tolentino B, Griffin JFT, de Lisle GW. Age susceptibility of red deer (Cervus elaphus) to paratuberculosis. Vet Microbiol. 2010;143:255–61.

37. Delgado L, Marin JFG, Munoz M, Benavides J, Juste RA, Garcia-Pariente C, et al. Pathological findings in young and adult sheep following experimental infection with 2 different doses of *Mycobacterium avium* subspecies *paratuberculosis*. Vet Pathol. 2013;50:857–66.

38. Philips JA, Ernst JD. Tuberculosis pathogenesis and immunity. Annu Rev Pathol-Mech. 2012;7:353–84.

39. Anonymous. Council Directive 86/609/EEC of 24 November 1986 on the approximation of Laws, regulations and administrative provisions of the Member States regarding the protection of animals used for experimental and other scientific purposes. Off J Eur Communities. 1986;29(L 358):1–28.

40. Anonymous. Bekanntmachung der Neufassung des Tierschutzgesetzes. Bundesgesetz-blatt, Teil I. 2006;2006(25):1206–22.

41. Englund S, Ballagi-Pordany A, Bolske G, Johansson KE. Single PCR and nested PCR with a mimic molecule for detection of *Mycobacterium avium* subsp. *paratuberculosis*. Diagn Micr Infec Dis. 1999;33:163–71.

42. Matthews JG. Diseases of the goat. 3rd ed. Oxford: Wiley-Blackwell; 2009.

43. Dennis MM, Reddacliff LA, Whittington RJ. Longitudinal study of clinicopathological features of Johne's disease in sheep naturally exposed to *Mycobacterium avium* subspecies *paratuberculosis*. Vet Pathol. 2011;48:565–75.

20

Anatomical basis for the development of a thoracic duct cannulation model without thoracotomy in Large White pigs

Hung-Hsun Yen[*], Christina M Murray and Helen MS Davies

Abstract

Background: To collect lymph draining the lungs provides a useful strategy for tracing pulmonary microvascular fluid and protein biology. A methodology that allows for *in vivo* sampling of efferent pulmonary lymph in real-time in sheep by cannulating the thoracic duct without entering the thoracic cavity was previously established. To develop a similar thoracic duct cannulation model without thoracotomy in pigs, we investigated the anatomy of the left cervico-thoracic regions of 15 Large White (Yorkshire or Yorkshire-dominated) piglets (aged 4–7 weeks).

Results: The thoracic duct, together with the left tracheal trunk, joined the cardiovascular system (the ampulla of the thoracic duct) at a site located craniomedial to the first rib on the left in 80 % (12/15) of the piglets.

Conclusions: As the location of the ampulla of the thoracic duct was consistent in most of the piglets, Large White piglets appear to be suitable for the development of a thoracic duct cannulation model without thoracotomy. The anatomical findings in this study will enable the development of further surgical procedures for cannulating the thoracic duct without thoracotomy, with minimal damage to local tissue, and without transecting any major blood vessels, nerves or muscle bellies. The establishment of a thoracic duct cannulation model for collecting *in vivo*, *in situ* efferent lymph, including pulmonary lymph, in pigs without entering the thoracic cavity would be invaluable for many immunological studies, studies on pulmonary immune responses in particular.

Keywords: Thoracic duct, Anatomy, Swine model

Background

The successful cannulation of the terminal part of the thoracic duct in the left pre-scapular region in sheep was initially described by Kassai et al. in 1972 (in Hungarian) [1]. In that study, they used the model to study *Dictyocaulus filaria* infection. In 2009, Yen et al. reported another successful preparation of a pulmonary lymph fistula through thoracic duct cannulation without thoracotomy using surgical approaches different to that of Kassai et al. [2]. These models provided a strategy for monitoring *in vivo*, *in situ* pulmonary pathology and immunobiology in real-time in sheep. It would be of great benefit to pulmonary studies if the model for *in vivo* real-time pulmonary lymph collection could be established in pigs. However, there are few references

for pigs that describe the anatomy of the thoracic duct at the point where it joins the cardiovascular system (the ampulla of the thoracic duct), its relationship to other anatomical structures and the anatomical variations within the same pig breed [3]. Further, photographic images showing genuine fresh tissues of the thoracic duct and associated anatomical structures in the pig are not available in the literature.

In pigs, pulmonary afferent lymph from the lungs drains into the tracheobronchial and cranial mediastinal lymph centres and then enters the thoracic duct [4]. Consequently, harvesting lymph from the thoracic duct provides a strategy to sample lymph that contains lymph draining the lungs and the local lymph centres. Changes to the composition of thoracic duct lymph may indicate functional processes occurring in the pulmonary system. However, thoracic duct lymph contains lymph draining several other body systems. Hence, changes in thoracic duct lymph composition may also result from the effects

---

* Correspondence: hyen@unimelb.edu.au
Faculty of Veterinary and Agriculture Science, The University of Melbourne, Parkville, VIC 3010, Australia

of processes in other body systems. When the lungs are the key target organs of pathogens or the corresponding treatments i.e. intra-bronchial delivery of treatments using a bronchoscope, changes in the composition of thoracic duct lymph should primarily come from the pulmonary lymph rather than from the other tissues.

In this study, we investigated the anatomy of the thoracic duct where it joins the cardiovascular system, and its relationship to the other major anatomical structures at the thoracic inlet in Large White piglets (also known as the Yorkshire or Yorkshire-dominated piglets) - a key pig breed usually accessible in the pig industry in Victoria, Australia and a number of other countries in the world. We believe that the results will be of help in identifying the lymphatic vessels and their relationships to the other structures at the thoracic inlet on the left side in pigs. These results provide the basis for the development of a pig model in which the thoracic duct and the tracheal trunk (left) are cannulated without thoracotomy for respiratory studies.

Results

We found that the anatomic positions of the thoracic duct and the left tracheal trunk where they joined the cardiovascular system were quite similar in all 15 of the Large White piglets in this study. In 12 of the 15 piglets (80 %), the thoracic duct and the left tracheal trunk joined the left external jugular vein craniomedial to the first rib on the left side. In three pigs, the ampulla of the thoracic duct was located close to the junction of the left external jugular vein and the left subclavian vein, more medial than craniomedial to the first rib on the left side. The left tracheal trunk was single at its proximal end cranial to its point of entry into the external jugular vein in all 15 Large White piglets. We did not find additional branches of the left tracheal trunk at its segment proximal to its point of entry into the external jugular veins in any pig. However, in one pig, the left tracheal trunk anastomosed with the thoracic duct (the ampulla of the thoracic duct) at the craniomedial thoracic inlet (Fig. 1).

In Fig. 2A, a short segment of the thoracic duct can be seen emerging from the thoracic cavity, and the junction of its ampulla with the left external jugular vein can be observed, located craniomedial to the first left rib. The ampullae of the left tracheal trunk and the efferent lymphatic of the left dorsal superficial cervical lymph node(s), which are located cranial to the ampulla of the thoracic duct, also inserted into the left external jugular vein (Fig. 2B). The magenta-colour of the thoracic duct was probably due to the presence of abundant red blood cells (RBCs) and their derivatives in the lymph since the animal had previously had severe abdominal

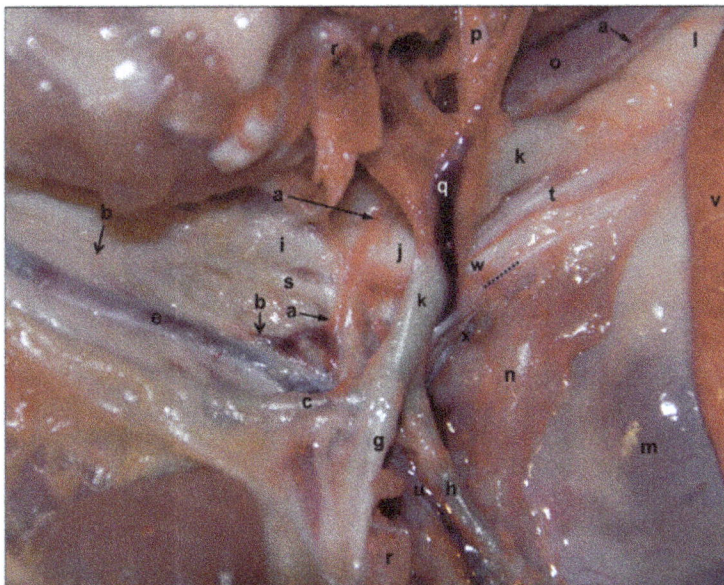

Fig. 1 The course of the thoracic duct and the tracheal trunk in the cervicothoracic region on the left. Dissections were performed on a 6-week old Large White pig cadaver to expose the craniolateral aspect of the left cervicothoracic region. The left forelimb was retracted craniolaterally. The tracheal trunk anastomosed with the thoracic duct (the ampulla of the thoracic duct) in this pig. The picture is positioned with cranial to the left. a: thoracic duct; b: left tracheal trunk; c: left superficial cervical artery; e: left external jugular vein; g: left axillary artery; h: left internal thoracic artery; i: left common carotid artery; j: bicarotid trunk; k: left subclavian artery; l: aorta; m: heart; n: thymus; o: oesophagus; p: left costocervical artery; q: left costocervical vein; r: the vertebral and sternal cutting edges of the first left rib; g: left costocervical vein; h: left internal thoracic artery; s: left vagosympathetic trunk t: left vagus nerve u: left internal thoracic vein; v: left cranial lobe of the lung; w: brachiocephalic trunk; x: cranial vena cava; dotted line: left phrenic nerve

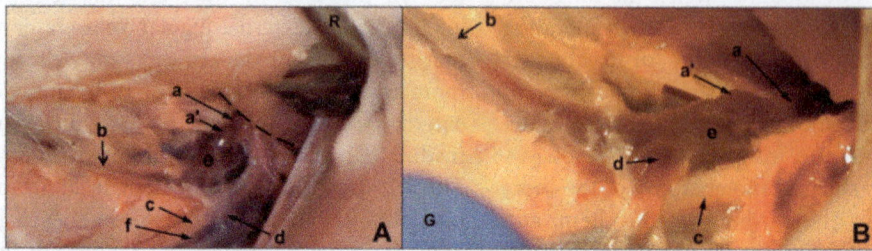

Fig. 2 Anatomic position of the thoracic duct and its ampulla at the cranial thoracic inlet on the left. The figures show the region cranial to the thoracic inlet on the left in a 7-week old Large White pig. The pictures are positioned with cranial to the left. **A**: The thoracic duct (a), emerging from the thoracic cavity, and its ampulla (a') that joins the external jugular vein craniomedially to the first rib (the dashed line marks the cranial border of the first rib) on the left could be identified. **B**: The dorsal craniolateral aspect of the left external jugular vein (e) at its junctions with the thoracic duct (a), left tracheal trunk (b), and the efferent lymphatic (d) of the left dorsal superficial cervical lymph nodes. c: left superficial cervical artery; f: left superficial cervical vein. (R: retractors; G: gloves)

haemorrhage due to sample collections associated with another study. In Fig. 2, clear and reddish lymph with an obvious boundary can be observed in the left tracheal trunk (b) proximal to the left external jugular vein (e). It is likely that there are valves located at the demarcation between the lymph with different colours.

Fig. 1 shows the course of the thoracic duct (indicated by ➡) and the tracheal trunk (labelled with →) in the cervicothoracic region on the left. Other major structures in this region are also identified and the relationship of the thoracic duct to these structures is clearly depicted. While an anastomosis of the left tracheal trunk and the thoracic duct was found in this animal, the ampulla of the thoracic duct was, as found in most of the specimens, located craniomedial to the first left rib.

While Figs. 1 and 2 show the colour of the thoracic ducts of pigs that underwent prior abdominal tissue collections, Fig. 3 shows the appearance of the thoracic duct of a normal pig dissected immediately after euthanasia. The red appearance of the thoracic ducts was a finding in all four pigs that were dissected immediately after euthanasia. No dissections on the bodies caudal to the diaphragm were performed on these pigs before approaching the thoracic ducts. In Fig. 3A, the left thoracic wall has been removed and the dorsal parts of the left lung retracted ventrally to expose a left lateral view of the thoracic duct running along the dorsal border of the aorta. In Fig. 3B, the diaphragm has been incised lateral and dorsal to the aortic hiatus and the left crus of the diaphragm retracted caudally to expose the cisterna chyli and its junction with the caudal end of the thoracic duct in the cranial sub-lumbar region of the abdominal cavity. The reddish colour of the thoracic duct became paler at about 40 min post-euthanasia as a result of more body fluid draining into the thoracic duct.

By identifying the cisterna chyli and its junction with the thoracic duct and tracking the course of the thoracic duct downstream to the cervicothoracic region, we also confirmed the course and position of the thoracic duct in the cranial thorax in these animals.

Discussion

In this paper we present photographs showing the course of the thoracic duct, the left tracheal trunk, and the efferent lymphatic of the left dorsal superficial cervical lymph node(s) at their points of entry to the left external jugular vein in fresh porcine specimens. These images also show the relationships between the lymphatic vessels and other anatomical structures in the cervicothoracic region on the left side in pigs. Findings in our study expand the understanding of the locations of the major lymphatic vessels in the left cervicothoracic region of pigs.

From our experience of studying lymphatic anatomy in sheep, dogs, and pigs, variations in the course and number of lymphatic vessels in different animals is not uncommon. Indeed, several references also identified the anatomical variations in lymphatic vessels [3, 5, 6]. The results of this study however, found that there was a single left tracheal trunk at its proximal end and point of entry in all 15 individual Large White pigs. These results therefore suggest that the anatomy of the left tracheal trunk at its proximal end where it enters the external jugular may be reasonably consistent in Large White pigs. It is possible however, that the sample number of pigs in the current study was not sufficiently high to observe uncommon variations. Results by Gomercic et al. for example, showed that Yorkshire pigs may sometimes have double tracheal trunks rather than the more commonly found single trunk [3].

As shown in Fig. 3, the colours of the thoracic ducts were found to be grossly reddish instead of translucent light yellowish in all four pigs that were euthanised specifically for this thoracic duct anatomy study. These results are compatible with previous observations [7, 8]. Nevertheless, the presence of large numbers of RBCs was not found in the tracheal trunks and the efferent lymphatic vessels of the dorsal superficial cervical lymph centres. The colours of these two lymphatic vessels were translucent and colourless to very light straw-coloured. Binns et al. also observed that the intestinal lymph of pigs

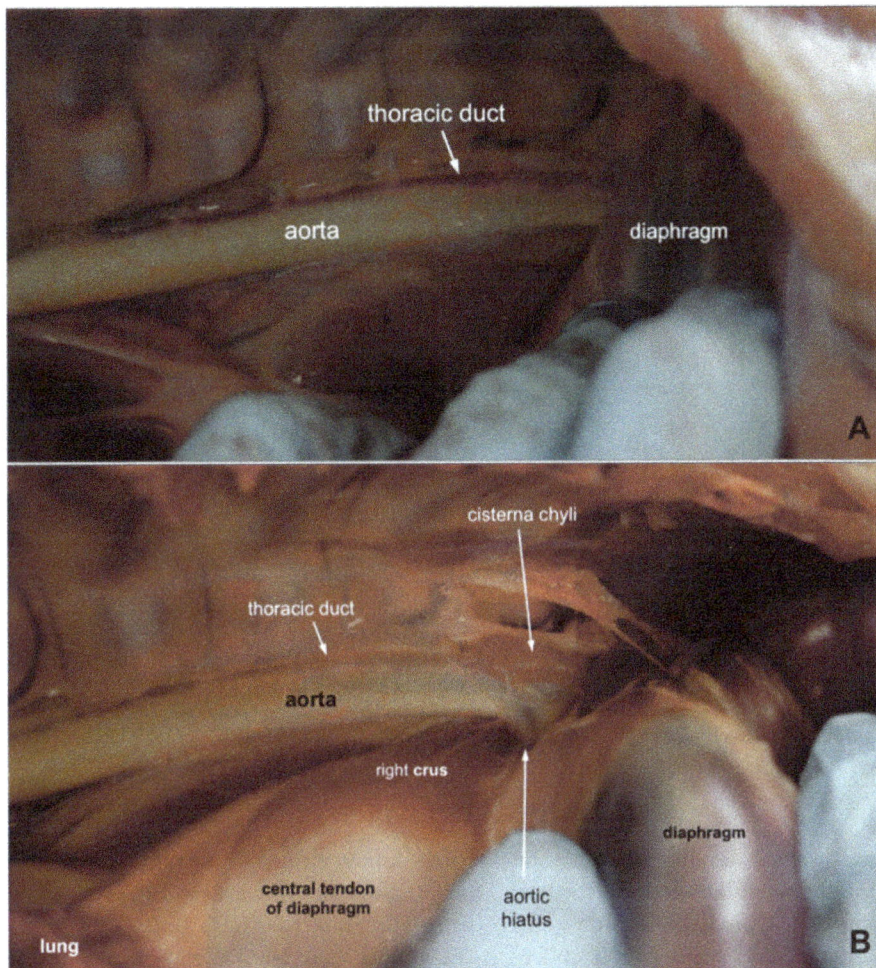

Fig. 3 The course of the thoracic duct and it junction with the cisterna chyli in the thoraco-abdominal junction on the left. Dissections were performed on a 7-week old Large White pig immediately after it was euthanised to expose the lateral aspect of the left thoraco-abdominal junction. The pictures are arranged with cranial to the left. **A**: The dorsal parts of the left lung were retracted ventrally to expose the thoracic duct that runs along the dorsal border of the aorta. The thoracic duct is red tinged probably due to the presence of large numbers of RBCs. **B**: The diaphragm has been incised lateral and dorsal to the aortic hiatus and the left crus of the diaphragm retracted caudally to expose the cisterna chyli and its junction with the caudal end of the thoracic duct in the cranial sub-lumbar region of the abdominal cavity. The reddish colour of the thoracic duct became paler due to influxes of more body fluid

was milky and not visibly bloody [7]. They speculated that the presence of large numbers of RBCs in the thoracic duct might result from the anastomoses of lymphatics and veins. The cause of these observed variations in RBC numbers in different lymphatics needs further investigation. Cannulation of individual lymphatic ducts for collection of lymph for measurement of blood cell numbers at different lymphatic sites could be a useful initial step.

Conclusions

The results of this study suggest that it is feasible to access the thoracic duct cranial to the thoracic inlet with minor tissue damage and without thoracotomy in Large White piglets. As shown in Fig. 2A, the junction of the thoracic duct and the external jugular vein was located craniomedial to the first rib on the left in 80 % of the 4 to 7-week-old Large White piglets. In this image, it is obvious that the connective tissue medial to the first rib is undamaged. This finding suggests that the thoracic duct can indeed be accessed without any surgical incision into the chest wall. With this high consistency in the thoracic duct location at the cranial thoracic inlet, the chances for approaching the thoracic duct successfully become more promising. A drawing annotating the positional relationships between the point of entry of the thoracic duct into the external jugular vein and the first rib and several nearby major blood vessels in the cervico-thoracic region on the left is presented in Fig. 4.

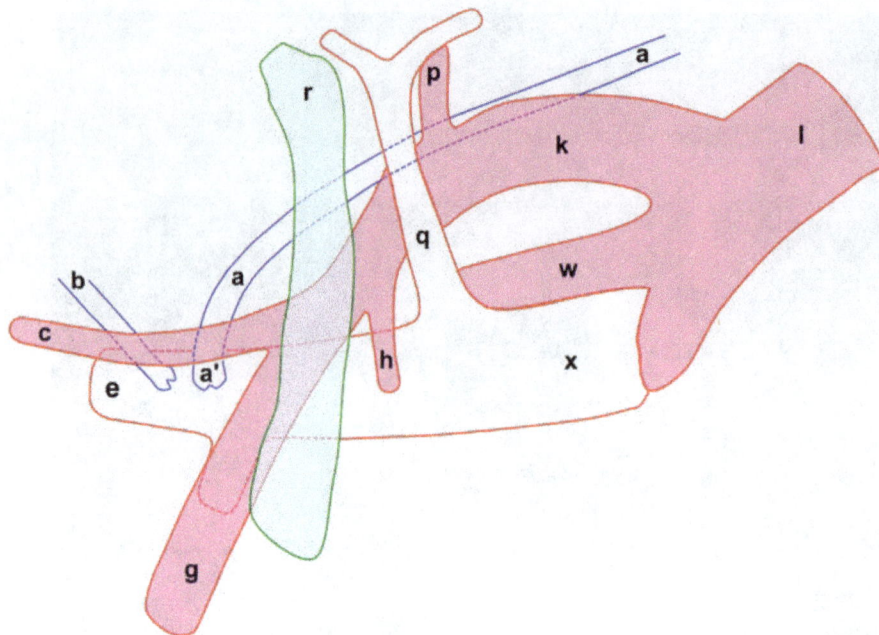

Fig. 4 Structural relationships of the thoracic duct and its entry into the external jugular vein cranial to the first rib on the left side. The point of entry (a') of the thoracic duct into the external jugular vein was located craniomedial to the first rib (r) on the left. The drawing is prepared with cranial to the left. a: thoracic duct; b: left tracheal trunk; c: left superficial cervical artery; e: left external jugular vein; g: left axillary artery; h: left internal thoracic artery; k: left subclavian artery; l: aorta; p: left costocervical artery; q: left costocervical vein; r: first left rib; w: brachiocephalic trunk; x: cranial vena cava

Based on these findings, we will develop a cannulation model, enabling both the thoracic duct and the tracheal trunk (left) to be catheterised without thoracotomy, for long-term efferent pulmonary and nasal lymph collection using Large White piglets. Long-term catheterisation of the thoracic duct in pigs allowing *in vivo*, *in situ*, and real-time lymph collection will be useful in biomedical research in the fields of pulmonology, gastro-enterology, pathobiology, pharmacokinetics and immunology studies [9]. Obtaining lymph supernatants of the draining tissues provides an approach to study the presence of, or changes in, molecules like exosomes, drugs and cytokines in studies such as those on the pharmacokinetics of medicines.

Methods
The cadavers of 15 Large White piglets about 4–7 weeks old were used for this study. The cadavers of 11 of the piglets were collected after they had been euthanised at the end of animal trials not associated with this study – that were conducted at the Faculty of Veterinary and Agricultural Science (FVAS) animal facility. Collections of multiple tissues in the abdominal cavities had been performed in these 11 pigs just before they were euthanised. Consequently, the presence of abundant RBCs in the thoracic duct was predicted in these specimens.

In addition to the 11 pig cadavers, four Large White piglets (aged 4–7 weeks) were housed in pens within the FVAS animal facility. These pigs were fed with commercial pellets and allowed access to water ad libitum. -They were euthanised by intravenous injection of Lethabarb (Pentobarbitone Na 325 mg/ml) into the right external jugular vein and dissected immediately following euthanasia. The University of Melbourne Animal Experimentation Ethics Committee approved all experimental procedures.

The dissection procedures were designed based on swine anatomical information from anatomical textbooks [10, 11] and modified from the surgical procedures in the previous study in sheep [2]. Dissections for approaching the thoracic duct were made through the caudal cervical region, craniomedial and slightly dorsal to the left shoulder joint. After the initial skin incision, and where possible, blunt dissection was mostly applied to avoid damaging the major blood vessels, lymphatics [11], and nerves in this region after skin incision. To generate enough space for deep dissections, blood vessel branches of the left superficial cervical artery and vein that coursed caudo-laterally to the suprascapular regions were ligated and transected. However, ligation and transection of other main blood vessels was generally not performed, in order to retain their relationships to the lymphatic vessels.

In most preparations, the left tracheal trunk, the efferent lymphatic of the dorsal superficial cervical lymph node(s), and the external jugular vein at the caudal cervical region were initially identified. The two lymphatic vessels were then followed downstream to the points of entry (ampullae) where they joined with the left external jugular vein. The thoracic duct - a large lymphatic vessel close to the first left rib that exits the thoracic cavity via the thoracic inlet - and its ampulla, which is beside the ampulla of the left tracheal trunk, were carefully isolated from the peripheral tissue. To confirm the identification of the thoracic duct and its relationship to the other anatomical structures adjacent to the thoracic inlet, the left chest wall was carefully removed to expose the thoracic duct in the thoracic cavity. We also dissected out part of the diaphragm to expose the junction between the thoracic duct and the cisterna chyli.

Abbreviations
FVAS: The faculty of veterinary and agricultural science; RBCs: Red blood cells.

Competing interests
The authors declare that they have no competing interests.

Authors' contributions
HHY conceived of the study, conducted dissections, took photos, analysed and interpreted the results, annotated the structures, and drafted the manuscript. CMM and HD analysed and interpreted the results, annotated the structures and helped to draft the manuscript. All authors read and approved the final manuscript.

Acknowledgements
The Early Career Research Grant, The University of Melbourne, supported this work. We thank Dr Prue Pereira-Fantini and Mr Magdy Sourial in the Murdoch Childrens Research Institute, Victoria, Australia for kindly providing the swine cadavers. The authors thank Mr Bob Geyer for his care of experimental animals. We also thank Dr Michiko Mirams for proofreading this manuscript.

References
1. Kassai T, Shnain A, Kadhim J, Altaif K, Jabbir M. Collection of lymph from sheep by the cannulation of the thoracic duct and an application of the method in hosts infected with Dictyocaulus filaria. Magyar Allatorvosok Lapja. 1972;27:691–6 (in Hungarian).
2. Yen HH, Wee JL, Snibson KJ, Scheerlinck JP. Thoracic duct cannulation without thoracotomy in sheep: a method for accessing efferent lymph from the lung. Vet Immunol Immunopathol. 2009;129(1–2):76–81.
3. Gomercic MD, Vukicevic TT, Gomercic T, Galov A, Fruk T, Gomercic H. The cisterna chyli and thoracic duct in pigs (Sus scrofa domestica). Vet Med. 2010;55(1):30–4.
4. Saar LI, Getty R. Porcine lymphatic system. In: Getty R, editor. Sisson and Grossman's The Anatomy of the Domestic Animals, vol. 2. Philadelphia, Pennsylvania, USA: W B Saunders Company; 1975. p. 1343–58.
5. Landolt CC, Matthay MA, Staub NC. Anatomic variations of efferent duct from caudal mediastinal lymph node in sheep. J Appl Physiol. 1981;50(6):1372–4.
6. Lascelles AK, Morris B. Surgical techniques for the collection of lymph from unanaesthetized sheep. Q J Exp Physiol Cogn Med Sci. 1961;46:199–205.
7. Binns RM, Hall JG. The Paucity of lymphocytes in the Lymph of Unanaesthetised Pigs. Br J Exp Pathol. 1966;47(3):275–80.
8. Ashitate Y, Tanaka E, Stockdale A, Choi HS, Frangioni JV. Near-infrared fluorescence imaging of thoracic duct anatomy and function in open surgery and video-assisted thoracic surgery. J Thorac Cardiovasc Surg. 2011;142(1):31–8. e31-32.
9. Chanoit G, Ferre PJ, Lefebvre HP. Chronic lymphatico-venous bypass: surgical technique and aftercare in a porcine model. Interact Cardiovasc Thorac Surg. 2007;6(6):705–7.
10. Nickel R, Schummer A, Seiferle E. The circulatory system, the skin, and the cutaneous organs of the domestic mammals / by August Schummer, Helmut Wilkens, Bernd Vollmerhaus, and Karl-Heinz Habermehl; translation by Walter G. Siller and Peter A. L. Wright. Berlin: Verlag Paul Parey, 1981; 1981.
11. Saar LI, Getty R. Porcine lymphatic system. In: Getty R, editor. Sisson and Grossman's The Anatomy of the Domestic Animals, vol. 1. Philadelphia, Pennsylvania, USA: W B Saunders Company; 1975. p. 1043–59.

21

Hypoxia following etorphine administration in goats (*Capra hircus*) results more from pulmonary hypertension than from hypoventilation

Leith Carl Rodney Meyer[1,2]*, Robyn Sheila Hetem[2], Duncan Mitchell[2] and Andrea Fuller[1,2]

Abstract

Background: Etorphine, a potent opioid agonist, causes pulmonary hypertension and respiratory depression. Whether etorphine-induced pulmonary hypertension negatively influences pulmonary gas exchange and exacerbates the effects of ventilator depression and the resultant hypoxemia is unknown. To determine if these effects occurred we instrumented twelve goats with peripheral and pulmonary arterial catheters to measure systemic and pulmonary pressures before and after etorphine administration. Concurrent cardiopulmonary and arterial blood gas variables were also measured.

Results: Etorphine induced hypoventilation (55% reduction to 7.6 ± 2.7 L.min^{-1}, $F_{(11,44)} = 15.2$ $P < 0.0001$), hypoxia (<45 mmHg, $F_{(11,44)} = 8.6$ $P < 0.0001$), hypercapnia (>40 mmHg, $F_{(11,44)} = 5.6$ $P < 0.0001$) and pulmonary hypertension (mean 23 ± 6 mmHg, $F_{(11,44)} = 8.2$ $P < 0.0001$). Within 6 min of etorphine administration hypoxia was twice ($F_{(11,22)} = 3.0$ $P < 0.05$) as poor than that expected from etorphine-induced hypoventilation alone. This disparity appeared to result from a decrease in the movement of oxygen (gas exchange) across the alveoli membrane, as revealed by an increase in the P(A-a)O$_2$ gradient ($F_{(11,44)} = 7.9$ $P < 0.0001$). The P(A-a)O$_2$ gradient was not correlated with global changes in the ventilation perfusion ratio ($P = 0.28$) but was correlated positively with the mean pulmonary artery pressure ($P = 0.017$, $r^2 = 0.97$), indicating that pulmonary pressure played a significant role in altering pulmonary gas exchange.

Conclusion: Attempts to alleviate etorphine-induced hypoxia therefore should focus not only on reversing the opioid-induced respiratory depression, but also on improving gas exchange by preventing etorphine-induced pulmonary hypertension.

Keywords: Hypoxia, Opioid, Respiratory depression, Oxygen diffusion

Background

Although opioids are effective in reducing pain and inducing anaesthesia, sedation or chemical immobilization, their use is not without complications or harmful side-effects. Of these side-effects, respiratory compromise is the most detrimental and well known [1-3]. Patients given opioids may develop hypercapnia, respiratory acidosis and hypoxia [4,5]. The respiratory compromise usually is attributed to respiratory depression, characterised by slowing of breathing frequency and decreased respiratory responses to hypercapnia, caused by the depressive effects of the opioids on the respiratory network and other neurons in the brain-stem [6,7]. Opioids also depress hypoxic and hypercapnic ventilator responses by acting on peripheral chemoreceptors [6,8].

We have reason to believe, though, that respiratory depression is not the sole cause of opioid-induced hypoxia. Serotonergics drugs improve respiratory rhythmogenesis through their effects on respiratory neurons [3,5,8]. However, when we used serotonergic drugs, acting on 5-HT1A and 5-HT4 receptors, to reverse etorphine-induced respiratory compromise, we found that their hypoxia-relieving effects were not related solely to their actions on respiratory neurons, but also their effects on pulmonary gas exchange [4,9]. We postulated that the improvements

* Correspondence: leith.meyer@up.ac.za
[1]Department of Paraclinical Sciences, Faculty of Veterinary Science, University of Pretoria, Onderstepoort 0110, South Africa
[2]Brain Function Research Group, School of Physiology, University of the Witwatersrand, 7 York Road, Parktown 2193, South Africa

in gas exchange were brought about by vasodilatory effects of these serotonergic drugs, which countered etorphine's vasoconstrictor effects in the pulmonary circulation [7].

We now have tested that postulate. We determined how etorphine, a potent opioid agonist widely used in chemical immobilization of wildlife [2], altered pulmonary arterial blood pressure and gas exchange, and established how much these effects contributed to etorphine-induced hypoxia. We measured blood gases, pulmonary pressures and other cardiorespiratory variables before and after etorphine administration in goats.

Methods

Twelve adult female mix breed goats (*Capra hircus*), weighing 33 ± 5 kg (mean $\pm$ SD), were used in this mechanistic study. They were housed together in temperature-controlled indoor pens (~22°C) in Johannesburg, at an altitude of 1753 m, on a 12 hour light/dark cycle (lights on 6:00). The goats were reared at this altitude and therefore adapted to lower inspired partial pressures of oxygen than at sea-level. They had water *ad libitum* and were fed on hay and sheep concentrate pellets. For six weeks before the start of data collection the goats were habituated to being restrained in sternal recumbency on a work table with a face mask over their muzzle, for a 5 min period every other day. The procedures were approved by the University of the Witwatersrand's Animal Ethics Screening Committee (clearance number 2008/49/04).

Goats were weighed 48 hours before, and starved for 24 hours before etorphine administration to reduce the risk of bloating and of regurgitation of ingesta. On the day of etorphine administration, each goat was restrained in sternal recumbency and its ears and left lateral neck area was shaved and swabbed with 5% chlorhexidine gluconate (Hibitane, Astra Zeneca, Johannesburg, South Africa) in 100% ethanol. A 22 gauge intravenous catheter (Introcan, B/Braun, Melsungen, Germany) was placed in one of the auricular arteries and connected via a fluid-filled arterial line to a pre-calibrated Deltran II pressure transducer (DPT-200, Utah Medical Products, Midvale, U.S.A.). Local anaesthetic (2 ml lignocaine, Bayer, South Africa) was injected subcutaneously around the left jugular vein before an 2.8 mm (outside diameter) introducer sheath (1350BF85, Edwards Life Sciences, Irene, South Africa) was inserted into the vein. A fluid-filled Swan-Ganz Catheter (Continuous Cardiac Output Thermodilution Catheter, 139HF75P, Edwards Life Sciences, Irene, South Africa), which was connected to another Deltran II pressure transducer, was inserted through this sheath and advanced through the vein and right heart. Under the guidance of the real-time pressure trace, the tip of the catheter was positioned in the pulmonary artery such that when the balloon of the catheter was inflated it "wedged" the artery. This placement enabled the measurement of

both pulmonary artery (averaged over 40s every minute) and pulmonary artery wedge (averaged over 10s every second minute) pressures. Through a three-way stopcock, a separate side-port of the Swan-Ganz catheter was connected to the pressure transducer to measure central venous pressure (averaged over 10s every other second minute). To standardise pressure readings the pressure transducers were placed at the level of the scapulohumeral joint (level of the heart base). The Swan-Ganz transducers were connected via blood pressure amplifiers (FE117, ADIntruments, Castle Hill, Australia) to a PowerLab Exercise Physiology System (ML870B80, ADIntruments, Castle Hill, Australia), which captured and displayed real-time data through LabChart software (Chart 5, ADIntruments, Castle Hill, Australia). The Swan-Ganz catheter also was connected to a Vigilance Monitor (Edwards Life Sciences, Irene, South Africa), which continuously measured pulmonary artery temperature and cardiac output based on thermodilution principles. Pulmonary artery temperature was used as the body temperature needed to calculate water vapour pressure in alveolar air and to allow for temperature-corrected blood gas measurements.

A clear canine anaesthetic face mask (J-298C, Jorgensen Laboratories, Loveland, USA) was placed over the muzzle of the goat and positioned so as to limit dead space. A gasket made from a latex glove formed a tight seal between the goat's muzzle and the face mask. The face mask was connected to a two-way valve which directed all the expired air into the PowerLab Exercise Physiology System, via a respiratory flow head (MLT1000L) linked to a spirometer (ML140) and a gas mixing chamber (MLA245), in which expired gas temperature was measured by a thermistor pod (ML309). The data from these modules were collected via the PowerLab 8/30 amplifier (ML870) and integrated with the Metabolic Module software to measure (at BTPS - body temperature and pressure saturated) minute ventilation (L.min^{-1}) and respiratory rate. Prior to each set of measurements the spirometer was calibrated using a 3 L calibration syringe.

Data were recorded from 4 min before the injection of etorphine hydrochloride (Captivon, Wildlife Pharmaceuticals, Whiteriver, South Africa) until 15 min after the injection. Etorphine was injected intramuscularly into the gluteus muscles using a 20G hypodermic needle at a dose of 0.1 mg.kg^{-1} (the drug was diluted in injectable water to standardise the volume injected to 1 ml) a dose shown in pilot studies to induce motionless immobilization for the 15 min of data recording and to have no long-term sequelae. Once immobile, the goats were positioned by a handler holding the horns so that the neck was aligned with the spinal column and the head was elevated above the thorax with the nose pointing downwards. This positioning allowed for unobstructed eructation of ruminal gas and an open upper airway. A 0.5 ml auricular arterial blood sample was drawn 2 min before, and at 2, 6, 10 and 14 min after etorphine injection (these time intervals were selected *a priori*); the catheter was flushed with 2 ml heparinized saline (5 iu.ml^{-1}, Heparin, Intramed, Johannesburg, South Africa) after each sample. Directly after each sample was drawn, the arterial partial pressure of oxygen (PaO$_2$), carbon dioxide (PaCO$_2$) and pH were measured on a pre-calibrated blood gas analyzer with pre-calibrated blood gas cassettes (Roche OPTI CCA Analyzer + OPTI cassette B, Kat Medical, Johannesburg, South Africa); data were reported at 37°C.

At the end of the recording period, all instruments were removed and the goats were returned to their pens, where the action of etorphine was antagonised by 2 mg.kg^{-1} naltrexone hydrochloride (Trexinol, Wildlife Pharmaceuticals, White River, South Africa) injected intramuscularly.

All measurements were made indoors, between 2 hours and 10 hours after lights-on, at an ambient dry-bulb temperature between 20°C and 22°C and relative humidity between 21% and 24%. Barometric pressures were measured to an accuracy of 0.1 mmHg, by the on-board barometer of the blood gas analyzer, which had been calibrated against a Fortin mercury barometer (On, F.D & Co Ltd, United Kingdom). Barometric pressure ranged from 628 mmHg to 634 mmHg. At that barometric pressure, the partial pressure of inspired oxygen was about 133 mmHg.

We used GraphPad Prism version 6 for Windows (GraphPad Software, San Diego, USA) for statistical analyses. All results are reported as mean ± SD, and a $P < 0.05$ was considered statistically significant. Partial pressure of alveolar oxygen (PAO$_2$) was determined by using the Alveolar Gas Equation (FiO$_2$ (Pb – PH$_2$O) – PaCO$_2$/RQ) where FiO$_2$ is the fractional inspired oxygen (0.209), Pb the measured barometric pressure (mmHg) and PH$_2$O the water vapour pressure of saturated air in the alveoli. PH$_2$O (mmHg) was calculated as 4.58 e{(17.27 × Tb)/(237.3 + Tb)} [10], where Tb is the body temperature. We assumed that the partial pressure of CO$_2$ in the alveoli was equal to the arterial partial pressure of CO$_2$ (PaCO$_2$) and used a RQ (respiratory quotient) value of 1, the norm in conscious healthy goats [11]. The alveolar-arterial oxygen partial pressure gradient P(A-a)O$_2$ was calculated as PAO$_2$ - PaO$_2$. Expected-PaO$_2$, a theoretical value of arterial partial pressure of oxygen that would be expected if the PaO$_2$ after etorphine administration was determined only by PAO$_2$, which would decrease when ventilation decreased, was calculated by assuming that P(A-a)O$_2$ remained at the value attained immediately before etorphine administration. Pulmonary vascular resistance was calculated by dividing the difference between the pulmonary artery and wedge pressure by the cardiac output. Global ventilation perfusion ratios were calculated by dividing ventilation by cardiac output.

A repeated measures two-way ANOVA followed by a Šídák's post-hoc test for multiple comparisons was used to test for differences between measured PaO$_2$ and expected PaO$_2$ across time following etorphine administration. A repeated measures one-way ANOVA followed by Dunnett's post-hoc test for multiple comparisons with a control was used to test for differences between values 2 min before etorphine administration and those after etorphine administration, for respiration rate, ventilation, heart rate, cardiac output, ventilation perfusion ratio, PaCO$_2$, P(A-a)O$_2$, systemic arterial pressures, pulmonary arterial pressures, pulmonary arterial wedge pressure and pulmonary vascular resistance at each time point that blood gases were measured (2, 6, 10 and 14 min) after etorphine administration. Pearson's correlations and linear regressions were used to test for linear relationships between mean (averaged over 12 animals) P(A-a)O$_2$, PaO$_2$, mean pulmonary artery pressure and other cardiorespiratory variables. Although the correlations were similar when pre-etorphine data were included, only post-etorphine administration data were included to avoid cloud regressions.

Results

Effects of etorphine on immobilization and cardiorespiratory function

Administration of etorphine induced immobilization within 2–3 min, following which the goats remained motionless and unresponsive to moderate sound (talking) and physical stimuli (blood sampling and the palpebral reflex test) for the 15 min of measurements. Before etorphine administration (–2 min) the goats had a respiratory rate of 35 ± 10 breaths.min^{-1} and minute ventilation was 13.7 ± 3.3 L.min^{-1}. Following etorphine administration, both respiratory rate (F$_{(11,44)}$ = 11.9 $P < 0.0001$) and ventilation (F$_{(11,44)}$ = 15.2 $P < 0.0001$) decreased significantly. Within 2 min of etorphine administration the respiratory rate decreased to 16 ± 7 breaths.min^{-1} and minute ventilation to 7.6 ± 2.7 L.min^{-1} (Figure 1A), levels close to which they remained throughout the immobilization. Heart rate, which was 108 ± 25 beats.min^{-1} before etorphine administration, did not change significantly following etorphine administration (F$_{(11,44)}$ = 4.1 $P = 0.30$). Cardiac output (3.9 ± 0.7 L.min^{-1} before etorphine administration) did not change immediately after etorphine administration, but decreased gradually from 3.8 ± 0.5 L.min^{-1} at 6 min to 3.4 ± 0.5 L.min^{-1} at the end of the immobilization (14 min), resulting in cardiac output being significantly lower overall, following etorphine administration (F$_{(11,44)}$ = 18.9 $P = 0.01$, Figure 1B). Global ventilation perfusion ratio across the lung, which was 3.5 ± 0.9 before etorphine administration, decreased to 2.0 ± 0.9 at 2 min, and remained low (2.1 ± 0.8) throughout the immobilization, so that,

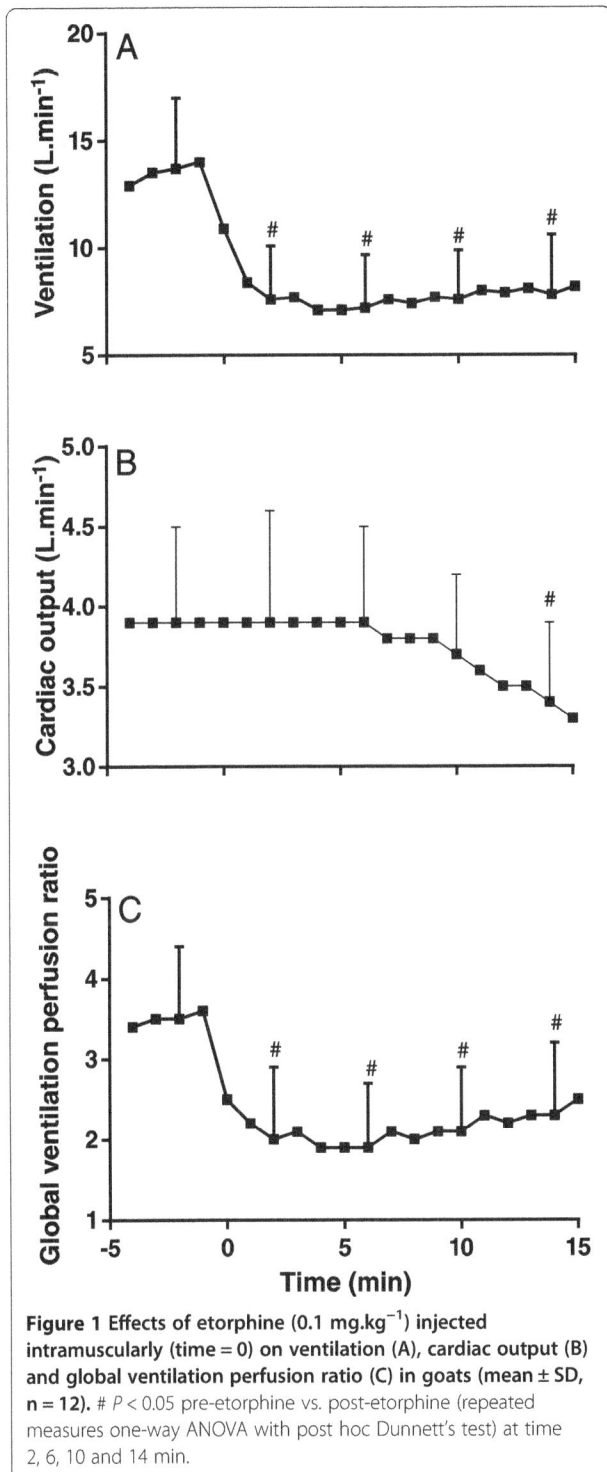

Figure 1 Effects of etorphine (0.1 mg.kg^{-1}) injected intramuscularly (time = 0) on ventilation (A), cardiac output (B) and global ventilation perfusion ratio (C) in goats (mean ± SD, n = 12). # $P < 0.05$ pre-etorphine vs. post-etorphine (repeated measures one-way ANOVA with post hoc Dunnett's test) at time 2, 6, 10 and 14 min.

overall, the ratio was significantly lower following etorphine administration ($F_{(11,44)} = 32.3$ $P < 0.0001$, Figure 1C).

Effects of etorphine on blood gases

Figure 2A shows the effect of etorphine on measured arterial partial pressure of oxygen (PaO$_2$). PaO$_2$ was 65 ± 6 mmHg before etorphine administration (−2 min) and

decreased to below 45 mmHg at 2 and 6 min after etorphine administration ($F_{(11,44)} = 8.6$ $P < 0.0001$), before gradually increasing again. The arterial partial pressure of carbon dioxide (PaCO$_2$) before etorphine administration was 31 ± 3 mmHg; after etorphine administration it increased ($F_{(11,44)} = 5.6$ $P < 0.0001$) to above 40 mmHg (9–12 mmHg increase) from 6 min to the end of the immobilization (Figure 2B). The alveolar arterial oxygen partial pressure difference (P(A-a)O$_2$) was 25 ± 5 mmHg before etorphine administration and increased after etorphine administration ($F_{(11,44)} = 7.9$ $P < 0.0001$), although it had returned to the pre-etorphine difference within 10 min after etorphine administration (Figure 2C).

Following etorphine administration, the calculated arterial partial pressure of oxygen that would be expected if the partial pressure of oxygen was influenced only by a decrease in ventilation, that is assuming that P(A-a)O$_2$ did not change, was lower than before etorphine administration ($F_{(11,44)} = 22.7$ $P < 0.0001$), and was greater than measured PaO$_2$ ($F_{(11,22)} = 3.0$ $P < 0.05$), though expected and measured values were the same after 10 min after etorphine administration (Figure 2A).

Effects of etorphine on the systemic and pulmonary vasculature

After etorphine administration, the systemic arterial pressures decreased (systolic $F_{(11,44)} = 6.8$ $P < 0.0001$; mean $F_{(11,44)} = 8.2$ $P < 0.0001$; diastolic $F_{(11,44)} = 8.6$ $P < 0.0001$), with decreases significant after 6 min (Figure 3A). Before the administration of etorphine (−2 min), pulmonary artery systolic pressure was 21 ± 5 mmHg, mean was 13 ± 4 mmHg and diastolic was 7 ± 4 mmHg (Figure 3B). Pulmonary artery pressures increased after etorphine administration (systolic $F_{(11,44)} = 6.8$ $P < 0.0001$, mean $F_{(11,44)} = 8.2$ $P < 0.0001$, diastolic $F_{(11,44)} = 8.6$ $P < 0.0001$), with systolic, mean and diastolic pressures all being significantly higher within 2 min after etorphine administration but returning to pre-etorphine values by the end of the immobilization. Pulmonary vascular resistance ($F_{(11,44)} = 2.6$ $P = 0.01$) and pulmonary artery wedge pressure ($F_{(11,44)} = 11.88$ $P < 0.0001$) were increased after etorphine administration from 2.9 ± 1.1 mmHg.min.L^{-1} and from 4.1 ± 2.9 mmHg respectively (Figure 3C), but only because values 3 min after etorphine administration were elevated significantly.

Factors influencing arterial partial pressure of oxygen

Although etorphine administration resulted in reduced ventilation and PaO$_2$, after etorphine administration there was no significant linear relationship between ventilation and the PaO$_2$ (Figure 4A, P = 0.16, r^2 = 0.70). In support of the poor influence of ventilation on PaO$_2$ after etorphine administration, we found that the arterial partial pressure of carbon dioxide (PaCO$_2$,

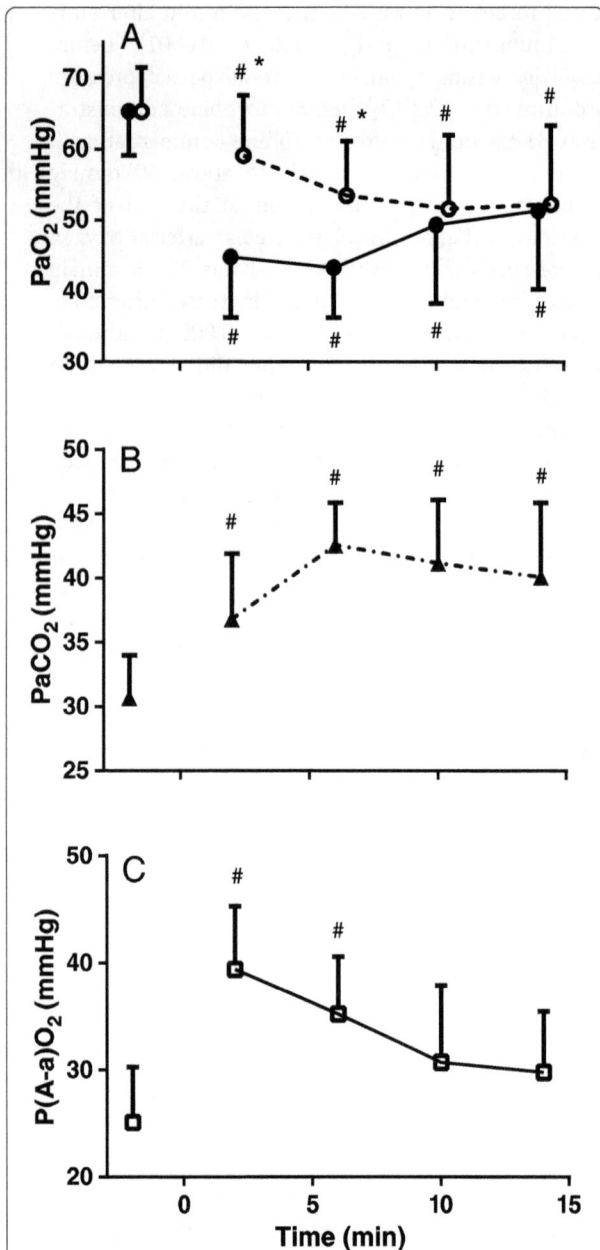

Figure 2 Effects of etorphine (0.1 mg.kg^{-1}) injected intramuscularly (time = 0) on measured arterial partial pressure of oxygen (PaO$_2$, solid symbols) and the theoretical value of arterial partial pressure of oxygen calculated assuming that alveolar-arterial oxygen partial pressure gradient P(A-a)O$_2$ remained constant (Expected-PaO$_2$, open symbols) (A), arterial partial pressure of carbon dioxide (B) and alveolar-arterial oxygen partial pressure gradient P(A-a)O$_2$ (C) in goats (mean ± SD, n = 12). # $P < 0.05$ pre-etorphine vs. post-etorphine (repeated measures two-way ANOVA with post hoc Sidak's multiple comparison test **(A)** and repeated measures one-way ANOVA with post hoc Dunnett's test **(B&C)**), * $P < 0.05$ PaO$_2$ vs. expected-PaO$_2$ (repeated measures two-way ANOVA with post hoc Sidak's multiple comparison test **(A)**) at time 2, 6, 10 and 14 min.

$P = 0.98$, r$^2 < 0.01$) and the calculated alveolar partial pressure of oxygen (PAO$_2$, $P = 0.99$, r$^2 < 0.01$), both variables associated with the magnitude of ventilation, were not correlated with PaO$_2$. Global pulmonary perfusion, measured as cardiac output ($P = 0.60$, r$^2 = 0.88$), also was not correlated to PaO$_2$. However, the relationship between global ventilation and perfusion (the ventilation perfusion ratio) after etorphine administration was correlated with the PaO$_2$ ($P = 0.04$, r$^2 = 0.92$, Figure 4B). Therefore, the changes in the PaO$_2$ appeared to be attributed mainly to intrapulmonary ventilation-perfusion mismatching rather than the pump action of breathing i.e. ventilation. That the main problem lay with altered oxygen movement across the alveoli membrane, not oxygen delivery, was confirmed by the large increase in the alveolar-arterial oxygen partial pressure gradient (P(A-a)O$_2$) soon after etorphine administration (Figure 2C). After etorphine administration, P(A-a)O$_2$ was linearly correlated with mean pulmonary artery pressure (Figure 4C, $P = 0.017$, r$^2 = 0.97$) and pulmonary vascular resistance (Figure 4D, $P = 0.023$, r$^2 = 0.95$), but not significantly correlated with global ventilation ($P = 0.59$, r$^2 = 0.17$), cardiac output ($P = 0.17$, r$^2 = 0.69$), global ventilation perfusion ratio ($P = 0.28$, r$^2 = 0.52$) or pressures in the left atrium as indicated by pulmonary artery wedge pressure ($P = 0.07$, r$^2 = 0.87$).

Pulmonary artery pressure after etorphine administration was correlated with pulmonary vascular resistance ($P = 0.04$, r$^2 = 0.52$), pulmonary artery wedge pressure (Figure 4E, $P = 0.0004$, r$^2 = 0.77$) and cardiac output (Figure 4F, $P = 0.003$, r$^2 = 0.47$), but not PAO$_2$ ($P = 0.61$, r$^2 = 0.15$). PAO$_2$ was also not correlated with pulmonary vascular resistance ($P = 0.28$, r$^2 = 0.51$).

Discussion

Intramuscular administration of 0.1 mg.kg^{-1} etorphine, a highly-potent opioid receptor agonist, induced rapid chemical immobilization and decreased the partial pressure of oxygen in arterial blood (Figure 2A). One cause of this exacerbated hypoxia could be hypoventilation, which opioid agonists are well known to induce (4–6). Our goats did develop hypoventilation (Figure 1A) with the expected concomitant hypercapnia (Figure 2B), but hypoventilation was not the only, nor even the primary, cause of the hypoxia. In the first six minutes after etorphine administration, when the hypoxia was most severe, the arterial partial pressure of oxygen was about half that which would have resulted from hypoventilation alone (Figure 2A). So not only was oxygen delivery to the alveoli compromised but so to was exchange of oxygen between alveoli and arterial blood. The alveolar-arterial oxygen partial pressure gradient (P(A-a)O$_2$) increased precipitously within 2 min of etorphine administration (Figure 2C). We identified one direct cause of the compromise of alveolar-

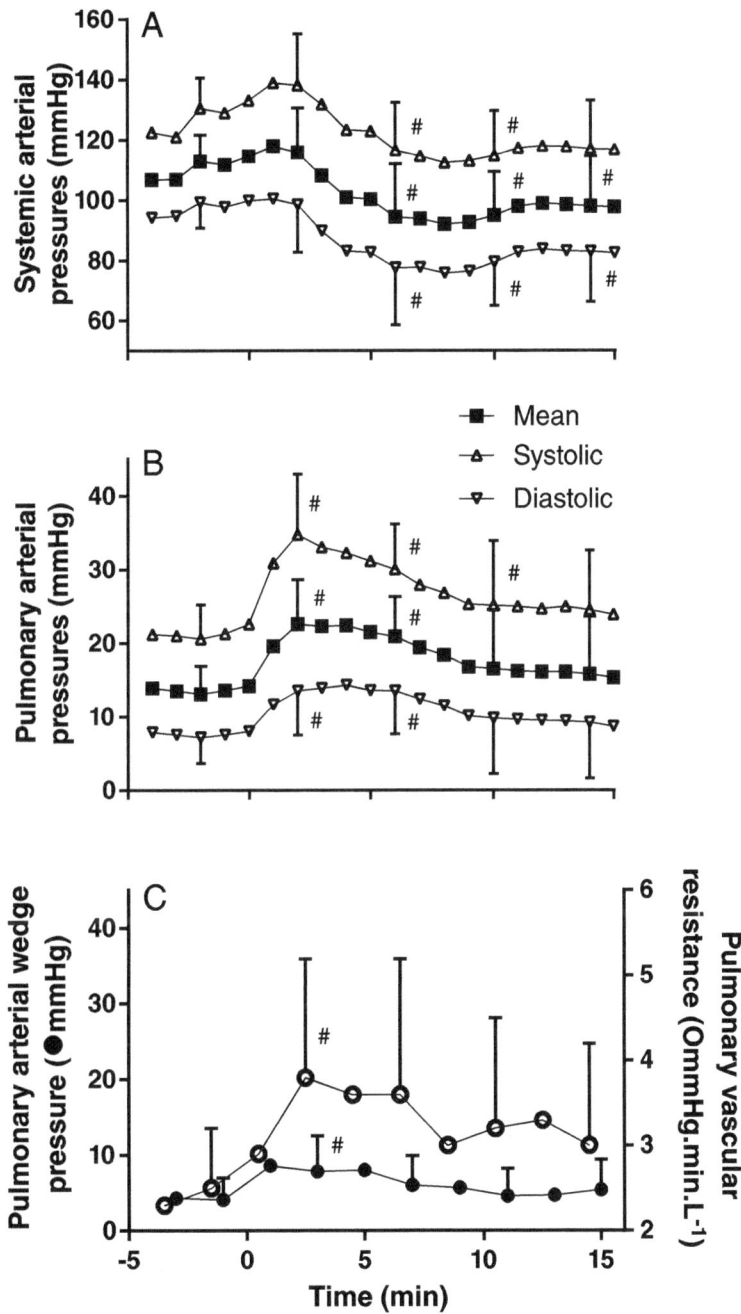

Figure 3 Effects of etorphine (0.1 mg.kg^{-1}) injected intramuscularly (time = 0) on systemic artery (A), pulmonary artery (B) and pulmonary artery wedge pressures and pulmonary vascular resistance (C) in goats (mean ± SD, n = 12). # $P < 0.05$ pre-etorphine vs post-etorphine (one-way ANOVA with post hoc Dunnett's test) at time 2, 6, 10 and 14 min.

arterial oxygen exchange: immediately after etorphine administration pulmonary vascular resistance also increased precipitously (Figure 3C) and pulmonary hypertension developed (Figure 3B). The alveolar-arterial oxygen partial pressure gradient (P(A-a)O$_2$) after etorphine administration was correlated strongly with mean pulmonary artery pressure (Figure 4C) indicating that the pulmonary hypertension likely played a major role in hindering oxygen

movement (gas exchange) across the alveoli membrane. It is reasonable to speculate that hypoxia could have been brought about by hydrostatic fluid shifts causing oedema of the interstitium, and possibly also the alveoli, so increasing diffusion distance and obstructing oxygen transfer into the blood.

Pulmonary hypertension can develop without pulmonary vascular resistance increasing, for example if global

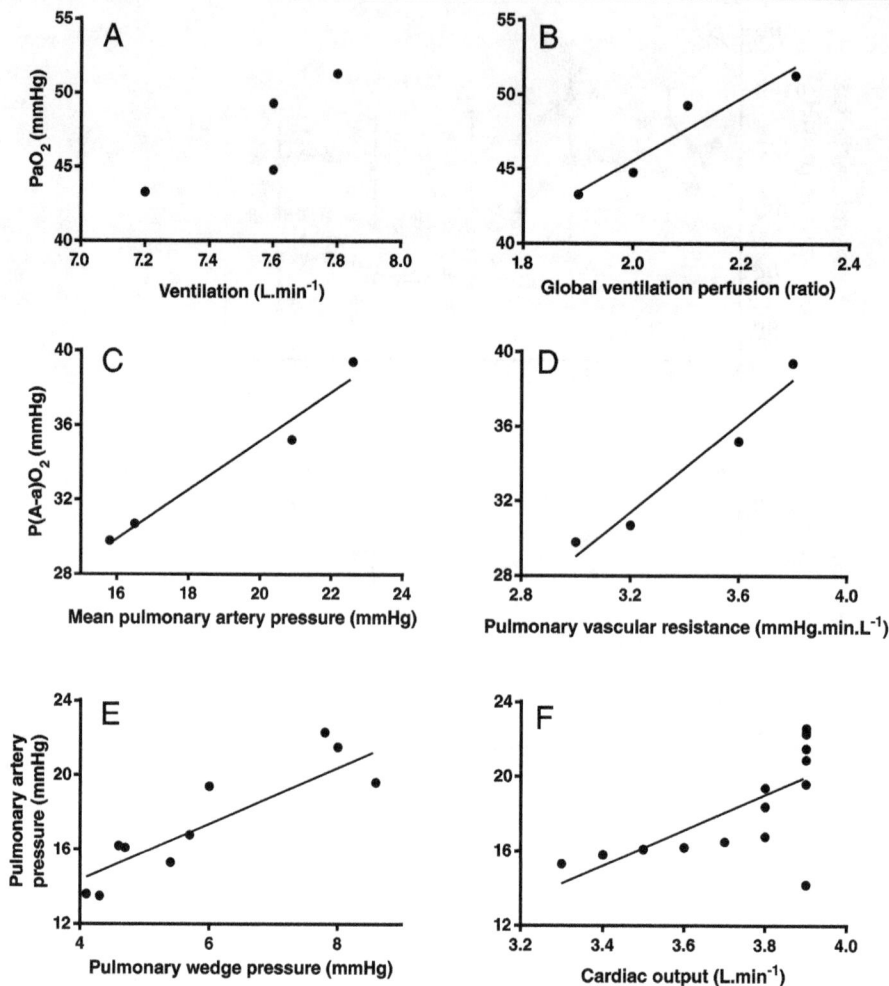

Figure 4 Mean arterial partial pressure of oxygen (PaO2) *vs.* mean ventilation (A, $r^2 = 0.7$, $P = 0.16$), mean arterial partial pressure of oxygen (PaO2) *vs.* mean global ventilation perfusion ratio (B, $r^2 = 0.92$, $P = 0.04$, $y = 21x + 3.6$), mean alveolar-arterial oxygen partial pressure gradient *vs.* mean of mean pulmonary artery pressure (C, $r^2 = 0.97$, $P = 0.017$, $y = 1.3x + 8.9$), mean alveolar-arterial oxygen partial pressure gradient *vs.* mean pulmonary vascular resistance (D, $r^2 = 0.95$, $P = 0.024$, $y = 11.9x - 6.5$), mean pulmonary artery pressure *vs.* mean pulmonary artery wedge pressure (E, $r^2 = 0.77$, $P = 0.004$, $y = 1.5x + 8.4$), mean pulmonary artery pressure *vs.* cardiac output (F, $r^2 = 0.47$, $P = 0.003$, $y = 9.5x - 17.2$). Data were averaged for 12 goats and r is Pearson's correlation coefficient.

pulmonary blood flow increases. In our goats, cardiac output, and therefore global pulmonary blood flow, had not changed at the time at which the hypoxia was most severe (Figure 1B). Although cardiac output was correlated with pulmonary artery pressures (Figure 4F) this relationship was poor and resulted mainly from the decrease in cardiac output and pulmonary artery pressures towards the end of the immobilization. Another possible cause of pulmonary hypertension is increase in left atrial pressure. In our goats, pulmonary artery wedge pressure, the surrogate for left atrial pressure, did increase following etorphine administration (Figure 3C) and mean pulmonary artery pressures did correlate positively with pulmonary artery wedge pressures (Figure 4E), so increases in pressure in the left atrium could have contributed to the pulmonary hypertension. However, changes

in pulmonary artery wedge pressure could not have entirely accounted for the almost two-fold increase in the mean pulmonary artery pressure, and we believe that the main contributor to the pulmonary hypertension must have been the increased pulmonary vascular resistance.

The most-likely cause of the increased pulmonary vascular resistance was pulmonary vasoconstriction. Pulmonary vasoconstriction following etorphine administration may result from activation of the sympathetic nervous system by etorphine [12], from the indirect effects of the hypoxia and hypercapnia [13] induced by etorphine [14,15], or by other unknown actions of etorphine on the pulmonary vasculature. However, generalised sympathetic activation appeared not to occur in our goats, as heart rate and systemic artery pressure did not increase. Hypoxic pulmonary vasoconstriction [16], brought about by etorphine-induced hypoventilation, may have contributed to the increased pulmonary artery pressures, but it did not appear to be the predominant factor, as changes in ventilation, as indicated by the partial pressures of alveolar oxygen and arterial carbon dioxide, were not correlated with the changes in pulmonary artery pressures and the partial pressure of alveolar oxygen was not correlated to pulmonary vascular resistance. The precise mechanisms underlying etorphine-induced and other possible opioid-induced pulmonary vasoconstriction still need to be elucidated.

If, indeed, etorphine administration induced pulmonary vasoconstriction, there is another possible contributor to the impaired oxygen transfer between alveoli and arterial blood, in addition to the impairment resulting from pulmonary hypertension. Less oxygen may have entered the arterial blood because there was less time for gas exchange to occur [16,17] after etorphine administration. Because pulmonary blood flow (cardiac output, Figure 1B) had not changed at the time at which pulmonary vascular resistance (Figure 3C) and, we presume, vasoconstriction were greatest, the speed of red cells traversing the narrowed pulmonary vessels would have increased. If arterial blood traversed the pulmonary capillary in less than 0.25 seconds, oxygen would not have enough time to diffuse and equilibrate in the blood [16].

Although we believe that pulmonary vasoconstriction and the resultant pulmonary hypertension were the main factors impairing oxygen exchange between alveoli and arterial blood, other factors may have been operating too. Following etorphine administration, there was a strong relationship between the PaO_2 and the global ventilation perfusion ratio (Figure 4B), but there was no significant relationship between global ventilation perfusion ratio and $P(A-a)O_2$. Additional ways in which the relationship between ventilation and blood oxygenation could be impaired include shunting, but we were unable to measure shunt fractions, or regional ventilation perfusion relationships in the lungs.

Etorphine not only had cardiovascular effects on the pulmonary circulation. Although we did not measure right atrial pressure, and therefore could not calculate systemic vascular resistance, we do know that, after etorphine administration, mean systemic arterial pressure dropped at a time at which cardiac output had not changed. The likely explanation was that etorphine's effects induced systemic vasodilation, in contrast to the pulmonary vasoconstriction that it induced. The modest increase in pulmonary artery wedge pressure, implying a modest increase in left atrial pressure, and the eventual decline in cardiac output, presumably indicate an effect of etorphine on the heart itself. We note, too, that there was no immediate change in heart rate following etorphine administration in spite of changes in systemic arterial pressure, possibly reflecting etorphine-induced impairment of the baroreceptor reflex.

We are not the first to report that etorphine, and other potent opioids like carfentanil, cause pulmonary hypertension [15], a response that has been implicated in the development of severe pulmonary oedema in animals [18,19]. Pulmonary hypertension and oedema also occur in humans who abuse heroin, morphine, opium and methadone [20]. As far as we are aware, the mechanisms by which acute opioid administration influences pulmonary oxygen exchange have not been explored previously. The effects of pulmonary hypertension on gas exchange have been studied in chronic pulmonary disease [21] and heart failure [22,23], where pulmonary hypertension can either have a protective or pathophysiological effects. Not all studies on the effects of opioids on the pulmonary vasculature are congruent; in the pulmonary vasculature of cats, Hakim *et al.* [20] found that morphine had vasoconstrictor effects whereas Kaye *et al.* [24] found vasodilator effects. The reasons for this disparity are not clear, but, intriguingly, in both studies the vasoactive effects described were antagonised by naloxone and chlorpheniramine or diphenhydramine, indicating that these effects were mediated or modulated by both opioid-receptor and histamine-receptor sensitive pathways [20,24].

In our study, acute etorphine administration led to pulmonary hypertension and systemic hypotension. The increased pulmonary artery pressures had a significant and important clinical impact on our goats. Traditionally hypoxia following etorphine administration has been attributed to its depressive effects on respiratory rhythmogenesis and control (i.e. opioid-induced respiratory depression). However, we have shown, for the first time, that the initial and most severe hypoxia caused by etorphine results mainly from the effects of pulmonary hypertension on alveoli gas exchange. Although these effects were temporary in our goats, their magnitude and timing is clinically significant as the first ten minutes after opioid administration is the time when the most lethal complications from etorphine immobilization can occur [4]. Whether similar pulmonary hypertension, causing a decrease in pulmonary gas exchange, results from administration of other opioids still needs to be investigated, particularly for those opioids used as immobilizing and anaesthetic induction agents.

Conclusion

Because etorphine-induced pulmonary hypertension played such an important role in the development and severity of hypoxia, methods of alleviating respiratory derangements from etorphine, and possibly other opioid agonists, should focus not only on reversing the opioid-induced central respiratory depression, but also on improving oxygen movement across the alveoli membrane, by preventing pulmonary vasoconstriction particular in areas of the lungs that are well ventilated.

Competing interests
The authors declare that they have no competing interests.

Authors' contributions
LCRM – Conceived the study, participated in its design, was involved in acquisition of the data, did the data analysis and interpretation and drafted the manuscript. RSH - Was involved in acquisition of the data, interpretation of the data and critically revised the manuscript for intellectual content. DM - Conceived the study, was involved in interpretation of the data and critically revised the manuscript for intellectual content. AF - Was involved in acquisition of the data, interpretation of the data and critically revised the manuscript for intellectual content. All the authors read and approved the final manuscript.

Acknowledgements
We thank Hugo Minnaar for his help with placing the Swan-Ganz Catheters, staff of the Central Animal Services of the University of the Witwatersrand for their animal management and support, and staff and students from the Brain Function Research Group for their help with animal handling and data collection. We also thank Wildlife Pharmaceuticals, South Africa, for their generous donation of etorphine (Captivon). This work was funded by a Faculty Research Committee Grant, University of the Witwatersrand, a Thuthuka Grant from the National Research Foundation, South Africa, and a Research Grant from the Wildlife Group of the South African Veterinary Association.

References

1. Shook JE, Watkins WD, Camporesi EM. Differential roles of opioid receptors in respiration, respiratory disease, and opioid-induced respiratory depression. Am Rev Respir Dis. 1990;142:895–909.
2. Swan GE. Drugs Used for the Immobilization, Capture, and Translocation of Wild Animals. In: McKenzie AA, editor. The Capture and Care Manual. Pretoria, South Africa: Wildlife Decision Support Services cc and The South African Veterinary Foundation; 1993. p. 17–23.
3. Dahan A, Aarts L, Smith TW. Incidence, reversal and prevention of opioid-induced respiratory depression. Anesthesiology. 2010;112:226–38.
4. Meyer LCR, Hetem RS, Fick LG, Mitchell D, Fuller A. Effects of serotonin agonists and doxapram on respiratory depression and hypoxemia in etorphine-immobilized impala (*Aepyceros melampus*). J Wildlife Dis. 2010;46:514–24.
5. Boom M, Nieters M, Sarton E, Aarts L, Smith TW, Dahan A. Non-analgesic effects of opioids: opioid-induced respiratory depression. Curr Pharm Design. 2012;18:5994–6004.
6. Pattinson KTS. Opioids and the control of respiration. Brit J Anaesth. 2008;100:747–58.
7. McCrimmon DR, Alheid GF. On the opiate trail of respiratory depression. Am J Physiol-Regul Inter Comp Physiol. 2003;285:R1274–5.
8. Kimura S, Haji A. Pharmacological strategy for overcoming opioid-induced ventilatory disturbances. Eur J Pharmacol. 2014;725:87–90.
9. Meyer LCR, Fuller A, Mitchell D. Zacopride and 8-OH-DPAT reverse opioid-induced respiratory depression and hypoxia but not catatonic immobilization in goats. Am J Physiol-Reg Inter Comp Physiol. 2006;290:R405–13.
10. Barenbrug AWT. Psychrometry and Psychrometric Charts. 3rd ed. Chamber of Mines of South Africa: Cape Town, South Africa; 1974.
11. Beker A, Gipson TA, Puchala R, Askar AR, Tesfai K, Detweiler GD, et al. Energy expenditure and activity of different types of small ruminants grazing varying pastures in the summer. J Appl Anim Res. 2010;37:1–14.
12. Roquebert J, Delgoulet C. Cardiovascular effects of etorphine in rats. J Auton Pharmacol. 1988;8:39–43.
13. Lumb AB, editor. Nunn's Applied Respiratory Physiology. 6th ed. Philadelphia, USA: Elsevier Butterworth Heinemann; 2005.
14. Heard DJ, Kollias GV, Buss D, Caligiuri R, Coniglario J. Comparative cardiovascular effects of intravenous etorphine and carfentanil in domestic goats. J Zoo Wildlife Med. 1990;21:166–70.
15. Heard DJ, Nichols WW, Buss D, Kollias GV. Comparative cardiopulmonary effects of intramuscularly administered etorphine and carfentanil in goats. Am J Vet Res. 1996;57:87–96.
16. West JB. Respiratory Physiology the Essentials. 9th ed. Baltimore: Lippincott William & Wilkins; 2012.
17. McKenzie A. The Capture and Care Manual. Wildlife Decision Support Services cc and The South African Veterinary Foundation: Pretoria, South Africa; 1993.
18. Shaw ML, Carpenter JW, Leith DE. Complications with the use of carfentanil citrate and xylazine hydrochloride to immobilize domestic horses. J Am Vet Med Assoc. 1995;6:833–6.
19. Hattingh J, Knox CM, Raath JP, Keet DF. Arterial blood pressure in anaesthetized African elephants. S Afr J Wildl Res. 1994;24:15–7.
20. Hakim TS, Grunstein MM, Michel RP. Opiate action in the pulmonary circulation. Pulm Pharmacol. 1992;5:159–65.
21. Agusti AGN, Rodriguez-Roisin R. Effect of pulmonary hypertension on gas exchange. Eur Respir J. 1993;6:1371–7.
22. Torchio R, Gulotta C, Greco-Lucchina P, Perboni A, Montagna L, Guglielmo M, et al. Closing capacity and gas exchange in chronic heart failure. Chest. 2006;129:1336.
23. Robertson HT. Gas exchange consequences of left heart failure. Comp Physiol. 2011;1:621–34.
24. Kaye AD, Hoover JM, Kaye AJ, Ibrahim IN, Fox C, Bajwa A, et al. Morphine, opioids, and the feline pulmonary vascular bed. Acta Anaesthesiol Scand. 2008;52:931–7.

22

A longitudinal survey of African swine fever in Uganda reveals high apparent disease incidence rates in domestic pigs, but absence of detectable persistent virus infections in blood and serum

Denis Muhangi[1*], Charles Masembe[2], Ulf Emanuelson[3], Sofia Boqvist[4], Lawrence Mayega[5], Rose Okurut Ademun[6], Richard P Bishop[7], Michael Ocaido[1], Mikael Berg[4] and Karl Ståhl[4,8]

Abstract

Background: African swine fever (ASF) is a fatal, haemorrhagic disease of domestic pigs, that poses a serious threat to pig farmers and is currently endemic in domestic pigs in most of sub-Saharan Africa. To obtain insight into the factors related to ASF outbreaks at the farm-level, a longitudinal study was performed in one of the major pig producing areas in central Uganda. Potential risk factors associated with outbreaks of ASF were investigated including the possible presence of apparently healthy ASF-virus (ASFV) infected pigs, which could act as long-term carriers of the virus. Blood and serum were sampled from 715 pigs (241 farms) and 649 pigs (233 farms) to investigate presence of ASFV and antibodies, during the periods of June-October 2010 and March-June 2011, respectively. To determine the potential contribution of different risks to ASF spread, a questionnaire-based survey was administered to farmers to assess the association between ASF outbreaks during the study period and the risk factors.

Results: Fifty-one (21 %) and 13 (5.6 %) farms reported an ASF outbreak on their farms in the previous one to two years and during the study period, respectively. The incidence rate for ASF prior to the study period was estimated at 14.1 per 100 pig farm-years and 5.6 per 100 pig farm-years during the study. Three pigs tested positive for ASFV using real-time PCR, but none tested positive for ASFV specific antibodies using two different commercial ELISA tests.

Conclusions: There was no evidence for existence of pigs that were long-term carriers for the virus based on the analysis of blood and serum as there were no seropositive pigs and the only three ASFV DNA positive pigs were acutely infected and were linked to outbreaks reported by farmers during the study. Potential ASF risk factors were present on both small and medium-scale pig farms, although small scale farms exhibited a higher proportion with multiple potential risk factors (like borrowing boars for sows mating, buying replacement from neighboring farms without ascertaining health status, etc) and did not implement any biosecurity measures. However, no risk factors were significantly associated with ASF reports during the study.

Keywords: African swine fever (ASF), Epidemiology, Incidence rate, Risk factors, Smallholder farmers

* Correspondence: mdenis@covab.mak.ac.ug
[1]Department of Wildlife and Aquatic Resources, College of Veterinary Medicine, Animal Resources and Biosecurity, Makerere University, P. O. Box 7062, Kampala, Uganda
Full list of author information is available at the end of the article

Background

ASF is a fatal, haemorrhagic, viral infection of pigs caused by ASFV, an *Asfivirus* and the only member of the family *Asfarviridae*, which poses a threat to both commercial and smallholder pig farmers. It is currently endemic in at least 26 countries in sub-Saharan Africa [1] as well as on the Island of Sardinia (Italy), the Caucasus, parts of Russia, and in eastern part of the European Union where it was introduced in 2014. The disease can have a severe socio-economic impact on people's livelihoods, food security and both regional and international trade [2].

In sub-Saharan Africa (SSA), the importance of pig production to food security and household incomes is growing and the numbers of pigs on the continent have increased almost threefold during the last decades [1, 3, 4]. This is as a result of a steady increase in demand for animal protein by a growing middle-class. Since most of the increase is taking place in smallholder or backyard husbandry systems with low levels of biosecurity, the growth of the sector creates disease prevention and control challenges [5]. A larger and denser pig population on the continent coupled with an increase in movements of pigs and pig products, as well as people, is most likely the main factor responsible for the upsurge of ASF in many new areas in SSA [1, 5]. The current ASF situation, with the rising numbers of endemically infected countries in SSA and Europe and more ASFV circulating globally constitutes a serious threat to ASF-free countries in Europe as well as Asia [6]. Further spill-over events from either Africa, the Caucasus or eastern Europe, as a result of increased movement of people and pig products, could lead to huge losses in international trade [5].

To date, three cycles involved in the transmission of ASF have been identified: the sylvatic cycle involving circulation of the virus between warthogs (*Phacochoerus africanus*) and soft ticks of the genus *Ornithodoros*, the tick-to-domestic pig cycle and lastly the domestic pig-to-pig cycle [7]. The sylvatic cycle is present in eastern and southern Africa and here, historically, it is considered the main source of outbreaks of ASF in domestic pigs [8]. Today, however, the disease has become endemic in the growing domestic pig populations in several countries in the region, including Uganda, with outbreaks mainly associated with movements of pigs and pig products [1]. A sufficiently large population provides a constant supply of naïve pigs, and is, in the low biosecurity setting dominating in SSA, therefore likely to allow maintenance of ASF without involvement of the sylvatic host. The presence of apparently healthy long-term carriers possibly shedding the virus as suggested by some authors [9–12] would further facilitate the indefinite perpetuation of the disease.

The aim of the study was to investigate the factors related to ASF outbreaks at farm-level, and maintenance of the disease in the domestic pig population, including the existence and possible role of apparently healthy ASFV infected pigs, which could act as long-term carriers of the virus.

Results

Farms sampled

A total of 715 pigs (241 farms) and 649 pigs (233 farms) were sampled at the first and second sampling time points, respectively. Despite one of the study's conditions being that the farmers were to keep pigs until the next visit for follow up, eight of the farmers were not available at the second sampling point. Of these, two had sold off all pigs as a result of suspected ASF on the farm. The rest either sold them off for reasons other than ASF or they were not available for interview at the second visit.

Four hundred seventy six (476) pigs on 161 farms from Masaka and 239 pigs on 80 farms were sampled from Rakai during the first sampling point (Fig. 1). Four hundred twenty two (422) pigs on 154 farms and 227 pigs on 79 farms from Masaka and Rakai, respectively were sampled during the second phase of the study (Fig. 1).

Awareness and knowledge of ASF

The vast majority of the farmers were aware of ASF and could correctly describe two to three of the most important clinical signs. ASF was generally described as a disease that has no cure or vaccine, and that kills large numbers of pigs fast. Pigs develop high fever, lose appetite and die within two days. Discoloration of the skin (turning blue or red) is also mentioned.

Incidence of ASF

A total of 51 (21 %) farms reported having had incidences of ASF one to two years preceding the first visit. Between the first and second visits, 13 (5.6 %) farms reported having experienced an outbreak of ASF (Fig. 1), with mortalities between 12–100 % (median 66 %). In one of the farms, ASF was confirmed as positive by RT-PCR in two out of the three pigs sampled. The incidence rates for ASF were estimated at 14.1 per 100 pig farm-years (95 % CI 7.7;23.5) and 5.6 per 100 pig farm-years (95 % CI 2.2;13.1) for the periods prior to and between the two visits, respectively. The difference in estimated incidence rates for the two periods was not statistically significant (*P*-value = 0.10).

ASFV DNA and antibody detection

Genomic DNA was successfully extracted from all the pooled samples. All the pigs in the initial round tested

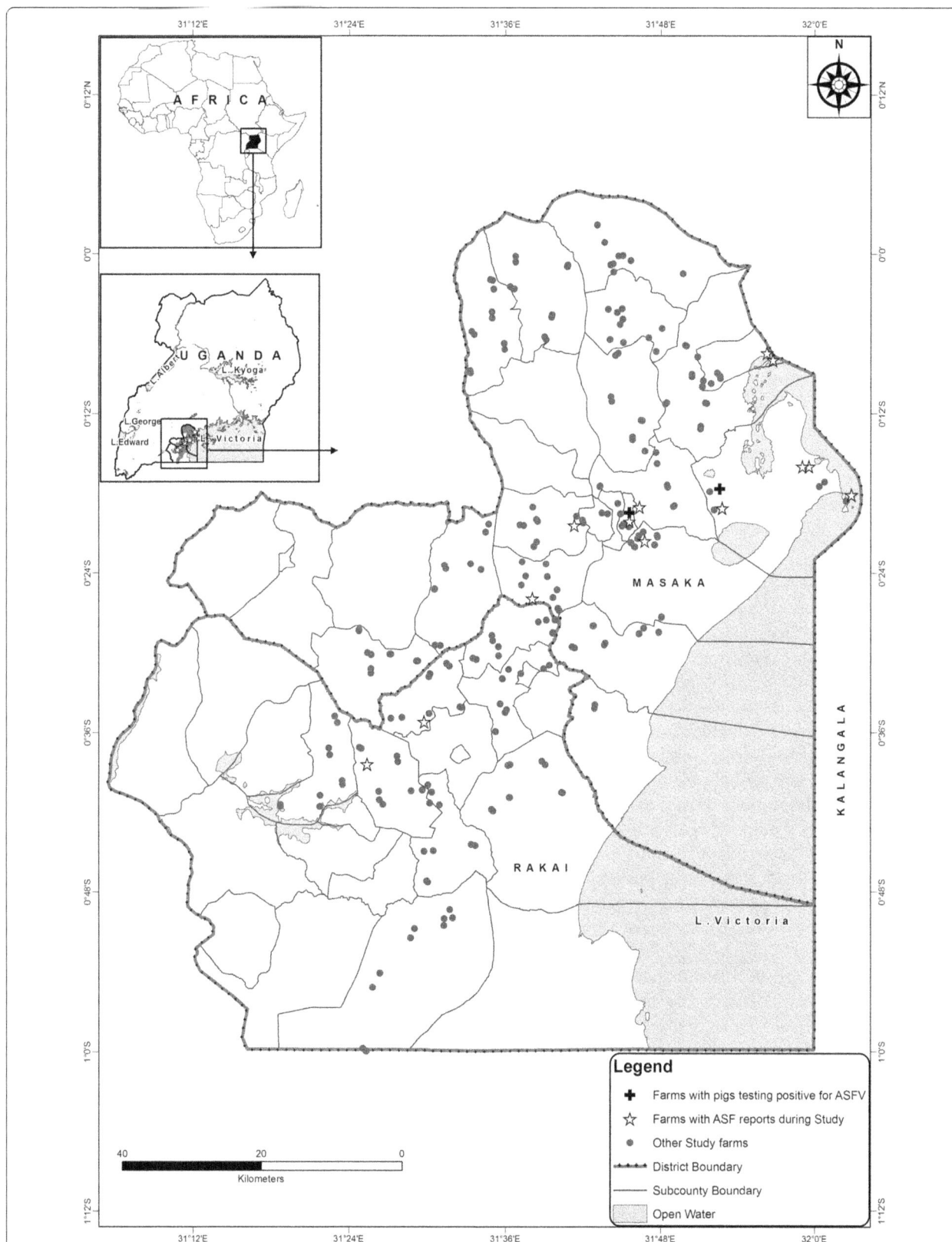

Fig. 1 Distribution of pig farms reporting ASF in Masaka and Rakai, Uganda. Map of the study area showing the pig farms sampled (n = 241) in Masaka and Rakai, Uganda (2010–2011). The highlighted farms (star symbol) are the farms where farmers reported ASF during the study and cross symbol are those confirmed positive by RT-PCR

negative for ASFV using RT-PCR. In the second sampling round, three pigs from two different farms tested positive (Ct values: 21.2, 37.9 and 38.8) (Fig. 1). These two farms were both located in areas where outbreaks of ASF had occurred. The corresponding true prevalences were estimated at 0 % (95 % CI 0; 0.6) and 0.5 % (95 % CI 0.1; 1.5) at the first and the second sampling-points, respectively.

Twenty-three sera were either antibody positive or doubtful on the first run using INGENASA. However, a re-run on all the positive sera (n = 5) using INGENASA and SVANOVIR ASFV-Ab ELISA tests, and all doubtful sera (n = 18) using SVANOVIR, resulted in none of the samples being positive for ASF antibodies with either of the two different ELISA tests used.

Differential diagnosis
In total 239 samples were analyzed for presence of antibodies and nucleic acids specific to CSFV and PRRSV, respectively. All samples tested negative for CSF and PPRS in ELISA as well as in RT-PCR. This is also reported as preliminary results in a student thesis [13].

Herd categories and risk factors
The numbers of farms according to size were 185 (78.7 %) and 50 (21.3 %) for small and medium-scale pig farms, respectively, with six missing values at first sampling. At second sampling, the numbers were 179 (76.5 %) and 49 (20.9 %) farms for the small-scale and medium-scale farms, respectively. Results from the questionnaire are presented in Tables 1 and 2. There were more farms with high proportions of improved breeds compared to those with local breeds of pigs. There were comparably more farms that borrowed boars from other farms for mating than those that did not, more farms sourcing replacement stock from neighbouring farms than those obtaining replacement stock generated on their own farms. For small-scale farms, those with none of the biosecurity measures (fences, controlled access to pens, foot-baths) were greater in number than those with at least one of the biosecurity measures in place (Table 1). The medium-scale farms had more farms that had at least one biosecurity measure than those that had none (Table 2). Feeding swill was common in both small and medium-scale farms.

The risk factor analysis of reported outbreaks of ASF during the study period did not produce any statistically significant predictors (Table 3).

Discussion
ASF has had a global upsurge, and has been reported in at least 26 countries in SSA alone during the last few years [1]. The disease is considered endemic in domestic pig populations in many of these countries, but data on

incidence rates is scarce. In our study population, more than 5 % of the farms reported incursions of ASF during the one-year study period (ASF between). Albeit based on farmer reports, this gives a rough estimate of the incidence rate of the disease in the population. Nine of the 13 affected farms were located in areas in which we confirmed ASF during this period (data not shown), supporting the accuracy of the reports. The estimated incidence rate for the period prior to the study (ASF prior) was numerically higher compared to ASF between, but the difference was not statistically significant. This latter estimate is likely to be less accurate than for ASF between, because it includes farmers' perception of time since last experience of ASF and was therefore excluded from analysis of risk factors. Record keeping among smallholder pig farmers in the region is generally poor [14].

Important differential diagnoses to ASF such as CSF and PRRS, have never been reported in Uganda or in neighboring countries [15], and our study also failed to demonstrate presence of or exposure to these diseases in the study population. Moreover, during the period 2010–2012, we investigated around 50 reported outbreaks of suspected ASF in Uganda, including several in the study area, and in all but two ASF was confirmed, clearly suggesting ASF as the most prevalent cause of disease with high mortality in pigs in the region. All samples (n = 80) from four of these outbreaks, including the two in which ASF was not confirmed, were also tested for CSF and PRRS with negative results in all but one sample which was weakly positive on PRRS ELISA [13]. Given that only one out of a total of 319 samples tested positive for PRRS antibodies, the weakly positive result was interpreted as false positive. Our case definition was based on farmer reports of outbreaks of disease with clinical signs suggestive of, but not pathognomonic to ASF, which could imply a risk for misclassification. However, given the level of awareness of ASF demonstrated by the farmers, the very dramatic clinical signs typically associated with ASF, and the probable absence of the most important differential diagnoses in the study population, this risk is considered low.

Bacterial diseases such as erysipelas, which do occur in the study area, are also often mentioned as differential diagnoses to ASF, due to similar clinical signs in the individual animal. However, in contrast to ASF, erysipelas is a curable disease that most often affects individual animals rather than entire herds, and was therefore not considered in the study.

Several authors have reported high prevalences of ASF, based on detection of ASFV DNA in blood, serum and/ or tissues using PCR in apparently healthy and often seronegative domestic pigs originating from locations

Table 1 Risk factors for small-scale farms for ASF reports between first and second sampling (n = 179), 2010–2011

Risk factor		[a] ASF between			
		No[b] (%)	Yes[b] (%)	NA[b] (%)	Total (n)
Awareness [c]	Not aware about ASF	67	0	33	3
	Aware about ASF	69	5	26	170
	NA [d]	33	0	67	6
Biosecurity measures [e]	At least one	70	3	28	40
	None	68	6	27	127
	NA	67	0	33	12
Borrow boar	No	59	0	41	27
	Yes	70	5	25	136
	NA	69	8	23	13
Breed	Local	67	4	28	67
	Improved	69	5	26	111
	NA	0	0	100	1
Duration of enterprises					
	Less or equal to 10 years	67	3	30	112
	Greater than 10 years	74	6	20	50
	NA	63	13	25	16
Ectoparasites control	No	74	0	26	27
	Yes	68	5	28	145
	NA	57	14	29	7
Feeding swill	No	72	9	19	47
	Yes	68	3	29	130
	NA	0	0	100	2
Labour	Family	69	4	26	160
	Hired	69	6	25	16
	NA	0	0	100	3
Pets present on farm	No	67	5	28	111
	Yes	68	4	28	57
	NA	82	0	18	11
Piglets housing	Piglets housing present	69	5	25	91
	Piglets not housed	71	2	27	83
	NA	0	20	80	5
Pigs housing	Pig housing present	66	5	29	111
	No pig housing	75	0	25	64
	NA	25	50	25	4

Table 1 Risk factors for small-scale farms for ASF reports between first and second sampling (n = 179), 2010–2011 *(Continued)*

Replacement stock	Own farm	73	5	23	66
	From neighbouring farms	67	4	29	106
	NA	43	14	43	7
Wild pigs (bush pigs) contact	No	72	5	22	98
	Yes	56	11	33	9
	NA	64	3	33	72

[a] ASF between- Reports of ASF on farms during the one year between the first and second sampling visits. This is the dependent variable and the row variables in the table are the independent variables

[b] The numbers in each of the cells under columns No, Yes and NA are relative proportions (percentages) of the total number of pigs (column Total, n) in each of the table rows

[c] Awareness encompasses those farms where farmers expressed having knowledge on the symptoms, spread, control and prevention measures for ASF

[d] Missing values

[e] Biosecurity measures considered were presence of a fence to the farm, controlled entrance to the pig pens (presence of gate/door) and presence of foot baths

from which no disease had been reported [9–11, 16]. Although the importance of this finding is debated [1], it has raised concern of a role of long-term carriers, which would not be detected through clinical or serological surveillance, in the maintenance of the disease in endemically infected populations. In this study, we did not find any evidence supporting a role of long-term carriers. No PCR positive animals were detected during the first sampling, only a few during the second, and no antibody positive animals during either of the samplings. The two farms with PCR positive animals were both located in areas that had recently reported ASF outbreaks, and in one of them, the farmer reported having had deaths on the farm as a result of ASF just prior to our visit. The three PCR positive animals were seronegative and it is likely that the absence of seroconversion reflected sampling at an early stage of infection before clinical signs had developed and an antibody response had been mounted. A neighbouring farm also reported having had ASF outbreak at the second sampling, which may suggest possible spread from either of the two farms given the management practices and risk factors mentioned earlier.

A number of studies have shown that pigs that survive ASF, may have persisting infection, with detectable virus only in lymphoid tissues, and not in blood or serum, up to 2–3 months after infection [17–19]. Moreover, it has been demonstrated that pigs that survive infection have detectable levels of antibodies that persist for at least 1–2 years, with a half-life estimated at 1.8 years [1, 19, 20]. A scenario with persistent infection only in lymphoid tissues in seronegative pigs has not been described to our knowledge. In this study, no pigs were sacrificed, and therefore

Table 2 Risk factors for medium-scale farms for ASF reports between first and second sampling (n = 49), 2010–2011

| | | [a]ASF between | | | |
		No[b] (%)	Yes[b] (%)	NA[b] (%)	Total (n)
Awareness [c]	Not aware about ASF	50	0	50	2
	Aware about ASF	85	4	11	46
	NA [d]	100	0	0	1
Biosecurity measures [e]	At least one	83	4	13	24
	None	85	5	10	20
	NA	80	0	20	5
Borrow boar	No	100	0	0	17
	Yes	78	4	19	27
	NA	60	20	20	5
Breed	Local	71	14	14	7
	Improved	85	2	12	41
	NA	100	0	0	1
Duration of enterprises	Less or equal to 10 years	85	3	12	34
	Greater than 10 years	75	8	17	12
	NA	100	0	0	3
Ectoparasites control	No	75	0	25	4
	Yes	86	2	12	43
	NA	50	50	0	2
Feeding swill	No	88	6	6	17
	Yes	81	3	16	32
	NA	0	0	100	1
Labour	Family	76	6	18	34
	Hired	100	0	0	9
	NA	100	0	0	6
Pets present on farm	No	84	4	12	25
	Yes	86	0	14	21
	NA	67	33	0	3
Piglets housing	Piglets housing present	80	5	15	40
	Piglets not housed	100	0	0	8
	NA	100	0	0	1
Pig housing	Pig housing present	82	5	14	44
	No pig housing	100	0	0	4
	NA	100	0	0	1
Replacement stock	Own farm	87	0	13	15
	From neighbouring farms	82	6	12	33
	NA	100	0	0	1

Table 2 Risk factors for medium-scale farms for ASF reports between first and second sampling (n = 49), 2010–2011 *(Continued)*

Wild pigs (bush pigs) contact	No	82	6	12	33
	Yes	100	0	0	1
	NA	87	0	13	15

[a] ASF between- Reports of ASF on farms during the one year between the first and second sampling visits. This is the dependent variable and the row variables in the table are the independent variables
[b] The numbers in each of the cells under columns No, Yes and NA are relative proportions (percentages) of the total number of pigs (column Total, n) in each of the table rows
[c] Awareness as a variable encompasses those farms where farmers expressed having knowledge on the symptoms, spread, control and prevention measures for ASF
[d] Missing values
[e] Biosecurity measures considered were presence of a fence to the farm, controlled entrance to the pig pens (presence of gate/door) and presence of foot baths

lymphoid or other tissues could not be tested, but because no antibody positive pigs were found, we do not believe this has affected our results.

To confirm that any positive animals found during the first sampling were persistently positive, as would be expected from long-term carriers, our ambition was to resample the same animals during the second sampling round. This was in many cases not possible. However, given that no animals were positive, neither on PCR nor on ELISA, during the first sampling round, and only three were PCR positive during the second (all closely linked with outbreaks directly affecting study farms), this did not affect the interpretation of our results nor the conclusion regarding presence or absence of potential long-term carriers in the study population.

The absence of detectable seropositivity in the study population is in accordance with several studies suggesting a very low seroprevalence of ASF in domestic pig populations in eastern Africa [21, 22]. The low seroprevalence, in spite of a relatively high incidence of ASF, reflects circulation of a highly virulent strain of ASFV with high mortality, but is likely also a result of the common practice of selling off pigs for slaughter as soon as an outbreak of ASF occurs, to salvage some income from the dying or in-contact pigs [1, 22]. A recent publication from Uganda, however, presents results from a combined slaughterhouse and on-farm study with sampling of apparently healthy pigs and reports a seroprevalence of above 50 %, indicating circulation of low virulent viruses and possibly development of natural resistance [12]. This is in vast contrast not only to our results, but also to those from the several other published studies from the region [10, 16, 21, 22]. The serological analyses in the aforementioned study [12], however, were performed using an in-house ELISA based on the semipurified ASFV antigen. This method is known

Table 3 Univariable logistic regression model on pig farms for ASF reports between the samplings (n = 233), 2010–2011

Independent variables		ASF between		
		OR	95 % CI	P-value
Awareness [a]	Not aware about ASF	1		
	Aware about ASF	-	-	-
Biosecurity measures [b]	None	1		
	At least one	1.01	(0.26;3.37)	0.99
Borrow boar	No	1		
	Yes	-	-	-
Breed	Local	1		
	Improved	0.92	(0.28;3.57)	0.90
Duration of enterprise				
	Less or equal to 10 years	1		
	Greater than 10 years	2.28	(0.61;8.55)	0.21
Ectoparasites control	No	1		
	Yes	-	-	0.99
Farm size	Small-scale	1		
	Medium-scale	2.16	(0.61;7.15)	0.21
Feeding swill	No	1		
	Yes	0.66	(0.20;2.31)	0.49
Labour	Family	1		
	Hired	1.78	(0.38;6.45)	0.41
Pets present on farm	No	1		
	Yes	0.64	(0.14;2.33)	0.53
Piglets housing	Piglets housing present	1		
	Piglets not housed	1.87	(0.52;8.77)	0.37
Pig housing	Pig housing present	1		
	No pig housing	-	-	0.99
Replacement stock	From own stock	1		
	From neighboring farms	1.63	(0.45;7.64)	0.49
Wild pigs (bush pigs) contact	No	1		
	Yes	2.04	(0.10;14.19)	0.53

ASF between - Reports of ASF on farms during the one year between the first and second sampling visits
OR odds tatio, CI confidence interval, ASF African swine fever
- indicates that the model was inestimable because of skewed data
[a]Awareness as a variable encompasses those farms where farmers expressed having knowledge on the symptoms, spread, control and prevention measures for ASF
[b]Biosecurity measures considered were presence of a fence to the farm, controlled entrance to the pig pens (presence of gate/door) and presence of foot baths

to give a certain proportion of false positive test results, especially with poorly preserved samples as is often the case under African conditions due to the hot climate and not always functioning cold chain. Therefore, unexpected positive results, such as in this case, should always be confirmed using an alternative test before conclusions can be drawn from the results [23, 24].

The vast majority of pig farms included in the study were small-scale (78.7 %) with a maximum of ten pigs while medium-scale farms (11–200 pigs) accounted for only 21.3 %. There were high proportions of farms with pigs and piglets that were not housed. There were differences in the relative importance of risk factors and the extent of use of biosecurity measures between medium-scale and small-scale farms (Tables 1 and 2). This difference in distribution of ASF risk factors and biosecurity measures between the two categories of farms agrees with the findings reported by Costard et al [25] in an earlier study in Madagascar. On both categories of small and medium-scale farms, farmers reported improper disposal of carcasses which included selling of dead/dying pigs for slaughter, throwing carcasses in bushes and giving pork from diseased pigs to neighbours (data not shown). These practices will certainly promote the spread of ASF through movement of the infected pigs, contaminated carcasses and pork products especially during ASF outbreaks. None of the risk factors were, however, significantly associated with ASF outbreaks between the two visits, probably partly due to low power of the study, imprecise identifications of the risk factors, and to some extent missing values (NA). However, the proportion of missing values was usually low (below 10 %), except for the question on contacts with wild pigs, and we believe that the missing answers would be non-differential thus only leading to a bias towards the null hypothesis.

Conclusions

Our results indicate a high incidence rate of ASF in the study area, and demonstrate that long-term carriers are not needed to explain the maintenance of the disease in the population. Potential ASF risk factors were present on both small and medium-scale pig farms, although small-scale farms exhibited a higher proportion with multiple potential risk factors and lacking any implementation of biosecurity measures. However, no risk factors were significantly associated with ASF reports during the study.

Methods

Study area and farm selection

A longitudinal study was carried out in the districts of Masaka and Rakai in central Uganda (Fig. 1). A total of 24 sub-counties were selected by targeting sub-counties with the largest number of pig farms as indicated by the district veterinary officers. A sampling frame of villages within selected sub-counties was generated, and five villages were randomly selected per sub-county. Two farmers within each of these villages were selected in consultation with the district veterinary officers. In some cases, the veterinary officers suggested new villages as replacements based on unavailability of pigs in some of the originally selected villages. A farm was only included in the sample if the farmer affirmed that he/she planned to keep pigs for the next one year and if the farm reared at least three pigs. The farms were visited twice, during June to October 2010 and during March to June 2011. All farms were geo-referenced (Fig. 1).

Data collection

Information was collected using a questionnaire with closed and open-ended questions, after getting informed consent. The questionnaire was initially discussed with the local veterinary personnel to make sure they all understood the questions similarly since they had to be translated into Luganda, the local language. The enumerators made sure that the questions were understood by the respondents. During the first visit, farmer awareness and knowledge of ASF was investigated. Also, the farmers were asked whether their pigs had had any incidences of infectious disease with clinical signs suggestive of ASF (that is mortality, fever, loss of appetite, reddened skin) on their farm in the previous 1–2 years. In addition, information on management practices, biosecurity measures and general information on the farms were taken (Tables 1 and 2). During the second visit, the farmers were asked specifically if they had had outbreaks of ASF since the previous visit and also to describe the outcome of these outbreaks in terms of clinical signs and mortality.

Sample collection

Permission was sought to sample three pigs from farms where interviews were conducted. Three pigs were chosen from each herd, restrained by the muzzle using a commercially available pig catcher and examined by a veterinarian. All the pigs sampled were at least three months of age. Sampling was done twice on the pig farms (*i.e.* at each visit at time periods as indicated above), with an ambition of including the same pigs in the two samplings. This, however, was in many cases not possible, because pigs had been sold or had died or the farmers could not be found at the time of the second sampling. Whole blood was taken from the jugular vein into appropriate vacutainers. Serum samples were similarly collected from each pig into appropriate serum vacutainers (BD, New Jersey). Whole blood was aliquoted into duplicate 2 ml cryovials (Cryo.s, Greiner Bio-one, Wemmel). Serum tubes were centrifuged at 2000 g for 10 mins to separate serum from clotted blood serum aliquoted into duplicate 2 ml cryovials. The aliquoting and centrifugation were done at the regional district laboratories every evening after farm visits. The duplicate cryovials were later transported on ice in cool boxes to the Molecular Genetics Laboratory in the College of Agriculture and Environmental Sciences, Makerere University for storage at -20 °C and -80 °C as working and long-term storage sample aliquots, respectively.

All handling of animals including sampling was carried out, or overseen, by District Veterinary office staff in accordance with their national mandate. The district veterinary office, under the Ministry of Agriculture Animal Industry and Fisheries (MAAIF) has the official mandate to carry out investigations related to animal disease in the country.

ASFV DNA detection

In order to check for the presence of ASFV nucleic acids, the samples were prepared for total DNA extraction. One hundred microlitres of anticoagulated blood from each pig sample for the three pigs per farm was collectively pooled and thoroughly mixed to make 300 µl. From this pool, 100 µl was used for total genomic DNA extraction using the DNeasy Blood & Tissue kit (Qiagen, Duesseldorf) following the manufacturer's protocol. In all extraction steps, a negative control was included. The extracted DNA was either immediately used in the RT-PCR assay, or stored at -20 °C until used. For the detection of ASFV DNA, a commercially available ASF RT-PCR Tetracore® assay (Tetracore Inc., Rockville, Maryland) was used according to the instructions of the manufacturer. The assay was optimized for use on a SmartCycler® (Cepheid Inc., Sunnyvale, California), a 10 kg portable instrument that is operated by a laptop computer [26].

For the pooled samples that tested positive, the entire procedure from DNA extraction to RT-PCR was repeated for individual pig blood samples to identify which of the three pigs was actually positive.

ASFV antibody detection

For the detection of antibodies against ASFV, a commercially available blocking ELISA (INGEZIM PPA Compac 11.PPA.K3, INGENASA, Spain), recommended by the OIE, was used in accordance with instructions from the manufacturer. It targets the VP73 viral protein and is reported to have a sensitivity and specificity of 95–98 % [27]. The positive and doubtful samples were re-tested for confirmation using the same INGENASA ELISA and the recently released SVANOVIR® ASFV-Ab (Boehringer Ingelheim Svanova, Uppsala, Sweden) indirect ELISA. The SVANOVIR® ASFV-Ab ELISA kit (screening plates) was used according to the instructions by the manufacturer.

Differential diagnosis

To reduce the risk of misclassification, a subset of the samples from the first sampling round was also tested for classical swine fever, the most important differential diagnosis to ASF. In addition, the same subset was tested for presence of porcine reproductive and respiratory syndrome (PRRS) virus, which in its most virulent form can cause a disease with clinical signs resembling ASF. For antibody detection, commercial ELISA kits were used (CSF Ab test and PRRS X3 antibody test, IDEXX Laboratories Inc., Maine, USA). For virus detection, commercially available CSF and PRRS RT-PCR kits were used (Tetracore Inc., Rockville, Maryland). All tests were run according to the instructions by the manufacturers.

Statistical analysis

Incidence rates for ASF in the study population were estimated based on the farmer reports of outbreaks 1–2 years prior to first sampling (ASF prior; 1.5 years taken as denominator) and of outbreaks between first and second sampling (ASF between; 1 year as denominator), respectively. A case was defined as a herd with a reported outbreak during the period of interest of an infectious disease with clinical signs suggestive of ASF, i.e. high mortality, high fever and loss of appetite, with or without discoloration of the skin, diarrhea, abortions etc.

A test of whether the two incidence estimates were significantly different was computed in R. Logistic regression models were used to assess the association between reports of outbreaks during the period of interest of an infectious disease with clinical signs suggestive of ASF (response variable) and management practices (independent variables). In this analysis, only outbreaks that occurred between first and second sampling were considered. None of the risk factors were associated with the response variable ($P > 0.25$) and no multivariable model was therefore attempted. Data was analysed using R statistical package (Version 2.15.2) for logistic regressions [28]. In this study, the farms were grouped into two categories basing on the number of pigs reared. They included; small-scale (1–10 pigs) and medium-scale pig farms (11–200 pigs).

Positive and negative test results based on RT-PCR and ELISA were entered into a Microsoft Excel spreadsheet (Microsoft Corporation, Redmond, Washington). Apparent and true prevalence were computed using epiR package in R (Version 2.15.3) and as earlier described [29] using sensitivity and specificity of 90 and 100 % respectively [26].

Abbreviations
ASF: African swine fever; ASFV: African swine fever virus; CSF: Classical swine fever; Ct: Cycle threshold; DNA: Deoxyribonucleic acid; ELISA:: Enzyme-linked immunosorbent assay; PCR: Polymerase chain reaction; PRRS: Porcine reproductive and respiratory syndrome; RT-PCR: Real time polymerase chain reaction.

Competing interests
The authors declare that they have no competing interests.

Authors' contributions
DM contributed to the conception of the idea, data collection, data analysis, laboratory studies, drafting and writing of the manuscript. CM contributed to data collection, laboratory studies and manuscript preparation. UE contributed to conception of the idea, data analysis and drafting of the manuscript. SB contributed to conception of the idea and writing of the manuscript. LM contributed to conception of the idea, design of the study and data collection and writing of the manuscript. ROA contributed to conception of the idea, data collection and writing of the manuscript. RPB contributed to conception of the idea, design and writing of the manuscript. MO contributed to conception of the idea and writing of the manuscript. MB contributed to conception of the idea, design and writing of the manuscript. KS contributed to the conception of the idea, data collection,

data analysis, laboratory studies, drafting and writing of the manuscript. All authors read and approved the final manuscript.

Authors' information

DM is a PhD holder (formerly PhD student) who worked with this team as part of his doctoral studies and is a researcher at Makerere University. CM is associate professor and researcher at Makerere University and has sufficiently researched on livestock diseases. UE is a Professor of veterinary epidemiology. SB has research interest in livestock diseases and veterinary public health and is associate professor at Swedish University of Agricultural Sciences (SLU). LM is a senior veterinary officer working under MAAIF and is conversant with ASF occurrence in the study area. ROA is senior veterinary officer at MAAIF's National Diseases Diagnostic Centre (NADDEC)'s laboratory, Uganda's livestock diseases diagnostic center. RPB is a researcher under International Livestock Research Institute (ILRI) and has previously researched on ASF in eastern Africa. MO is a professor of veterinary medicine with research interests in tick-borne diseases in both domestic animals and wildlife. MB is a professor of veterinary virology based at SLU. KS is associate professor and deputy state epizootiologist at the National Veterinary Institute (SVA) in Uppsala, Sweden, with expertise in infectious diseases epidemiology and disease control.

Acknowledgements

We acknowledge the Swedish research council FORMAS (Grant No. 221-2009-1984) and the Swedish international development cooperation agency, Sida (Grant No. 75007369) through the Embassy of Sweden in Kampala under the framework of Sida-Mak bilateral research support program phase 3 to the vet sub-program (awarded in 2010) who provided the financial support for this study. We also acknowledge the contribution from our collaborating institutions like Swedish University of Agricultural Sciences (SLU), National Veterinary Institute (SVA), International Livestock Research Institute (ILRI), Makerere University, and MAAIF in Uganda. Our gratitude also goes to Ms. Susan Ndyanabo who assisted in running some experiments at the molecular genetics laboratory, College of Agriculture and Environmental Sciences, Makerere University and to all the field veterinarians in Masaka and Rakai, who worked with us in collecting samples and data for this study.

Author details

[1]Department of Wildlife and Aquatic Resources, College of Veterinary Medicine, Animal Resources and Biosecurity, Makerere University, P. O. Box 7062, Kampala, Uganda. [2]Department of Biological Sciences, College of Natural Sciences, Makerere University, P. O. Box 7062, Kampala, Uganda. [3]Department of Clinical Sciences, Swedish University of Agricultural Sciences, P. O. Box 7054, SE-750 07 Uppsala, Sweden. [4]Department of Biomedical Sciences and Veterinary Public Health, Swedish University of Agricultural Sciences, P. O. Box 7028, SE-750 07 Uppsala, Sweden. [5]District Veterinary Office, under the Ministry of Agriculture, Animal Industry and Fisheries, Masaka, Uganda. [6]Ministry of Agriculture, Animal Industry and Fisheries, P. O. Box 102, Entebbe, Uganda. [7]International Livestock Research Institute (ILRI), P.O. Box 30709, GPO 00100 Nairobi, Kenya. [8]Department of Disease Control and Epidemiology, National Veterinary Institute (SVA), SE-751 89 Uppsala, Sweden.

References

1. Penrith ML, Vosloo W, Jori F, Bastos ADS. African swine fever virus eradication in Africa. Virus Res. 2013;173:228–46.
2. FAO. FAO takes a close look at the threat of African swine fever introduction into Eastern Europe. In: EMPRES Transboundary Animal Diseases Bulletin. vol. 36. Rome, FAO (available at http://www.fao.org/docrep/013/i1958e/i1958e00.pdf) 2010.
3. FAOSTAT: [http://faostat3.fao.org/home/index.html]. 2011.
4. Kagira J, Kanyari PN, Maingi N, Githigia S, Ng'ang'a JC, Karuga J. Characteristics of the smallholder free-range pig production system in western Kenya. Trop Anim Health Prod. 2010;42(5):865–73.
5. FAO. African Swine Fever (ASF) Recent developments and timely updates - Worrisome dynamics: Steady spread towards unaffected areas could have

disastrous impact. In: Edited by Focus on No. 6 [electronic bulletin]. Rome, FAO (available at http://www.fao.org/docrep/016/ap372e/ap372e.pdf); 2012.
6. Sánchez-Vizcaíno JM, Arias M. African Swine fever virus. In: Zimmerman JJ, Karriker LA, Ramirez A, Schwartz KJ, Stevenson GW, editors. Diseases of swine. 10th ed. Ames, Iowa: Blackwell Publishing Professional; 2012. p. 396–404.
7. Penrith ML, Thomson GR, Bastos ADS. African swine fever. In: Coetzer JAW, Tustin RC, editors. Infectious diseases of livestock with special reference to Southern Africa. Cape Town: Oxford University Press; 2004. p. 1087–119.
8. Jori F, Vial L, Penrith ML, Pérez-Sánchez R, Etter E, Albina E, et al. Review of the sylvatic cycle of African swine fever in sub-Saharan Africa and the Indian Ocean. Virus Res. 2013;173(1):212–27.
9. Owolodun OA, Obishakin ET, Ekong PS, Yakubu B. Investigation of African swine fever in slaughtered pigs, Plateau state, Nigeria, 2004–2006. Trop Anim Health Prod. 2010;42(8):1605–10.
10. Gallardo C, Okoth E, Pelayo V, Anchuelo R, Martı´n E, Simo´ n A, et al. African swine fever viruses with two different genotypes, both of which occur in domestic pigs, are associated with ticks and adult warthogs, respectively, at a single geographical site. J Gen Virol. 2011;92:432–44.
11. Fasina FO, Shamaki D, Makinde AA, Lombin LH, Lazarus DD, Rufai SA, et al. Surveillance for African swine fever in Nigeria, 2006–2009. Transbound Emerg Dis. 2010;57:244–53.
12. Atuhaire DK, Afayoa M, Ochwo S, Mwesigwa S, Mwiine FN, Okuni JB, et al. Prevalence of African swine fever virus in apparently healthy domestic pigs in Uganda. BMC Vet Res. 2013;9:263.
13. Andersson M. African swine fever in Uganda- description of a recent outbreak and studies of possible differential diagnoses. Uppsala, Sweden: Swedish University of Agricultural Sciences; 2011. Retrieved from http://stud.epsilon.slu.se/2407/1/andersson_m_110401.pdf.
14. Muhanguzi D, Lutwama V, Mwiine FN. Factors that influence pig production in Central Uganda - Case study of Nangabo Sub-County. Wakiso district Vet World. 2012;5(6):346–51.
15. OIE: WAHID interface animal health information [http://www.oie.int/wahis_2/public/wahid.php/Diseaseinformation/Diseasedistributionmap]. 2014.
16. Okoth E, Gallardo C, Macharia JM, Omore A, Pelayo V, Bulimo DW, et al. Comparison of African swine fever virus prevalence and risk in two contrasting pig-farming systems in South-West and Central Kenya. Prev Vet Med. 2013;110(2):198–205.
17. Wilkinson PJ. The persistence of African swine fever in Africa and the Mediterranean. Prev Vet Med. 1984;2:71–82.
18. de Carvalho Ferreira HC, Weesendorp E, Elbers AR, Bouma A, Quak S, Stegeman JA, et al. African swine fever virus excretion patterns in persistently infected animals: a quantitative approach. Vet Microbiol. 2012;160(3–4):327–40.
19. Penrith ML, Thomson GR, Bastos AD, Phiri OC, Lubisi BA, Du Plessis EC, et al. An investigation into natural resistance to African swine fever in domestic pigs from an endemic area in Southern Africa. Rev Sci Tech. 2004;23(3):965–77.
20. Sanchez Botija C. Peste Porcina Africana- Nuevos desarollos. Rev sci tech Off int Epiz. 1982;1(4):991–1029.
21. Gallardo C, Ademun AR, Nieto R, Nantima N, Arias M, Martín E, et al. Genotyping of African swine fever virus (ASFV) isolates associated with disease outbreaks in Uganda in 2007. Afr J Biotechnol. 2011;10(17):3488–97.
22. Muwonge A, Munang'andu HM, Kankya C, Biffa D, Oura C, Skjerve E, et al. African swine fever among slaughter pigs in Mubende district, Uganda. Trop Anim Health Prod. 2012;44:1593–8.
23. OIE. African swine fever. In: Manual of diagnostic tests and vaccines for terrestrial animals (mammals, birds and bees). Chapter 2.8.1. Paris, France: World Organisation for Animal Health; 2012.
24. Cubillos C, Gómez-Sebastian S, Moreno N, Nuñez MC, Mulumba-Mfumu LK, Quembo CJ, et al. African swine fever virus serodiagnosis: a general review with a focus on the analyses of African serum samples. Virus Res. 2013;173(1):159–67.
25. Costard S, Porphyre V, Messad S, Rakotondrahanta S, Vidon H, Roger F, et al. Multivariate analysis of management and biosecurity practices in smallholder pig farms in Madagascar. Prev Vet Med. 2009;92(3):199–209.
26. Zsak L, Borca MV, Risatti GR, Zsak A, French RA, Lu Z, et al. Preclinical diagnosis of African swine fever in contact-exposed swine by a real-time PCR assay. J Clin Microbiol. 2005;43(1):112–9.
27. Etter EMC, Seck I, Grosbois V, Jori F, Blanco E, Vial L, et al. Seroprevalence of African Swine Fever in Senegal, 2006. Emerg Infect Dis. 2011;17:1.

28. R Core Team. R: A Language and Environment for Statistical Computing. In. Edited by R Foundation for Statistical Computing. Vienna, Austria: R Foundation for Statistical Computing; ISBN 3-900051-07-0; http://www. R-project.org/; 2012.

29. Reiczigel J, Földi J, Ózsvári L. Exact confidence limits for prevalence of a disease with an imperfect diagnostic test. Epidemiol Infect. 2010;138(11):1674–8.

Permissions

List of Contributors

Hua Zhang
College of Veterinary Medicine, Nanjing Agricultural University, Nanjing, Jiangsu 210095, China

Zhenlei Zhou
College of Veterinary Medicine, Nanjing Agricultural University, Nanjing, Jiangsu 210095, China

Jingwen Luo
College of Veterinary Medicine, Nanjing Agricultural University, Nanjing, Jiangsu 210095, China

Jiafa Hou
College of Veterinary Medicine, Nanjing Agricultural University, Nanjing, Jiangsu 210095, China

Cristina López
Pharmacology, Department of Biomedical Sciences, Institute of Biomedicine (IBIOMED), University of León, Campus de Vegazana s/n, 24071 León, Spain

Juan José García
Pharmacology, Department of Biomedical Sciences, Institute of Biomedicine (IBIOMED), University of León, Campus de Vegazana s/n, 24071 León, Spain

Matilde Sierra
Pharmacology, Department of Biomedical Sciences, Institute of Biomedicine (IBIOMED), University of León, Campus de Vegazana s/n, 24071 León, Spain

María José Diez
Pharmacology, Department of Biomedical Sciences, Institute of Biomedicine (IBIOMED), University of León, Campus de Vegazana s/n, 24071 León, Spain

Claudia Pérez
Department of Animal Health, University of León, Campus de Vegazana s/n, 24071 León, Spain

Ana Maria Sahagún
Pharmacology, Department of Biomedical Sciences, Institute of Biomedicine (IBIOMED), University of León, Campus de Vegazana s/n, 24071 León, Spain

Nélida Fernández
Pharmacology, Department of Biomedical Sciences, Institute of Biomedicine (IBIOMED), University of León, Campus de Vegazana s/n, 24071 León, Spain

Yun Feng
College of Life Science, Capital Normal University, Beijing 100048, Peoples' Republic of China

Yu Ding
College of Life Science, Capital Normal University, Beijing 100048, Peoples' Republic of China

Juan Liu
College of Life Science, Capital Normal University, Beijing 100048, Peoples' Republic of China

Ye Tian
College of Life Science, Capital Normal University, Beijing 100048, Peoples' Republic of China

Yanzhou Yang
Key Laboratory of Fertility Preservation and Maintenance, Ministry of Education, Key Laboratory of Reproduction and Genetics in Ningxia, Department of Histology and Embryology, Ningxia Medical University, Ningxia 750004, Peoples' Republic of China

Shuluan Guan
College of Life Science, Capital Normal University, Beijing 100048, Peoples' Republic of China

Cheng Zhang
College of Life Science, Capital Normal University, Beijing 100048, Peoples' Republic of China

Anna Tauro
Fitzpatrick Referrals, Halfway Lane, Eashing, Godalming GU7 2QQ, Surrey, UK

Diane Addicott
Murrayfield, Lockerbie, UK

Rob D Foale
Dick White Referrals, Six Mile Bottom, Suffolk, UK

Chloe Bowman
Adelaide Veterinary Specialist and Referral Centre (AVSARC), Norwood Adelaide, South Australia

Caroline Hahn
Royal (Dick) School of Veterinary Studies, University of Edinburgh, Roslin, UK

Sam Long
Adelaide Veterinary Specialist and Referral Centre (AVSARC), Norwood Adelaide, South Australia

Jonathan Massey
CIGMR, The University of Manchester, Manchester, UK

Allison C Haley
The University of Georgia, College of Veterinary Medicine, Athens, USA

Susan P Knowler
The University of Surrey, Guildford, Surrey, UK

Michael J Day
University of Bristol, Langford, Bristol, UK

Lorna J Kennedy
CIGMR, The University of Manchester, Manchester, UK

Clare Rusbridge
Fitzpatrick Referrals, Halfway Lane, Eashing, Godalming GU7 2QQ, Surrey, UK
The University of Surrey, Guildford, Surrey, UK

Carinne Puech
INRA, UMR1309 CMAEE, Montpellier F-34398, France
CIRAD, UMR CMAEE, Montpellier F-34398, France

Laurence Dedieu
CIRAD, DGD-RS-Dist, Montpellier F-34398, France

Isabelle Chantal
CIRAD, UMR Intertryp, Montpellier F-34398, France

Valérie Rodrigues
INRA, UMR1309 CMAEE, Montpellier F-34398, France
CIRAD, UMR CMAEE, Montpellier F-34398, France

Martin Peters
Chemisches und Veterinäruntersuchungsamt Westfalen, Zur Taubeneiche 10-12, 59821 Arnsberg, Germany

Irene Reber
Institute of Genetics, Vetsuisse Faculty, University of Bern, Bremgartenstrasse 109a, 3001 Bern, Switzerland

Vidhya Jagannathan
Institute of Genetics, Vetsuisse Faculty, University of Bern, Bremgartenstrasse 109a, 3001 Bern, Switzerland

Barbara Raddatz
Department of Pathology, University of Veterinary Medicine Hannover, Bünteweg 17, 30559 Hannover, Germany

Peter Wohlsein
Department of Pathology, University of Veterinary Medicine Hannover, Bünteweg 17, 30559 Hannover, Germany

Cord Drögemüller
Institute of Genetics, Vetsuisse Faculty, University of Bern, Bremgartenstrasse 109a, 3001 Bern, Switzerland

Jo L Hardstaff
University of Liverpool- Institute of Infection and Global Health, The Farr Institute@HeRC, 2nd Floor - Block F, Waterhouse building, Liverpool L69 3GL, UK

Barbara Häsler
Leverhulme Centre for Integrative Research on Agriculture and Health, Royal Veterinary College, Hawkshead Lane, North Mymms, Hatfield, Hertfordshire AL9 7TA, UK

Jonathan R Rushton
Department of Production and Population Health, Royal Veterinary College, Hawkshead Lane, North Mymms, Hatfield, Hertfordshire AL9 7TA, UK

Andrew S Bowman
The Ohio State University College of Veterinary Medicine, 1920 Coffey Road, Columbus, OH 43210, USA

Roger A Krogwold
USDA, APHIS, Veterinary Services, Pickerington, OH 43147, USA

Todd Price
North Central Veterinary Service, Sycamore, OH 44882, USA

Matt Davis
Hord Livestock Company, Bucyrus, OH 44820, USA

Steven J Moeller
The Ohio State University College of Agriculture, Columbus, OH 43210, USA

Meredyth L Jones
Large Animal Clinical Sciences, Texas A&M University College of Veterinary Medicine & Biomedical Sciences, College Station, TX 77843, USA

Kevin E Washburn
Large Animal Clinical Sciences, Texas A&M University College of Veterinary Medicine & Biomedical Sciences, College Station, TX 77843, USA

Virginia R Fajt
Veterinary Physiology and Pharmacology, Texas A&M University College of Veterinary Medicine & Biomedical Sciences, College Station, TX 77843, USA

Somchai Rice
Pharmacology Analytical Support Team (PhAST), Veterinary Diagnostic Laboratory, Iowa State University College of Veterinary Medicine, Ames, IA 50011, USA

Johann F Coetzee
Pharmacology Analytical Support Team (PhAST), Veterinary Diagnostic Laboratory, Iowa State University College of Veterinary Medicine, Ames, IA 50011, USA

Veterinary Diagnostic and Production Animal Medicine, Iowa State University College of Veterinary Medicine, Ames, IA 50011, USA

Rui Zhang
Department of Microbiology, Western College of Veterinary Medicine, University of Saskatchewan, Saskatoon, SK, Canada
Present address: Department of Basic Veterinary Medicine, College of Veterinary Medicine, China Agricultural University, Beijing, China

Douglas H Thamm
Flint Animal Cancer Center, Colorado State University, Fort Collins, CO, USA

Vikram Misra
Department of Microbiology, Western College of Veterinary Medicine, University of Saskatchewan, Saskatoon, SK, Canada

Rowena MA Packer
Department of Clinical Science and Services, Royal Veterinary College, Hertfordshire, UK

Mette Berendt
Department of Veterinary Clinical and Animal Sciences, Faculty of Health and Medical Sciences, University of Copenhagen, Frederiksberg, Denmark

Sofie Bhatti
Department of Small Animal Medicine and Clinical Biology, Faculty of Veterinary Medicine, Ghent University, Ghent, Belgium

Marios Charalambous
Cornell University College of Veterinary Medicine, Ithaca, New York, USA

Sigitas Cizinauskas
The Referral Animal Neurology Hospital "Aisti", Vantaa, Finland

Luisa De Risio
Animal Health Trust, Lanwades Park, Newmarket, UK

Robyn Farquhar
Fernside Veterinary Centre, Hertfordshire, UK

Rachel Hampel
Department of Clinical Science and Services, Royal Veterinary College, Hertfordshire, UK

Myfanwy Hill
Department of Clinical Science and Services, Royal Veterinary College, Hertfordshire, UK

Paul JJ Mandigers
Department of Clinical Sciences of Companion Animals, Utrecht University, Utrecht, The Netherlands

Akos Pakozdy
University Clinic for Small Animals, Clinical Department for Companion Animals and Horses, University of Veterinary Medicine, Vienna, Austria

Stephanie M Preston
Department of Clinical Science and Services, Royal Veterinary College, Hertfordshire, UK

Clare Rusbridge
School of Veterinary Medicine, Faculty of Health & Medical Sciences, University of Surrey, Surrey, UK

Veronika M Stein
Department of Small Animal Medicine and Surgery, University of Veterinary Medicine Hannover, Buenteweg 9, 30559 Hannover, Germany

Fran Taylor-Brown
Department of Clinical Science and Services, Royal Veterinary College, Hertfordshire, UK

Andrea Tipold
Department of Small Animal Medicine and Surgery, University of Veterinary Medicine Hannover, Buenteweg 9, 30559 Hannover, Germany

Holger A Volk
Department of Clinical Science and Services, Royal Veterinary College, Hertfordshire, UK

J Alex Pasternak
Vaccine and Infectious Disease Organization (VIDO), University of Saskatchewan, 120 Veterinary Road, Saskatoon, SK S7N 5E3, Canada

Siew Hon Ng
Vaccine and Infectious Disease Organization (VIDO), University of Saskatchewan, 120 Veterinary Road, Saskatoon, SK S7N 5E3, Canada

Rachelle M Buchanan
Vaccine and Infectious Disease Organization (VIDO), University of Saskatchewan, 120 Veterinary Road, Saskatoon, SK S7N 5E3, Canada

Sonja Mertins
Klinikum der Universität zu Köln, Institut für Medizinische Mikrobiologie, Immunologie und Hygiene, Goldenfelsstraße 19-21, 50935 Köln, Germany

George K Mutwiri
Vaccine and Infectious Disease Organization (VIDO), University of Saskatchewan, 120 Veterinary Road, Saskatoon, SK S7N 5E3, Canada

Volker Gerdts
Vaccine and Infectious Disease Organization (VIDO), University of Saskatchewan, 120 Veterinary Road, Saskatoon, SK S7N 5E3, Canada

Heather L Wilson
Vaccine and Infectious Disease Organization (VIDO), University of Saskatchewan, 120 Veterinary Road, Saskatoon, SK S7N 5E3, Canada

Yifei Yang
Laboratory of Animal Pathology and Public Health, College of Veterinary Medicine, China Agricultural University; Key Laboratory of Zoonosis of Ministry of Agriculture, China Agricultural University, Beijing 100193, China

Ruihan Shi
Laboratory of Animal Pathology and Public Health, College of Veterinary Medicine, China Agricultural University; Key Laboratory of Zoonosis of Ministry of Agriculture, China Agricultural University, Beijing 100193, China

Ruiping She
Laboratory of Animal Pathology and Public Health, College of Veterinary Medicine, China Agricultural University; Key Laboratory of Zoonosis of Ministry of Agriculture, China Agricultural University, Beijing 100193, China

Jingjing Mao
Laboratory of Animal Pathology and Public Health, College of Veterinary Medicine, China Agricultural University; Key Laboratory of Zoonosis of Ministry of Agriculture, China Agricultural University, Beijing 100193, China

Yue Zhao
Laboratory of Animal Pathology and Public Health, College of Veterinary Medicine, China Agricultural University; Key Laboratory of Zoonosis of Ministry of Agriculture, China Agricultural University, Beijing 100193, China

Fang Du
Laboratory of Animal Pathology and Public Health, College of Veterinary Medicine, China Agricultural University; Key Laboratory of Zoonosis of Ministry of Agriculture, China Agricultural University, Beijing 100193, China

Can Liu
Laboratory of Animal Pathology and Public Health, College of Veterinary Medicine, China Agricultural University; Key Laboratory of Zoonosis of Ministry of Agriculture, China Agricultural University, Beijing 100193, China

Jianchai Liu
Department of Veterinary Medicine, Laboratory of Animal Histology and Anatomy, College of Agriculture, Hebei University of Engineering, Handan, Hebei 056021, China

Minheng Cheng
Laboratory of Animal Pathology and Public Health, College of Veterinary Medicine, China Agricultural University; Key Laboratory of Zoonosis of Ministry of Agriculture, China Agricultural University, Beijing 100193, China

Rining Zhu
Laboratory of Animal Pathology and Public Health, College of Veterinary Medicine, China Agricultural University; Key Laboratory of Zoonosis of Ministry of Agriculture, China Agricultural University, Beijing 100193, China

Wei Li
Laboratory of Animal Pathology and Public Health, College of Veterinary Medicine, China Agricultural University; Key Laboratory of Zoonosis of Ministry of Agriculture, China Agricultural University, Beijing 100193, China

Xiaoyang Wang
Laboratory of Animal Pathology and Public Health, College of Veterinary Medicine, China Agricultural University; Key Laboratory of Zoonosis of Ministry of Agriculture, China Agricultural University, Beijing 100193, China

Majid Hussain Soomro
Laboratory of Animal Pathology and Public Health, College of Veterinary Medicine, China Agricultural University; Key Laboratory of Zoonosis of Ministry of Agriculture, China Agricultural University, Beijing 100193, China

Marcin R Tatara
Department of Animal Physiology, University of Life Sciences in Lublin, ul. Akademicka 12, 20-950 Lublin, Poland
II Department of Radiology, Medical University of Lublin, ul. Staszica 16, 20-081 Lublin, Poland

Witold Krupski
II Department of Radiology, Medical University of Lublin, ul. Staszica 16, 20-081 Lublin, Poland

Krzysztof Kozłowski
Department of Poultry Science, University of Warmia and Mazury in Olsztyn, ul. Oczapowskiego 5, 10-719 Olsztyn, Poland

Aleksandra Drażbo
Department of Poultry Science, University of Warmia and Mazury in Olsztyn, ul. Oczapowskiego 5, 10-719 Olsztyn, Poland

Jan Jankowski
Department of Poultry Science, University of Warmia and Mazury in Olsztyn, ul. Oczapowskiego 5, 10-719 Olsztyn, Poland

In-Cheol Cho
National Institute of Animal Science, Rural Development Administration, Jeju 690-150, Republic of Korea

Yong-Sang Park
College of Veterinary Medicine, Jeju National University, Jeju 690-756, Republic of Korea

Jae-Gyu Yoo
National Institute of Animal Science, Rural Development Administration, Jeju 690-150, Republic of Korea

Sang-Hyun Han
Educational Science Research Institute, Jeju National University, Jeju 690-756, Republic of Korea

Sang-Rae Cho
National Institute of Animal Science, Rural Development Administration, Jeju 690-150, Republic of Korea

Hee-Bok Park
Division of Animal and Dairy Science (Brain Korea 21 plus Program), Chungnam National University, Daejeon 305-764, Republic of Korea

Kyong-Leek Jeon
College of Veterinary Medicine, Jeju National University, Jeju 690-756, Republic of Korea

Kyoung-Ha Moon
College of Veterinary Medicine, Jeju National University, Jeju 690-756, Republic of Korea

Han-Seong Cho
College of Veterinary Medicine, Jeju National University, Jeju 690-756, Republic of Korea

Tae-Young Kang
College of Veterinary Medicine, Jeju National University, Jeju 690-756, Republic of Korea

Miguel Salgado
Department of Biochemistry and Microbiology, Faculty of Sciences, Universidad Austral de Chile, Edificio Instapanel, Campus Isla Teja, CC 567 Valdivia, Chile

Barbara Otto
Department of Biochemistry and Microbiology, Faculty of Sciences, Universidad Austral de Chile, Edificio Instapanel, Campus Isla Teja, CC 567 Valdivia, Chile

Manuel Moroni
Department of Animal Pathology, Faculty of Veterinary Sciences, Universidad Austral de Chile, Valdivia, Chile

Errol Sandoval
Department of Biochemistry and Microbiology, Faculty of Sciences, Universidad Austral de Chile, Edificio Instapanel, Campus Isla Teja, CC 567 Valdivia, Chile

German Reinhardt
Department of Biochemistry and Microbiology, Faculty of Sciences, Universidad Austral de Chile, Edificio Instapanel, Campus Isla Teja, CC 567 Valdivia, Chile

Sofia Boqvist
Department of Biomedical Sciences and Veterinary Public Health, Swedish University of
Agricultural Sciences, Box 7028, SE-750 07 Uppsala, Sweden

Carolina Encina
Department of Biochemistry and Microbiology, Faculty of Sciences, Universidad Austral de Chile, Edificio Instapanel, Campus Isla Teja, CC 567 Valdivia, Chile

Claudia Muñoz-Zanzi
Division of Epidemiology and Community Health, School of Public Health, University of Minnesota, Minneapolis, Minnesota, USA

José Manuel Alvarez-Mercado
Departamento de Parasitología, Facultad de Medicina Veterinaria y Zootecnia, Universidad Nacional Autónoma de México. Cd. Universitaria, C.P. 04510 México, DF, Mexico

Froylán Ibarra-Velarde
Departamento de Parasitología, Facultad de Medicina Veterinaria y Zootecnia, Universidad Nacional Autónoma de México. Cd. Universitaria, C.P. 04510 México, DF, Mexico

Miguel Ángel Alonso-Díaz
Centro de Enseñanza Investigación y Extensión en Ganadería Tropical, Facultad de Medicina Veterinaria y Zootecnia, Universidad Nacional Autónoma de México, Km. 5.5, Carretera Federal Tlapacoyan-Martínez de la Torre, C.P. 93600 Veracruz, Mexico

Yolanda Vera-Montenegro
Departamento de Parasitología, Facultad de Medicina Veterinaria y Zootecnia, Universidad Nacional Autónoma de México. Cd. Universitaria, C.P. 04510 México, DF, Mexico

José Guillermo Avila-Acevedo
Lab. de Fitoquímica, UBIPRO, Facultad de Estudios Superiores Iztacala, UNAM, Avenida de los Barrios 1, C.P. 54090 Edo. de México, Mexico

Ana María García-Bores
Lab. de Fitoquímica, UBIPRO, Facultad de Estudios Superiores Iztacala, UNAM, Avenida de los Barrios 1, C.P. 54090 Edo. de México, Mexico

Tatjana Sattler
Large Animal Clinic for Internal Medicine, University of Leipzig, An den Tierkliniken 11, 04103 Leipzig, Germany
Institute for Veterinary Disease Control, AGES, Robert-Koch-Gasse 17, 2340 Mödling, Austria

Eveline Wodak
Institute for Veterinary Disease Control, AGES, Robert-Koch-Gasse 17, 2340 Mödling, Austria

Friedrich Schmoll
Institute for Veterinary Disease Control, AGES, Robert-Koch-Gasse 17, 2340 Mödling, Austria

Heike Köhler
Institute of Molecular Pathogenesis, Friedrich-Loeffler-Institut, Federal Research Institute for Animal Health, Jena, Germany

Anneka Soschinka
Institute of Molecular Pathogenesis, Friedrich-Loeffler-Institut, Federal Research Institute for Animal Health, Jena, Germany
Tierärztliche GmbH Hagenow, Hagenow, Germany

Michaela Meyer
Institute of Molecular Pathogenesis, Friedrich-Loeffler-Institut, Federal Research Institute for Animal Health, Jena, Germany
Tierarztpraxis Dr. Peitzmeier, Hille, Germany

Angela Kather
Institute of Molecular Pathogenesis, Friedrich-Loeffler-Institut, Federal Research Institute for Animal Health, Jena, Germany
Institute of Immunology, Jena University Hospital, Jena, Germany

Petra Reinhold
Institute of Molecular Pathogenesis, Friedrich-Loeffler-Institut, Federal Research Institute for Animal Health, Jena, Germany

Elisabeth Liebler-Tenorio
Institute of Molecular Pathogenesis, Friedrich-Loeffler-Institut, Federal Research Institute for Animal Health, Jena, Germany

Hung-Hsun Yen
Faculty of Veterinary and Agriculture Science, The University of Melbourne, Parkville, VIC 3010, Australia

Christina M Murray
Faculty of Veterinary and Agriculture Science, The University of Melbourne, Parkville, VIC 3010, Australia

Helen MS Davies
Faculty of Veterinary and Agriculture Science, The University of Melbourne, Parkville, VIC 3010, Australia

Leith Carl Rodney Meyer
Department of Paraclinical Sciences, Faculty of Veterinary Science, University of Pretoria, Onderstepoort 0110, South Africa
Brain Function Research Group, School of Physiology, University of the Witwatersrand, 7 York Road, Parktown 2193, South Africa

Robyn Sheila Hetem
Brain Function Research Group, School of Physiology, University of the Witwatersrand, 7 York Road, Parktown 2193, South Africa

Duncan Mitchell
Brain Function Research Group, School of Physiology, University of the Witwatersrand, 7 York Road, Parktown 2193, South Africa

Andrea Fuller
Department of Paraclinical Sciences, Faculty of Veterinary Science, University of Pretoria, Onderstepoort 0110, South Africa
Brain Function Research Group, School of Physiology, University of the Witwatersrand, 7 York Road, Parktown 2193, South Africa

Denis Muhangi
Department of Wildlife and Aquatic Resources, College of Veterinary Medicine, Animal Resources and Biosecurity, Makerere University, P. O. Box 7062, Kampala, Uganda

Charles Masembe
Department of Biological Sciences, College of Natural Sciences, Makerere University, P. O. Box 7062, Kampala, Uganda

Ulf Emanuelson
Department of Clinical Sciences, Swedish University of Agricultural Sciences, P. O. Box 7054, SE-750 07 Uppsala, Sweden

Sofia Boqvist
Department of Biomedical Sciences and Veterinary Public Health, Swedish University of Agricultural Sciences, P. O. Box 7028, SE-750 07 Uppsala, Sweden

Lawrence Mayega
District Veterinary Office, under the Ministry of Agriculture, Animal Industry and Fisheries, Masaka, Uganda

Rose Okurut Ademun
Ministry of Agriculture, Animal Industry and Fisheries, P. O. Box 102, Entebbe, Uganda

Richard P Bishop
International Livestock Research Institute (ILRI), P.O. Box 30709, GPO 00100 Nairobi, Kenya

Michael Ocaido
Department of Wildlife and Aquatic Resources, College of Veterinary Medicine, Animal Resources and Biosecurity, Makerere University, P. O. Box 7062, Kampala, Uganda

Mikael Berg
Department of Biomedical Sciences and Veterinary Public Health, Swedish University of Agricultural Sciences, P. O. Box 7028, SE-750 07 Uppsala, Sweden

Karl Ståhl
Department of Biomedical Sciences and Veterinary Public Health, Swedish University of Agricultural Sciences, P. O. Box 7028, SE-750 07 Uppsala, Sweden
Department of Disease Control and Epidemiology, National Veterinary Institute (SVA), SE-751 89 Uppsala, Sweden

9 781682 861219